HEALTH COMMUNICATION

HEALTH COMMUNICATION

Lessons from Family Planning and Reproductive Health

Phyllis Tilson Piotrow,
D. Lawrence Kincaid,
Jose G. Rimon II,
and Ward Rinehart
*with the editorial assistance
of Kristina Samson*

Foreword by Everett M. Rogers

*Under the auspices of the Center for Communication Programs,
Johns Hopkins School of Public Health*

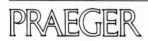

Westport, Connecticut
London

Library of Congress Cataloging-in-Publication Data

Health communication : lessons from family planning and reproductive
    health / Phyllis Tilson Piotrow ... [et al.] ; foreword by Everett
M. Rogers.
        p. cm.
    "Under the auspices of the Center for Communication Programs,
Johns Hopkins School of Public Health."
    Includes bibliographical references and index.
    ISBN 0–275–95577–X (alk. paper).—ISBN 0–275–95578–8 (pbk. :
alk. paper)
    1. Communication in birth control—Developing countries.
I. Piotrow, Phyllis Tilson.
HQ766.5.D44F368   1997
363.9′6′091724—DC21   97–19235

British Library Cataloguing in Publication Data is available.

Library of Congress Catalog Card Number: 97–19235
ISBN: 0–275–95577–X
ISBN: 0–275–95578–8 (pbk.)

First published in 1997

Praeger Publishers, 88 Post Road West, Westport, CT 06881
An imprint of Greenwood Publishing Group, Inc.

Printed in the United States of America

∞™

The paper used in this book complies with the
Permanent Paper Standard issued by the National
Information Standards Organization (Z39.48–1984).

10 9 8 7 6 5 4 3 2 1

To all those who work in this field and the people who seek their help.

Contents

Illustrations

TABLES

FIGURES

BOXES

Foreword

The last 50 years have seen communication study applied to become a powerful force for public education and behavior change. With the growth of mass media and the scientific methods to measure its impact, communication now plays a crucial role in social change, especially in the nations of Latin America, Africa, and Asia. It promises to play an even larger role in the future.

As a scientific discipline, communication developed from sociology, social psychology, and political science and was applied in schools of journalism and speech. This book, *Health Communication: Lessons from Family Planning and Reproductive Health*, illustrates how communication has been applied and advanced in an important new field of public health.

Health Communication centers on the lessons learned about effective family planning communication over the past 15 years, during which Population Communication Services (PCS) has been involved with national family planning programs in some 50 developing nations. PCS is a program in the Center for Communication Programs of the Johns Hopkins University's School of Hygiene and Public Health. Staffed by over 100 professionals, PCS works closely with governments, nongovernmental organizations, and commercial firms in developing countries to help design, implement, and evaluate family planning communication programs.

Today, every national family planning program in the world incorporates a communication component with a staff and budget. It was not always so. Prior to 1982, when PCS was established with funding from the United States Agency for International Development (USAID), the field of family planning communication was underfunded, undervalued by policy-makers, and largely devoid of strategic thinking. In 1973 I authored a book titled *Communication Strategies for Family Planning*. There was not a great deal to write about.

The greatest contribution of PCS, in my opinion, has been to identify and develop communication strategies and to evaluate these strategies in well-designed research. For example, PCS has been one of the leading organizations in the world in utilizing the Enter-Educate approach, the notion of embedding educational content about family planning in such entertainment media as radio and television soap operas, street theater, and popular music.

This book describes how PCS and its partners designed and tested logos (the Green Umbrella in Bangladesh and the Yellow Flower in Uganda, for example) in order to integrate the various components of a family planning/reproductive health program. These logos appear on clinics, nurses' uniforms, and packets of oral contraceptives and condoms. This book shares the lessons learned from PCS-assisted projects throughout the developing world: the Green Star campaign in Tanzania, the Blue Circle in Indonesia, the Gold Star in Egypt, and the *jiggasha* (networks) approach in Bangladesh.

PCS has capitalized on the amazing growth of audiences for radio and television broadcasting. For example, the number of television sets in developing nations grew from 13 million in 1955 to 707 million in 1995! Broadcasting is a component in many PCS projects, providing a powerful lever for behavior change with a reasonable and affordable cost-benefit.

A basic reason for the general success of projects assisted by PCS is the extensive use of formative evaluation research to pretest logos, Enter-Educate media messages, and campaign materials. The effects of almost every project are evaluated, often in ingenious designs. For instance, this book describes the use of "mystery clients," individuals who visit family planning clinics disguised as regular clients but whose real task is to observe how clients are treated. Mystery clients were used to determine the effectiveness of the GATHER approach (greet, ask, tell, help choose, explain, and return/refer), developed by PCS to train clinic staff to be more sensitive to clients' needs (such as asking clients about their own preferences and helping them to make informed choices). PCS evaluations have often been interrupted time-series field experiments, in which a communication campaign's effects are measured over time by the increase in, say, the number of family planning users before, during, and after a communication intervention.

This book is filled with rich examples of effective family planning communication from all over the world. Not surprisingly, family planning communication has been an essential component in successful national family planning programs in nations like Indonesia, Egypt, and Bangladesh. PCS has advanced not only the applied specialty of family planning communication but also our basic understanding of human communication.

I recommend *Health Communication* to scholars, students, and program officials who want to know how human fertility behavior can be changed through strategic communication. Here, writ large, is the inside story of how adequate funding over a sustained period, applied by a dedicated staff of able people using strategies based on research, is helping to solve one of the world's gravest problems.

Everett M. Rogers
Department of Communication and Journalism
University of New Mexico

Preface

The theme of this book is simple but profound: Systematic communication strategies can improve health behavior. The power of communication today stems from two recent developments: the rapid growth of communication media and the notable increase in our understanding of communication processes.

The power of communication is clear. Communication influences how people vote. Communication determines what people buy. Communication affects what people wish for and what they aspire to become. Communication shapes how people conduct their daily lives, even their sexual behavior.

In the field of public health, substantial evidence shows that:

- people want to know more about their health;
- people want to talk more about health to friends and family, hear about it through mass media, and discuss it with competent, caring service providers;
- people are willing to change their health behavior; and
- public health communication programs are helping people make these changes.

The issue is no longer whether health communication can influence behavior. Now the issue is how to sharpen our understanding of communication to do a better job. This understanding will grow quickly as more health professionals recognize that communication is an investment and not an extravagance.

In family planning and reproductive health, the value of that investment is clear. Family planning saves lives. Family planning improves the quality of life and health for women, children, families, communities, and nations. And family planning costs very little. People want family planning, but programs need to tell people what family planning methods are available and where, how to use them, and what to expect.

This book is about the theory and practice of family planning communication. The theory comes from many sources, including sociology, psychology, political science, communication science, and medicine. The practice, as described here, comes from 15 years of health communication work through the Population Communication Services (PCS) project and other activities of the Center for Communication Programs in the School of Hygiene and Public Health of the Johns Hopkins University.

Funded primarily by the United States Agency for International Development (USAID), PCS has included among its partners many dedicated organizations and individuals in countries around the world who are working effectively in health communication. PCS partners also include the Academy for Educational Development (AED); the Program for Appropriate Technology in Health (PATH); Porter, Novelli and Associates; Saffitz, Alpert and Associates; and, most recently, the Center for Development and Population Activities (CEDPA), Save the Children, and Prospect Associates.

This book reviews the development of family planning communication and compiles what we have learned from working in some 50 countries around the world. While this book focuses on our experience in family planning communication, the lessons apply to a broad range of health issues, from diet to drug abuse, from child survival to accident prevention. Policy-makers may find the book useful to gain the confidence to invest more in health communication capabilities. Health communication planners may see it as a resource for developing more effective strategies. Health communicators may find value in the tools and techniques described for developing health communication materials. Researchers may find ideas about evaluating communication programs and improving them as a result. Trainers, teachers, and students may find this book a useful text for studying the state of the art of health communication. Graduate schools of public health and communication may see implications for collaboration and curriculum development in higher education. To accompany the book, a videotape of highlights of family planning communication projects assisted by Johns Hopkins is available from the Center for Communication Programs.

In writing this book, the authors hope to encourage all those who care about health and communication to explore health communication issues more deeply. The health challenges of the next century are formidable. From HIV/AIDS to environmental pollution, they threaten the health and welfare of billions of people. These challenges cut across national boundaries and demand increasing resources. Addressing these challenges requires both political will and professional wisdom. Effective communication demands a high level of commitment and teamwork among donor agencies, government agencies, nongovernmental organizations, commercial enterprises, and communities. Working together to make the world a healthier place, we can all do better. We can learn from both our mistakes and our successes. In fact, we may find some wisdom to the basic truth that to change others, we may have to change ourselves first.

Acknowledgments

This book is a product of 15 years of work on family planning and related health communication with colleagues and counterparts in over 50 countries around the world. The institutions that have worked with the Johns Hopkins Center for Communication Programs are listed in the Appendix. The individuals we have worked with in this field are, we are happy to say, almost as numerous as the stars we see in the sky. And for us they are the real stars in this effort, because without them there would have been no programs and no book. To all of these individuals and organizations, our heartfelt appreciation for the collaborative efforts that have helped to make health communication the force that it is today.

Special thanks go to officials in the United States Agency for International Development, both in the Office of Population in Washington, D.C., and in the USAID missions overseas. They have shared with us a vision of what can be accomplished through strategic communication. They have also provided the resources and support to make that vision a reality in many countries. In particular, thanks to R. T. Ravenholt, J. Joseph Speidel, Steven Sinding, Duff Gillespie, Elizabeth Maguire, James Shelton, and Margaret Neuse for their recognition of the value of effective communication; and to Anne Aarnes, Roy Jacobstein, Clayton Vollan, Earle Lawrence, Chloe O'Gara, Sandra de Castro Buffington, and Joanne Grossi for their judicious guidance as technical advisors for the Population Communication Services project. Keys MacManus and Joyce Holfeld also provided helpful advice at various times.

We also want to thank the foundations that have generously responded to our appeals for project assistance, including the Compton Foundation, the Cowell Foundation, the Levinson Foundation, the Packard Foundation, the Public Welfare Foundation, and the Winslow Foundation. In addition, many of the developing-country students who have helped in our work were partially supported through William H. Draper, Jr. Fellowships supported by the Draper Family, the Dillon Fund, the Educational Foundation of America, the Hewlett Foundation, the

Kempner Fund, the Rockefeller Foundation, the Share-It-Now Foundation, the Swensrud Foundation, and others.

Within the Johns Hopkins School of Public Health, we are grateful for the support of Deans D. A. Henderson and Alfred Sommer, who have encouraged the Center for Communication Programs to make a significant contribution. We have also benefited from the unfailing help of Herbert Hansen, Donna Helm, Anne Muller, Patricia Friend, and Frederick DeKuyper. We especially appreciate the continuing support of the Chairmen of the Department of Population Dynamics, initially John F. Kantner and, for most of this period, W. Henry Mosley.

The entire staff of the Center for Communication Programs has contributed to this book, directly or indirectly, including particularly the program staff of Population Communication Services and many of the Center's overseas representatives. For their contributions to the text, special thanks go to Pamela Allen, Patrick Coleman, Peggy D'Adamo, Elizabeth DuVerlie, Robert Foreman, Bill Glass, Lauren Goodsmith, Karen Heckert, Lamia Jaroudi, Miriam Jato, Young Mi Kim, Karungari Kiragu-Gikonyo, Adrienne Kols, Susan Krenn, Robert Lande, Philippe Langlois, Susan Leibtag, Cheryl Lettenmaier, Gary Lewis, Benjamin Lozare, Marsha McCoskrie, Alice Payne Merritt, Rita Meyer, Nicole Pelsinsky, Andrew Plumer, Patricia Poppe, Bryant Robey, Walter Saba, J. Douglas Storey, Ian Tweedie, Carol Underwood, Tom Valente, Edson Whitney, James Williams, Sung Hee Yun, and, finally, Johanna Zacharias, who served as editor for most of the preparation of the book. Robert J. Riccio managed its final production.

We also appreciate the valuable insights of Everett M. Rogers, Craig Lefebvre, and Gary Saffitz.

The authors are particularly grateful to those who turned our unruly drafts into an orderly manuscript. Kristina Samson, indispensable in her role as editorial assistant and researcher, organized the process and checked all the facts and references.

Norma Booth, our cheerleader and counselor, very competently prepared the manuscript from start to finish. Peter Hammerer formatted the book.

Many have contributed to this process and helped to improve the book. For all their help, we are grateful; for any errors and misinformation, we are responsible.

Chapter 1

Public Health, Family Planning, and Communication

Human reproduction is the key not only to human survival but also to the continuing health of billions of men and women and their present and future children. Yet human reproduction has always been among the most sensitive and challenging areas of public health. Indeed, some would argue that reproduction is not a public health issue at all but rather should be left to individual conscience, religious guidance, personal choice, or family privacy.

Nevertheless, issues relating to reproduction are becoming increasingly prominent on the public health agenda. In matters of reproduction and sexual behavior, private behavior has public consequences. Those consequences are important. Especially when individual private behavior may be multiplied by 3 billion—roughly the number of men and women of reproductive age in the world today—what an individual or couple may consider "nobody's business but my own" becomes everyone's concern.

In fact, since long before there was such a concept as "public health," society has sought to regulate the sexual and reproductive behavior of individuals for the good of the whole. Such regulation has long manifested itself in social and family structure, social norms, traditions, and law (Fee, 1987; Rosenkrantz, 1972; Winslow, 1923). Only in this century, however, have organized public efforts developed to help individuals and couples meet their own needs to protect their reproductive health, control their fertility, and, as a result, serve society's needs at the same time (Chaudhuri, 1983; Critchlow, 1995; Donaldson & Tsui, 1990; M. Green, 1993; Knowles, 1991; Watson, 1977). Today the public health agenda includes national and international programs to address the health and demographic impacts of high fertility, to reduce teenage pregnancies, to promote safe motherhood, to increase child survival, to halt the spread of HIV/AIDS and other sexually transmitted diseases, and to avert domestic violence against women and children. These are high priority issues.

Even as the agenda expands, however, many challenges remain in designing, implementing, and evaluating public health programs that address private behavior. How, for example, can publicly funded, government-supervised programs acceptably and effectively influence the number of children people want and have? How can public health programs—which have achieved some of their greatest successes through community-wide application of advanced technology, such as water and sanitation programs, use of pesticides, and compulsory immunization—achieve comparable success in changing the behavior of individuals and couples in the private spheres of sexual, reproductive, and family life?

As public health programs worldwide face these challenges, the research findings and program experience of the last half century with regard to changes in human fertility are highly relevant. Family planning programs have played a crucial role in reducing average family size worldwide to just under three children per woman (2.96) (United Nations [UN], 1996). The lessons learned from these programs are applicable to many other public health programs where changes in individual behavior are required for better health.

The spread of family planning represents a major shift in individual and social behavior. Communication has been crucial to this shift. Unlike other areas of public health, where community-wide application of new technology has played the major role, in the field of reproductive health individual decision-making prevails. Even though technological advances have been important, individuals still decide whether and which of the available family planning technologies they will use, how effectively they will use them, and for how long. Communication at all levels—personal, family, community, and mass media—therefore plays a major role in that decision-making.

COMMUNICATION AND FAMILY PLANNING

Communication is the key process underlying changes in knowledge of the means of contraception, in attitudes toward fertility control and use of contraceptives, in norms regarding ideal family size, and in the openness of local cultures to new ideas and aspirations and new health behavior. This communication can occur both spontaneously, within and between social groups of a society, and deliberately, by means of the planned interventions of governmental and nongovernmental organizations and commercial enterprises. This planned communication can initiate change, accelerate changes already under way, or reinforce change that has already occurred.

Communication can spread knowledge, values, and social norms. Such knowledge includes the idea of fertility control itself as well as knowledge about specific methods of contraception and how they are used. For example, communication can convey the advantages and disadvantages of smaller families or the beneficial and harmful consequences of specific contraceptives. Communication also can introduce new values or change the priorities of existing values. For example, communication can endorse equality between the sexes and a greater role for women in reproductive and sexual decisions. Communication also makes it possible to learn about the behavior of others—for example, which and how many of one's relatives, friends, and neighbors are practicing family planning. The perception of what everyone else is doing influences what people accept as normative, acceptable behavior.

The assumptions and expectations conveyed by modern communication media can help make family planning a legitimate topic of public discussion and a legitimate practice. Discussion of formerly taboo topics, such as some aspects of reproductive health, in community meetings and on television and radio can greatly reduce the embarrassment of talking with friends or family members about family planning. Finally, purposefully designed messages in the mass media can change the way that people perceive modern contraceptives and can present models of family planning as a positive behavior with rewarding consequences.

The purpose of this book is to focus on the lessons that have been learned over the last two decades about the design, implementation, and evaluation of family planning communication programs. The book draws primarily on the experience of the Population Communication Services (PCS) program at the Johns Hopkins University School of Public Health, one of the largest, oldest, and most comprehensive programs in this field. This chapter gives a brief summary of the background of family planning communication before and at the beginnings of comprehensive national programs. It is followed by a systematic overview of the process of developing communication programs designed to influence human reproductive behavior and particularly to increase use of family planning. Chapter 2 describes the theoretical and conceptual understanding of individual behavior change that guides program design and the process by which these concepts are incorporated into operational programs. Chapters 3 through 8 describe the lessons learned about each phase of communication program development from analysis and strategic design through evaluation and planning for continuity and sustainability. Chapter 9 identifies some of the challenges that lie ahead for family planning and other reproductive and family health communication programs in the 21st century.

Most of the lessons learned from the Population Communication Services project apply to other fields of public health as well. They apply especially to activities that require informed individual choice and changes in personal behavior. But they also apply wherever systematic communication efforts, favorable community norms, and supportive government policies are important to achieving public health goals—in other words, throughout public health.

FERTILITY CHANGE AND IDEATIONAL FACTORS

By the late 19th century, even before public health programs began to address the issues of high fertility and reproductive health, fertility was declining in much of Europe and the United States. Why did this happen in the absence of specific programs or modern contraceptives? For decades the standard explanation for declining fertility was based on a *socioeconomic* model called the demographic transition theory, which attributes fertility decline to a decrease in parental demand for children induced by the structural economic changes of modernization, including urbanization and industrial employment, and by decreasing mortality (Notestein, 1946; T. W. Schultz, 1974; Caldwell, 1987).[1]

More recently, another model has been proposed, an *ideational* model (Cleland, 1985; Retherford, 1985; Cleland & Wilson, 1987). It attributes declining fertility to the diffusion of new ideas, new behavior, and new technology. The ideational model emphasizes the importance of communication in stimulating behavior change—communication via mass media, community activities, and interpersonal discussion that introduces individuals and communities to new ideas and opportunities. As a result, what was previously unknown becomes familiar, and what was previously taboo can become a community norm.

These two models are often seen as competing, but in fact they have different and often complementary emphases. The socioeconomic model emphasizes the changing circumstances that require couples or households to adapt. The ideational model emphasizes how the idea of fertility control spread and came to be adopted as a feasible and socially acceptable means of adapting to various economic or social circumstances.

While the relative weight that should be given to each model remains controversial, there is much evidence that supports the ideational model and documents the impact of communication on behavior changes. This evidence comes both from demographic studies of 18th and 19th century European fertility and from analysis of internationally comparable fertility surveys since the 1970s in developing countries. In the European transition to lower fertility:

- fertility declines occurred most rapidly within similar linguistic and cultural groups, where communication was relatively easy, as in England (Coale & Watkins, 1986);
- fertility declines were frequently not related to socioeconomic conditions or economic thresholds (Coale & Watkins, 1986); and
- fertility declines sometimes preceded and sometimes followed declines in infant and child mortality (van de Walle & Knodel, 1980).

In analyses of data from developing countries, contraceptive prevalence and fertility declines both are closely related to the strength of national family planning programs (Freedman & Berelson, 1976; Lapham & Mauldin, 1985; Mauldin & Ross, 1991; Ross & Frankenberg, 1993; International Bank for Reconstruction and Development, 1993). Strong programs have strong communication components that include mass media, community outreach, and interpersonal communication. For example, Bangladesh is one of the poorest countries in the world, but by 1996, 45 percent of married women of reproductive age were using modern family planning, largely as a result of a national program delivering information and supplies to women in their homes (Population Reference Bureau, 1996; Robey, Piotrow, &

Salter, 1994; Robey, Ross, & Bhushan, 1996; Ross & Mauldin, 1996). The Bangladesh contraceptive prevalence rate is now close to those of more developed countries such as Bolivia, Egypt, and Morocco. In short, while socioeconomic development, including especially education of women, is clearly an important factor in fertility declines, increased attention to the role of ideational factors and thus communication has provided a new perspective and new opportunities to strengthen family planning programs.

FAMILY PLANNING COMMUNICATION IN NATIONAL PROGRAMS

National family planning programs began in the mid-20th century and have evolved rapidly to meet the information and service needs of their clients. The communication component of these programs also has evolved as new knowledge and new technologies have become available.[2]

The initial stage of program organization continued through the 1960s and has been described as the "clinic era" of family planning (Rogers, 1973; Stycos, 1973). It was based on the standard medical care model, which assumed that "patients" would seek contraceptive services if they were simply made available in existing or new clinics. The clinic approach assumes implicitly that a sufficient portion of the population is already well informed and motivated to act. The model of communication implied by this approach is captured by the phrase "build it and they will come." In the clinic era of family planning programs, highly motivated patients did come, often over long distances, when they heard about the services by word of mouth or, occasionally, through the mass media.

For a majority of the population, however, this was not enough. For many traditionally oriented people, visiting public clinics to discuss a taboo subject violated their own norms of proper behavior. For others, the benefits of family planning were not obvious or not obviously worth the time and costs of obtaining a contraceptive method at an inconvenient or inhospitable clinic. Health care providers, however, saw little reason to turn to communication to encourage clinic visits. In fact, because family planning was considered to be primarily a medical matter in the hands of physicians, the idea of actively promoting these services ran counter to norms of professional medical practice.

The "clinic era" gave way to the "field era," which began in the late 1960s. The field era constituted an active rather than passive approach to family planning and related communication (Rogers, 1973). Clinics were (and still are) an important component, but community extension agents—family planning field workers—took responsibility for informing and motivating people through home or community visits. The field era was derived from the extension agent approach to agricultural development. At that time, field work was supported by a variety of information sources—posters, leaflets, radio broadcasts, mobile vans with films, and so forth—that informed the public about the availability of family planning methods and services.

By the early 1970s general knowledge of family planning had already begun reaching levels as high as 70 to 85 percent of married women of reproductive age, and two new contraceptive technologies were introduced, the intrauterine device (IUD) and oral contraceptives—the Pill. The so-called KAP gap began to emerge, the statistical phenomenon in which survey respondents reported high levels of knowledge (K) of and positive attitudes (A) toward family planning but still relatively low levels of practice (P) (Freedman, 1984).

Two major reviews of family planning communication were published in the early 1970s. They provide a benchmark to measure both the status of these early programs and progress over the subsequent 25 years. In 1971 Wilbur Schramm's review, *Communication in Family Planning*, was published by the Population Council. In 1973 Everett Rogers' ground-breaking *Communication Strategies for Family Planning* appeared. Both of these expert reviews covered the experience of population programs from the early 1950s to the early 1970s. Schramm examined communication programs in 11 countries, only 5 of which had official family planning policies: India, Iran, Kenya, South Korea, and Taiwan. Rogers examined the level of communication inputs in 20 national programs.

At that time only 5 of the 20 were considered "successful" national programs—Hong Kong, Mauritius, Singapore, South Korea, and Taiwan. Contraceptive prevalence attributable to government programs ranged from 19 to 25 percent among married women of reproductive age in the countries with programs labeled "successful." All five of these countries had three important components: availability of clinical services, home visits by field workers, and substantial use of mass media (Lapham & Mauldin, 1972; Rogers, 1973).

In the 15 countries that Rogers labeled "unsuccessful" in the early 1970s, one or more of these components was either missing or only partially in place. In such countries as Colombia, Egypt, Indonesia, Kenya, Pakistan (then including Bangladesh), and Thailand, programs all were evaluated as "unsuccessful" because there was no evidence of fertility decline and because contraceptive prevalence rates attributable to government programs were low, ranging from less than 1 percent in Indonesia to 13 percent in Thailand. Kenya was the only sub-Saharan African country with a family planning program even mentioned, but it, too, was rated "unsuccessful" at that time (Lapham & Mauldin, 1972 & 1984; Mauldin & Ross, 1991; Rogers, 1973).

Schramm's review of family planning communication consisted primarily of a description of the *channels* of communication being used, categorized as either personal or public communication. He found "relatively little difference, from country to country, in what is said by family planning programs to their publics" (Schramm, 1971). At that time, he observed, radio was the "chief mass medium" of family planning campaigns, primarily in the form of 20- to 60-second spot announcements. Radio novellas or story forms of presentation were just beginning to be used at that time, in Hong Kong and South Korea. Interviews and talks with doctors were common. Communication experts were just beginning to recommend that personal appeals related to family welfare might be more effective than collective or patriotic appeals (Keeny, 1965). But at that time, Schramm found hardly any careful testing of alternative messages or any pretesting of the messages being used. Television ownership was still too rare for the medium to be considered very useful for promoting family planning in most developing countries.

Recommendations for communication programs at that time addressed mainly the quantity and frequency of reach to specific audiences (Bogue & Johnson, 1969). Wilder (quoted in Rogers, 1973, p. 269) described the typical communication activity of national family planning agencies at that time: "We have enough money to do some publicity. Let's have a series of six posters on family planning. The chief artist prepares sketches for the posters. He has spent his life learning how to draw and paint in an artistic and pleasing way, but usually he knows little about the nature of family planning or the objectives of the communication campaign. He has little knowledge of the audience for his posters, or the kinds of messages that they can understand, or what they would be interested in." Furthermore, when such posters were printed and distributed, no one assessed who, if anyone, actually saw them or what effect they had on the public.

Communication programs lacked any coherent strategy. Rogers (1973) lamented that in effect the dominant communication strategy was what he called the "large volume error": "If I produce lots of messages, my responsibility is finished." In fact, the overriding theme of his review was that "communication efforts for family planning goals would be much more effective if explicit attention were given to communication strategies" (p. 28).

THE ROLE OF MASS MEDIA

Both reviews were ambivalent on the effectiveness of mass media, and they relied more on prevailing theory than on the empirical data that were beginning to surface. Rogers (1973, p. 266), for example, applied his well-known generalization from previous research on diffusion of innovations. He concluded that mass media channels in family planning programs "are relatively more important at the knowledge function, and interpersonal channels are relatively more important at the persuasion function in the innovation-decision process." Schramm (1971, p. 32) offered a similar modest assessment: "Ten years of family planning experience . . . have led to the conclusion that public information can create a climate of knowledge and attitudes that will make it easier for the field and clinical staffs to recruit new acceptors."

Even in their own reviews, however, both experts presented evidence suggesting that mass media were not only legitimizing and stimulating discussion but also were triggering behavior change. Impressive results were reported for campaigns using radio. As Schramm (1971, p. 32) noted, a "considerable" number of survey respondents said information from the mass media motivated their clinic visits (as high as 38 percent in South Korea) or increased the number of couples adopting contraceptives (40 percent increase in Pakistan).

The problem then and now is how to interpret these kinds of impact data. At that time they were treated as isolated discrepancies from the dominant paradigm of limited and diffuse mass media effects. Schramm, for example, concluded that the case for mass media impact was "not clear" and tended to be based on "anecdotal evidence" from case studies. He called for rigorous experimental designs that could reach more definitive conclusions about mass media effects on family planning behavior. Research designs used at that time for the evaluation of mass media programs did not allow for definitive conclusions, he observed.

A major reason that broadcast mass media were not considered important in the early 1970s was that they were not yet very accessible in most developing countries. At the time "most developing countries [had] little television, but transistor radio receivers [were] appearing in even the most remote places" (Schramm, 1971, p. 4). Even ownership of radios, the most efficient mass media channel, was still rare compared with today, however. Television was virtually nonexistent for most populations in developing countries.

In summary, Schramm's and Rogers' reviews of family planning communication 25 years ago revealed the following weaknesses in program-based family planning communication:

- little evidence of coherent communication planning and strategic design to achieve specific objectives;
- a lack of multimedia communication campaigns integrated with other program components, such as the service delivery system;
- an overemphasis on trying to make audiences aware of family planning, under the erroneous assumption that awareness and knowledge automatically lead to persuasion and adoption;
- attempts to communicate the same messages to everyone, rather than segmenting audiences according to their varying needs for information and contraception;
- lack of any systematic pretesting of messages with members of intended audiences;
- no systematic application of scientific theories regarding how communication changes behavior; and
- lack of rigorous evaluation research to determine what effect communication was having, why, and with whom.

Moreover, both authors were ambivalent about assigning the mass media any major role in influencing individual behavior.

THE CHANGING ENVIRONMENT FOR FAMILY PLANNING AND COMMUNICATION

Since the early 1970s substantial changes have occurred in family planning programs, in global communication, and in the communication component of family planning programs. In historical terms, the speed of these changes has been so rapid that they can be considered not merely evolutionary but rather, more accurately, revolutionary.

By the mid-1990s more than 168 countries had adopted national population and development policies (United Nations Population Fund [UNFPA], 1995). Most of these policies include extensive family planning information and service programs. Three international conferences of governments have focused world attention on population issues, those held in Bucharest in 1974, Mexico City in 1984, and Cairo in 1994. Within the developing world, current annual expenditures on family planning programs are estimated at about US$4 to $5 billion, including both government and personal expenditures. International donor funding for these programs increased from $165 million in 1971 to $1.2 billion in 1994 (Conly, 1996). The United Nations contribution through the United Nations Population Fund increased from $9.5 million in 1971 to almost $300 million in 1995 (Conly, 1996). United States government support to developing-country programs increased from $96 million in 1971 to $585 million in 1995. The value of just the contraceptive shipments funded by the United States Agency for International Development (USAID) increased from $3.6 million annually in the early 1970s to almost $50 million in the mid-1990s, while United Nations shipments in 1994 totalled more than $80 million (Conly, 1996).

These changes in political and economic support are clearly reflected in the impact of family planning programs. Twenty-five years later, most of the 15 countries that were identified in the early 1970s as unsuccessful have developed strong family planning programs (Ross & Mauldin, 1996). According to a 1994 analysis of family planning programs in more than 90 developing countries by the Futures Group and the Population Council, programs in Bangladesh, Thailand, and Indonesia were rated among the 10 strongest in the world; programs in Colombia, Egypt, and Kenya were rated as moderately strong (Ross & Mauldin, 1996). Between 1970 and 1990 the total fertility rates of these countries dropped—by as much as 4.0 children per woman in Thailand and 2.1 in Indonesia. Contraceptive prevalence rates for most of the programs that once were labeled unsuccessful are now well above the level of programs that were labeled successful 25 years ago (see Table 1.1). All of the now-successful countries have had strong national family planning programs in which communication played an important role (Ross & Mauldin, 1996).

Restrictions on communication about family planning have eased as well. Although religious and other controversies about specific family planning methods continue to influence media coverage in some countries, one noteworthy sign of the changing times is the massive national family planning program in Iran, where Muslim religious leaders have now endorsed family planning, including vasectomy, and where contraceptive prevalence has reached an estimated 65 percent (MacFarquhar, 1996). Among regions of the developing world, contraceptive prevalence is highest in the predominantly Catholic countries of Latin America and the Caribbean, averaging over 50 percent. Radio and television regularly include news, public interest spots, and advertisements related to family planning despite lingering religious opposition.

Table 1.1
Then and Now: Changes in Contraceptive Prevalence Rates (CPR)
in 20 Developing Countries, Circa 1970 and 1996

Country (Year National Family Planning Program Began)	CPR in 1970 Due to Government Programs[a]	CPR Circa 1970[b]	CPR in 1996[c]
National Family Planning Program Called "Successful" in 1973			
Singapore (1965)	25	60	65
Taiwan (1964)	25	44	75
South Korea (1961)	24	33	79
Mauritius (1965)	19	19+	75
Hong Kong (1956)	19	50	81
National Family Planning Program Called "Unsuccessful" in 1973			
Colombia (1967)	6	18	72
Egypt (1965)	6	9	48
India (1952)	8	14	41
Indonesia (1968)	0.5	9	55
Iran (1967)	8	NA	65
Kenya (1965)	2	NA	33
Malaysia (1966)	8	9	56
Morocco (1965)	1	3	42
Nepal (1966)	2	3	23
Pakistan (1960)[d]	12	6	12
Bangladesh	e	4[f]	45
Philippines (1970)	8	16	40
Sri Lanka (1965)	7	32	66
Thailand (1968)	13	14	66
Tunisia (1964)	6	NA	50
Turkey (1967)	3	9	63

Note: "Successful programs" were defined in 1973 (Rogers, 1973) as programs that had produced any decline in age-specific fertility rates. "Unsuccessful programs" had not.

CPR = contraceptive prevalence rate as percentage of married women of reproductive age.

NA = not available.

[a]Data on CPR due to government programs only are from Rogers, 1973 based primarily on Lapham and Mauldin, 1972 and supplemented by Nortman, 1972.

[b]Data for Singapore (1973), India (1970), Malaysia (1966), Nepal (1966), Philippines (1968), Sri Lanka (1975), Thailand (1969), and Turkey (1968), are from United Nations, 1989; all others, for 1970, are from Lapham and Mauldin, 1972.

[c]All 1996 data are from Population Reference Bureau, 1996.

[d]12% CPR due to government programs reflects both East and West Pakistan. 6% total CPR circa 1970 is for East Pakistan. East Pakistan became Bangladesh in 1971. 12% CPR in 1996 is for Pakistan only.

[e]In 1970 Bangladesh was part of Pakistan, and its CPR is reflected in the 1970 Pakistan data.

[f]Bangladesh CPR is based on 1969 data, as reported by the U.S. Bureau of the Census (McDevitt, 1996).

Figure 1.1
Developing-World Radio and Television Receivers, 1955–1995

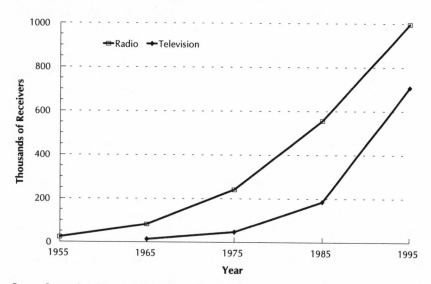

Source: International Broadcasting Audience Research Library/British Broadcasting Company, 1996.

Another dramatic change in the last 25 years has been the global telecommuni-cations revolution. The number of radio and television receivers in developing countries has grown exponentially since 1955 (see Figure 1.1). Between 1965 and 1995 the number of radios in developing countries grew more than tenfold, from 82 million to 997 million. The number of television sets grew from only 13 million to 707 million (International Broadcasting Audience Research Library/British Broadcasting Company [IBAR/BBC], 1996). About 2 billion radios and 1.5 billion television sets are projected for the year 2000. Certainly in the area of communica-tion, one of the biggest differences between family planning and other public health programs 25 years ago and today is the increased capacity to reach people by means of mass media, especially television.

From a demographic standpoint, these dramatic changes—reinforced by other factors—have resulted in a world population in 1995 that is approximately 420 million less than it would otherwise have been. Based on data available in 1973, demographers projected that the population in developing countries would be 4.953 billion people if fertility rates remained unchanged (UN, 1977). As it turned out, by 1995 the population in the developing world was only 4.533 billion (Population Reference Bureau [PRB], 1996), a difference of almost half a billion people. This difference was a result of the reduction in the population growth rate that has occurred over the last 25 years, from 2.2 percent in the 1970s to 1.9 percent by the mid-1990s. While some of this change was due to economic and social development as well as geographic and cultural factors, the family planning program efforts of governments and private organizations played a major role. Bongaarts (1995, p. 26) estimated that strong voluntary family planning programs helped reduce fertility on average by about one birth per woman in the developing world, which "amounts to fully 43 percent of the observed fertility decline between the early 1960s and the late 1980s." Nevertheless, about 90 million people, almost as much as the population of Mexico, Nigeria, or northern Europe, are still being added to the world's population each year. Most of this increase takes place in developing countries, where family size still averages 3.4 children (4.0, excluding China) (PRB, 1996).

THE ROLE OF POPULATION COMMUNICATION SERVICES

Recognizing the urgent need for family planning and the increasingly important role of communication in family planning programs, USAID began as early as the 1970s to address communication issues. By 1976, about 11 percent of U.S. population assistance was devoted to communication (PRB, 1976). In addition to support for broad-based programs, such as the work of the International Planned Parenthood Federation (IPPF) and the Pathfinder Fund, USAID initiatives in communication included support for the following:

- the East-West Communications Institute at the University of Hawaii, which served as a clearinghouse for communication materials, a training center, and a source of curriculum modules for communication training;
- the University of Chicago, where Professor Donald Bogue provided long- and short-term training for a generation of communication specialists;
- special-audience activities carried out by such organizations as the American Home Economics Association, World Action for Youth, and World Education, Inc., to reach different constituencies worldwide;
- the Airlie Foundation in Virginia, which operated the InterAmerican Dialogue Center and produced more than 100 films on population and health issues;
- the Population Information Program, originally at George Washington University and transferred to the Johns Hopkins University in 1978, which publishes *Population Reports* and which established POPLINE, the computerized bibliographic database for the population field;
- social marketing programs operated by Population Services International, the Futures Group, and others, first to sell needed supplies through retail outlets at subsidized prices and later to bring marketing and advertising skills to health promotion; and
- pilot projects through the HEALTHCOM project at the Academy for Educational Development to test and evaluate the impact of communication in other areas of public health, such as child survival.

By the early 1980s it was clear that a more comprehensive, systematic effort was needed in the field of family planning and population communication. The Population Communication Services (PCS) project was the result. Awarded by USAID in 1982 to the Johns Hopkins University School of Public Health as a result of a competitive procurement, Population Communication Services has become an acknowledged leader in family planning communication. Annual budgets have increased from about $2 million in 1983 to more than $20 million in 1997, reflecting the international community's response to a readily accessible source of professional communication skills, funding support, and technical assistance for family planning programs throughout the developing world.

PCS works in close partnership with dozens of government agencies, private nongovernmental organizations, and commercial firms in more than 50 countries. Thousands of individuals have shared in carrying out the programs described in succeeding chapters, learning the lessons spelled out here, and applying them to improve programs. These partners and collaborators are listed in the Appendix. The PCS team has also included the Academy for Educational Development (AED); the Program for Appropriate Technology in Health (PATH); Porter, Novelli and Associates; Saffitz, Alpert and Associates, Inc.; and, since 1995, the Center for Development and Population Activities (CEDPA), Save the Children, and Prospect Associates. Together with counterparts and colleagues worldwide, the PCS project represents a major commitment to the field of family planning communication.

In functional terms, the PCS team provides a broad range of assistance, including support for:

- communication needs assessments;
- workshops, seminars, and conferences;
- specific products such as posters, brochures, films, and videos;
- training in communication skills and management;
- technical assistance to all types of communication and community-mobilization projects;
- development of national communication strategies and campaigns; and
- evaluation of communication interventions.

Over the last 15 years, from 1982 to 1997, the PCS team has carried out approximately 70 national needs assessments, organized almost 500 training events, implemented more than 260 projects, fielded about 1,400 technical assistance trips, and prepared over 500 published articles and professional presentations or major reports.

In 1988 the Center for Communication Programs was formed at the Johns Hopkins School of Public Health, bringing together PCS, the Population Information Program, and a number of other family planning and health related communication programs. These other programs of the Center include health communication programs, similar to the work of PCS, with Pathfinder International in Egypt and Uganda, the Futures Group in Ghana, John Snow International in Morocco, and Management Sciences for Health in Senegal and Haiti. Several of these programs are discussed in the book.

The importance of the PCS project lies not only in the quantity of its work to date—although that provides a massive research base for study of the field—but also and especially in the quality, innovativeness, and direction of these activities over the last decade. As a 1989 external evaluation of PCS noted:

A.I.D.'s overriding aim in creating the JHU/PCS Project was to develop a source of creative leadership to meet new IEC [Information, Education, and Communication] opportunities that have arisen as a result of political or technological changes. The consensus in the field is that the Project has succeeded in this respect.... Overall, JHU/PCS has been very successful in reaching its stated objectives. Through its activities, JHU/PCS has given coherence and integrity to the IEC function in national family planning programs in LDCs [Less Developed Countries]. It has succeeded in defining the field of IEC, and, through its several innovative approaches, changed this definition in directions that are more useful and that contribute to the increased effectiveness of family planning programs. (McWilliam & Rogers, 1989, p. 9)

In fact, the PCS project has responded to the need, identified by Everett Rogers in the 1970s, for a strategic approach to communication issues (Rogers, 1973). Thus, as family planning programs have moved from the "clinic era" of the 1960s through the "field era" of the 1970s, so also family planning communication programs have changed and evolved. Above all, they have now become strategic programs (see Chapter 4). In other words, *they are designed on the basis of scientifically collected data to achieve measurable objectives that reach and involve specific audiences and that position health practices persuasively as a benefit in the minds of the intended audience.* They also are designed to leave, upon their conclusion, trained practitioners and effective institutions to continue this work in the future.

The strategic development and use of communication is a major contribution of PCS and its partners to the family planning field. Strategic thinking lies at the heart of effective communication. This strategic approach to communication has helped to change communication programs from a "spare wheel," called upon when other approaches fail, to a "steering wheel" that can provide direction for program activities.[3]

Some of the key elements of strategic communication include:

- a science-based approach to communication that builds on conceptual models in behavioral sciences, social learning, persuasion theory, and social marketing to achieve realistic objectives. Some of these models are discussed in Chapter 2.
- emphasis on audience involvement and participation throughout the project planning, implementation, and evaluation process—in effect, a dialogue between program managers and their intended audiences that includes focus-group research, pretesting, sample surveys, interactive counseling approaches, exit interviews, and even participatory mass media formats. Listening to and obtaining feedback from the audience are built into each step of the program development process.
- recognition that behavior change is as much a societal process as it is an individual decision-making process. Therefore communication programs need to reach multiple audience segments—including family members, elders, young people, health care providers, community leaders, news and entertainment media, and policy-makers—and to identify and evaluate changes at the levels of the individual, couple, family, village, and nation.
- use of mass media and multimedia channels not only to increase awareness and to influence community norms but also to provide specific information, legitimization,

and cues to action for individual behavior. New horizons in mass media and electronic communication such as E-mail and the Internet also offer new opportunities to inform and influence health behavior.

- appreciation of the crucial role of entertainment, through mass media and at the community level, to capture the attention, the interest, and, above all, the emotions of an audience and thus to make learning, to quote Aristotle, "the liveliest pleasure" (Aristotle, trans. 1987). The Enter-Educate approach—which combines educational health messages with entertaining songs, drama, and comedy—has dramatically increased the number of people reached by family planning messages and has helped to bring family planning out of the clinic and directly into the popular culture.
- an increasing focus on sustainability for communication activities, both through sharing or leveraging costs with other donors and through institution-building and skills development. Many projects have demonstrated that high-quality communication helps to pay for itself and that high-quality programs generate a can-do spirit that sustains subsequent programs.

These six elements characterize the latest stage in family planning communication—"the strategic communication era." The lessons from this era and the ways in which they can be systematically applied to improve family planning and other types of public health information are spelled out in the following chapters. Applying the lessons of the past and the technology of the future, strategic communication offers even greater potential for improvements in health behavior and reproductive health and for lowering fertility rates in the next 25 years than have been achieved in the last 25.

NOTES

1. The term "modernization" is a source of confusion because of its multiple uses and meanings. To economists it is a trend toward increased per capita economic production due to application of new technology. Lerner (1963), a sociologist, identified four major components of modernization: industrialization, urbanization, education, and mass media development. Inkeles and Smith (1974), social psychologists, defined modernity as an increase in an individual's sense of subjective efficacy, societal participation, and innovativeness.

2. Originally, the term Information, Education, and Communication, or IEC, was adopted as a compromise to avoid the need for consensus on any one of the three terms, each of which has different connotations and academic origins. Over the last 25 years, however, the term "communication" has gradually become the general concept that encompasses the other two.

3. The spare wheel/steering wheel analogy was first made by UNICEF Deputy Director in Latin America Luis Rivera in the late 1980s to distinguish "program communication" from "program support communication." JHU/PCS has built on this definition of program communication to emphasize the concept of "strategic communication."

Chapter 2

Conceptual Frameworks for Strategic Communication

EXPANDING THE ROLE OF COMMUNICATION

One of the biggest obstacles to the effective use of communication in early family planning programs was thinking about communication in too narrow a manner. Communication was originally conceptualized as a simple one-way transmission of messages from a source to a receiver with the intention of producing some effect (Rogers, 1973). The intended effect was usually limited to making the receiver aware of some point of view, new product, or course of action. Neither the social process of communication nor the influence of communication on behavior received enough consideration. This was the concept underlying the "large volume" approach that was common to family planning communication programs before the 1980s (see Chapter 1). Attention was given to the production of materials rather than to their content; to technical quality rather than to how different audience members would interpret the meaning of the content within their particular social context.

Just as family planning communication has changed in response to the evolution of family planning programs (see Chapter 1), so also family planning communication has changed as the concept of communication has evolved. By the 1990s, the conceptual framework for communication had expanded dramatically. The key program elements of strategic communication identified in Chapter 1 —audience participation, recognition of behavior change as both a social and an individual process, use of mass media, and development of entertainment for educational purposes—are rooted in new conceptual frameworks of communication and behavior change.

AUDIENCE PARTICIPATION

The first step in this reconceptualization began in the late 1970s, when communication was defined as a two-way, interactive process involving two or more individuals or groups in which all participants both encode (create and share) and decode (perceive and interpret) information until the goals of each are adequately achieved. In other words, the definition and practice of communication shifted from *monologue* to *dialogue*. A convergence model of communication was developed by D. Lawrence Kincaid to capture this new participatory orientation (1979).

Thus communication was redefined as "a process in which the participants create and share information with one another in order to reach a mutual understanding" (Kincaid, 1979; Rogers & Kincaid, 1981). Mutual understanding builds the foundation for mutual agreement, which in turn makes collective action possible. In the convergence model of communication, the emphasis shifts to the iterative process of information sharing over time, to the ways in which participants interpret and understand that information, and to the dynamic process of feedback and adaptive behavior. In the process, there is convergence of both the ideas and the behavior of the participants. The distinction between sender and receiver disappears because all participants have the opportunity to be both senders and receivers.

The practical implications of this shift in thinking about communication are readily apparent. Program officials who attempt to bypass or shortcut this process by simply sending out whatever messages make sense or appeal to them should expect to have limited (and unknown) impact on their audience. Communication in this way sometimes even has effects on the audience contrary to those intended. One of the main lessons learned over the last 25 years is that *effective communication begins with the audience, the client, or the consumer and continues over time as a process of mutual adjustment and convergence.*

Audiences have different ways of thinking, different vocabulary, even different ways of interpreting drawings and photographs from those of the experts and officials who initiate communication programs. The attitudes and predispositions—even the thought processes—of potential audiences need to be taken into account when communication is designed to address them. Messages need to be (1) based on information obtained from audience members themselves and (2) pretested with them to make sure they were correctly designed. Only then can program managers have any degree of confidence that audience members will interpret family planning messages in the way that they were intended.

Small group discussions or in-depth interviews give audience members the opportunity to express themselves to program officials first, before communication programs are designed. Effective program managers pay attention to this valuable experience when designing their messages and then return to other members of the same audience to pretest their messages to see if they have been produced correctly. If this communication design process is followed, then the probability that family planning communication will be effective greatly increases. This is the communication theory underlying market research and such formative research techniques as focus-group discussions, audience surveys, and message pretesting. In other words, communication research is a systematic dialogue with members of the intended audience.

SOCIAL MARKETING THEORY AND PRACTICE

At approximately the same time that the concept of communication was being expanded to recognize more interaction with the audience, a new and similar concept was introduced from the field of commerce and advertising—social marketing. First proposed by Kotler and Zaltman in 1971, social marketing was defined by Kotler as "the design, implementation, and control of programs calculated to influence the acceptability of social ideas and involving considerations of product, planning, pricing, communication, distribution, and marketing research" (Kotler & Zaltman, 1971, p. 5).

Social marketing focused primarily on influencing consumer behavior by emphasizing the "four Ps"—product, price, place, and promotion. Initially, in the field of family planning, this meant promoting and selling over-the-counter contraceptive products, such as condoms, at subsidized prices that were affordable to a defined population (Altman & Piotrow, 1980). But each of the four elements gradually expanded. Thus social marketing could promote not only a specific product such as a condom but also a practice such as breastfeeding or nonsmoking. Price could mean the psychological cost of adopting a practice that others frowned upon. Place could refer to any distribution channels, commercial or otherwise, that would reach the intended client or consumer. And promotion could range from point-of-purchase information in pharmacies to billboards, mass media, or any form of advertising and even community entertainment events (Kotler & Roberto, 1989; Lefebre & Flora, 1988; Manoff, 1985). In fact, by 1995 the definition of social marketing had expanded to include not only most voluntary public health programs but also many other social issues. Thus, in the words of Alan Andreason, social marketing is broadly defined as "the application of commercial marketing technologies to the analysis, planning, execution, and evaluation of programs designed to influence the voluntary behavior of target audiences in order to improve their personal welfare and that of their society" (Andreason, 1995, p. 7). As a result, while communication experts saw social marketing as one component of communication, social marketers began to see health communication as one component of social marketing, sparking a controversy that still flourishes (Buchanan, Reddy, & Hossain, 1994; Hastings & Haywood, 1991).

Social marketing programs expanded rapidly during the 1980s and early 1990s. In fact, one might even call that period "the social marketing era" in family planning. Largely under the aegis of Population Services International and of the

Social Marketing for Change (SOMARC) program of the Futures Group social marketing organizations sell condoms, and, sometimes in addition, oral contraceptives, IUDs, injectable contraceptives, oral rehydration salts, and even mosquito nets. As the threat of AIDS spread worldwide, social marketing became a major strategy in developing countries for selling condoms to men, who were rarely reached by clinical or field services. By the mid-1990s, 54 social marketing programs were under way in 50 countries, providing 13.9 million couple-years of contraceptive protection and serving 9 percent of couples of reproductive age in developing countries (Harvey, 1996).

Social marketing has brought a useful discipline and focus to family planning programs and to the communication component of these programs. Emphasis on audience research, audience segmentation into identified markets, and the establishment of a market niche for specific methods reinforced the new emphasis on addressing the concerns and unmet needs of the audience. Moreover, calling on the professional skills of the commercial communication industry, such as market research firms, advertising agencies, and public relations organizations, stimulated creativity in health communication.

But social marketing, although a useful addition to clinics and field outreach, does not meet everyone's family planning needs. Some clients cannot pay even subsidized prices; some may substitute social marketing products for commercial brands; many will need advice and counseling from health professionals; and some methods—particularly voluntary female sterilization and vasectomy—do not lend themselves well to social marketing. Nor does social marketing theory satisfy the growing need for a strategic approach to health communication at all levels, that is, for a national strategy of health communication in each country. Thus the present era, in which clinic, field, and marketing approaches all play a role in national health strategies, can best be described as "the strategic communication era," both for programs and for communication.

BEHAVIOR CHANGE AS A PROCESS

With increasing attention focused on the audience, as individuals, as clients, and as customers, and on the exchanges between providers and clients, health communicators began turning to theories of communication and behavior change that emphasize process. These theories help to explain the process that individuals go through as they exchange information and as they interpret and react to different messages.

Various models for this process developed in different fields. In the late 1940s Hovland and colleagues developed the first mass communication impact model that described the communication process as a hierarchy, leading from cognition to affective response (like or dislike, attitude) to behavior or action (Hovland, Lumsdain & Sheffield, 1949). In the field of marketing and advertising, the model specified four stages in an individual's change: attention, interest, desire, and action (AIDA). This was soon expanded to six steps: attention, interest, comprehension, impact, attitude, and sales (Palda, 1966). This evolving model closely resembled the classic model of the diffusion of innovations developed in rural sociology during the 1940s and 1950s (Ryan & Gross, 1943; Rogers, 1962) and which now includes five stages: knowledge, persuasion, decision, implementation, and confirmation (Rogers, 1983 & 1995).

In addressing communication as a process, models in different fields identified specific pathways to behavior change. The convergence concept of communication used in the revised diffusion model specifies five individual steps in the process—perception, interpretation, understanding, agreement, and action—but it adds three social outcomes: mutual understanding, mutual agreement, and collective action (Kincaid, 1987; Rogers & Kincaid, 1981). Also, a 12-step input-output communication/persuasion model was developed by social psychologists to describe the persuasion process (McGuire, 1989). The most recent model of health behavior change comes from the field of psychotherapy. It consists of five stages of personal change: precontemplation, contemplation, preparation, action, and maintenance of new behavior (Prochaska, DiClemente, & Norcross, 1992). This model has been applied to individual and group counseling for alcohol and drug addiction. The striking similarity of these models across such diverse scientific and applied disciplines suggests that a "stage" model is also appropriate for family planning communication.

Other behavioral change models emphasize different stimuli for behavior change but are compatible with the concept of a gradual, step-by-step process. Social comparison and influence theories, for example, emphasize the effect of social interaction on individual behavior (Festinger, 1954; Latane, 1981; Moscovici, 1976). Network analysis illustrates how communication networks can provide a source of new ideas and a stimulus for behavior change (Rogers & Kincaid, 1981; Valente, 1995). Some theories, such as Fishbein and Ajzen's theory of reasoned action, emphasize the role of cognitive factors in behavior change (Fishbein & Ajzen, 1975). Still other theories have explored the power of emotion to influence behavior (Zajonc, 1984). Each of these theories offers insights that can be relevant to individuals or societies as they shift behavior patterns and to public health programs as they deliberately try to influence health behavior. (See Box 2.1 for a summary of relevant theories relating to communication effects on behavior.)

THE STEPS TO BEHAVIOR CHANGE FRAMEWORK

To design strategic communication programs that are appropriate for family planning and reproductive health, Population Communication Services developed a theoretical framework termed the Steps to Behavior Change (SBC). This framework is an adaptation of diffusion of innovations theory and the input/output persuasion model, enriched by social marketing experience and flexible enough to use other theories within each of the steps, or stages, as appropriate. It consists of five major stages of change: knowledge, approval, intention, practice, and advocacy. These five stages and sixteen steps are shown in Box 2.2.

Box 2.1
Theories of Communication Impacts on Behavior
Over the last 50 years social scientists have advanced various theories of how communication can influence human behavior. These theories and models provide family planning communicators with indicators and examples of what influences behavior, in what ways, and under what conditions and offer foundations for planning, executing, and evaluating communication projects. Theories particularly relevant to health communication include:

Stage/Step Theories *Diffusion of innovations theory*, by B. Ryan and N. Gross, 1943, traces the process by which a new idea or practice is communicated through certain channels over time among members of a social system. The model describes the factors that influence people's thoughts and actions and the process of adopting a new technology or idea (Rogers, 1962 & 1983; Ryan & Gross, 1943 & 1950; Valente, 1995). *The input/output persuasion model*, by W. J. McGuire, 1969, emphasizes the *hierarchy of communication effects* and considers how various aspects of communication, such as message design, source, and channel, as well as audience characteristics, influence the behavioral outcome of communication (McGuire, 1969 & 1989). *Stages of change theory*, by psychologists J. O. Prochaska, C. C. DiClemente, and J. C. Norcross, 1992, identifies psychological processes that people undergo and stages they reach as they adopt new behavior. Changes in behavior result when the psyche moves through several iterations of a spiral process: from precontemplation through contemplation, preparation, and action, to maintenance of the new behavior (Prochaska et al., 1992).

Cognitive Theories *Theory of reasoned action*, by M. Fishbein and I. Ajzen, specifies that adoption of a behavior is a function of intent, which is determined by a person's attitude (beliefs and expected values) toward performing the behavior and by perceived social norms (importance and perception that others expect the behavior) (Fishbein & Ajzen, 1975). *Social cognitive (learning) theory*, by A. Bandura, specifies that audience members identify with attractive characters in the mass media who demonstrate behavior, engage emotions, and facilitate mental rehearsal and modeling of new behavior. The behavior of models in the mass media also offers vicarious reinforcement to motivate audience members' adoption of the behavior (Bandura, 1977 & 1986).

Social Process Theories *Social influence, social comparison*, and *convergence theories* specify that one's perception and behavior are influenced by the perceptions and behavior of members of groups to which one belongs and by members of one's personal networks. People rely on the opinions of others, especially when a situation is highly uncertain or ambiguous and no objective evidence is readily available. Social influence can have vicarious effects on audiences by depicting in television and radio programs the process of change and eventual conversion of behavior (Festinger, 1954; Kincaid, 1987 & 1988; Latane, 1981; Moscovici, 1976; Rogers & Kincaid, 1981; Suls, 1977).

Emotional Response Theories *Theories of emotional response* propose that emotional response precedes and conditions cognitive and attitudinal effects. This implies that highly emotional messages in entertainment (see Chapter 4) would be more likely to influence behavior than messages low in emotional content (Clark, 1992; Zajonc, 1984; Zajonc, Murphy, & Inglehart, 1989).

Mass Media Theories *Cultivation theory of mass media*, proposed by George Gerbner, specifies that repeated, intense exposure to deviant definitions of "reality" in the mass media leads to perception of that "reality" as normal. The result is a social legitimization of the "reality" depicted in the mass media, which can influence behavior (Gerbner, 1973 & 1977; Gerbner et al., 1980).

Box 2.2
Steps to Behavior Change
Knowledge
1. Recalls family planning messages.
2. Understands what family planning means.
3. Can name family planning method(s) and/or source of supply.
Approval
4. Responds favorably to family planning messages.
5. Discusses family planning with personal networks (family, friends).
6. Thinks family, friends, and community approve of family planning.
7. Approves of family planning.
Intention
8. Recognizes that family planning can meet a personal need.
9. Intends to consult a provider.
10. Intends to practice family planning at some time.
Practice
11. Goes to a provider of information/supplies/services.
12. Chooses a method and begins family planning use.
13. Continues family planning use.
Advocacy
14. Experiences and acknowledges personal benefits of family planning.
15. Advocates practice to others.
16. Supports programs in the community.

The SBC framework shows how individuals and groups progress from knowledge to sustained behavior change and advocacy. It emphasizes that behavior change—and thus communication intended to influence behavior—is a process. It recognizes that behavior change is the goal but that people usually move through several intermediate steps before they change their behavior. Furthermore, it suggests that people at different stages constitute distinct audiences. Thus they usually need different messages and sometimes different approaches, whether interpersonal communication, community mobilization, or mass media.

This SBC framework has been refined by advances in theory and by practical experience in implementing communication programs. These modifications recognize the following:

- Not all individuals go through each step of the process in the same order, at the same speed, or at the same time. For example, some women recognize a personal need to limit family size before they ever hear of family planning methods. Other women learn about and approve of family planning but wait a long time before they begin to practice it. Most women and men increase their knowledge of family planning gradually, not all in one step, as they are exposed to different sources of information, and as they try one method, learn about its advantages and disadvantages in practice, discontinue, and then try another.
- As knowledge and approval reach high levels in more advanced programs, emphasis shifts to later steps, such as identifying effective cues to action, maximizing access to

and quality of services, identifying and removing barriers to change, reinforcing current users, and creating opportunities for advocacy.

- Social norms and public policies influence individual behavior change. Therefore political leaders, policy-makers, and local people of influence are part of the audience for most mass media communication, most community mobilization activities, and much interpersonal communication.

- Advocacy for behavior change, through public acknowledgment, promotion by satisfied users, and support for programs, is the final stage of behavior change. Once the benefits of family planning or any other health practice are confirmed by experience, a person's public advocacy of the practice to others cements conviction and sustains the new behavior. Advocacy also helps other people move through the steps by offering them a behavioral model and confirming community norms. Advocacy is positive feedback to the process of behavior change.

In summary, the communication process is characterized by a sequence of intermediate outcomes and feedback. Progress from one step to the next increases the probability of behavior change and continuation. Family planning and other forms of health communication are an adaptive social process, in which changes in a population have positive feedback effects that can accelerate the rate of change. Public policy and communication programs influence both individual and social change, establishing new community norms and, over time, providing support for stronger and more effective policies and programs.

MEETING THE AUDIENCE'S COMMUNICATION NEEDS WITH THE SBC FRAMEWORK

How does the communication expert apply this theoretical framework about behavior change to operational programs? Survey research can identify different segments of the population in terms of their current stage of change. For example, a certain percentage may still never have heard of family planning, while others are already using some method. The rest of the audience will fall somewhere between these two points in certain proportions. For example, some women will approve of contraceptive use, have positive attitudes, and desire to avoid pregnancy but will not have taken any action yet. These women have what is called "an unmet need" for family planning (see Chapter 3) (Robey, Ross, & Bhushan, 1996; Westoff & Bankole, 1995). The reasons for this unmet need vary, but often an unmet need for family planning can be traced to an unmet need for communication.

Building on the behavior change models and theories discussed above, practical guides have been developed that make it easier to develop communication programs that are participatory and effective. One such practical guide used in Johns Hopkins programs is termed the Seven Cs of Effective Communication (J. R. Williams, 1992) (see Chapter 5, Lesson 1). Corresponding to specific steps to behavior change, the Seven Cs suggest the type of information most needed at each stage of change.

MASS MEDIA, ENTERTAINMENT, AND MEDIA ADVOCACY

Even without any modern communication media, people communicate, exchange ideas, and alter their behavior. But the unprecedented growth of mass media—first print, then radio, now television and computer communication—has raised new possibilities for rapid global communication and thus new theories about how people may react and change as a result of mass media.

By the early 1970s expectations that mass media could have a direct effect on mass behavior had faded. In fact, a "limited effects" view of mass media was dominant in the United States (Klapper, 1960; McQuail, 1994). Klapper (1960) concluded that mass media by themselves—apart from reinforcing the status quo—do not act as the sole cause of audience effects but rather as a contributory agent through a set of mediating factors and influences. Research in the United States was showing that important individual differences in gender, age, education, and psychological predisposition led to selective exposure, attention, retention, and perception of mass media messages (Klapper, 1960). The notion of a homogeneous "mass" audience was being replaced by the notion of a heterogeneous audience comprised of different types of individuals and different subcultures, each with different ways of looking at the world. Thus the concept of audience segmentation emerged, consistent with theories of behavior change and marketing that could guide political, consumer, and other types of mass media campaigns and focus resources where the potential for change was the greatest.

Research on a U.S. presidential campaign in the 1940s led to the "two-step flow" hypothesis of mass media effects: that the media had direct effects on opinion leaders, who then had indirect effects on other members of the audience by means of interpersonal communication (Katz & Lazarsfeld, 1955). By the end of the 1970s the accepted view of mass media was that they were effective for increasing awareness but that only interpersonal communication could persuade or motivate action (Rogers, 1983).

One of the first theories to propose that mass media may have more powerful effects was Noelle-Neumann's (1993) "spiral of silence" theory of opinion formation. Her research on political campaigns in Germany in the 1960s and 1970s concluded that the more frequently the dominant or majority opinion is disseminated by the mass media, the more likely it is that individuals with contrary opinions will remain silent, thus accelerating the effects of the media (in a spiraling process). The theory assumes that individuals have a fear of isolation and hence try to identify with and express the majority opinion or perceived consensus. The theory implies that, for a new, minority opinion to become accepted, the ideal condition would be for the majority to remain silent while the minority opinion receives more public expression via the mass media. This leads the audience to perceive that the minority opinion may actually be the majority position (social norm). If the majority remains relatively silent, the minority opinion could eventually prevail. This outcome is similar to what Gerbner's (1973) cultivation theory of mass media would predict: even if the message is distinctive and deviates from "reality," its persistent exposure on television can lead to its adoption (perception) as the consensual view of society. This is sometimes called the "legitimizing effect" of the mass media.

At about this same time Katz, Blumler, and Gurevitch (1974; Blumler & Katz, 1974) were proposing a "uses and gratifications" approach to mass media, which treated audience members as active selectors of media content rather than as passive receivers. Entertainment was considered to be one of the main functions of mass media, along with surveillance (news), correlation (interpretation of reality), and cultural transmission (values and norms).

Then Ball-Rokeach and Defleur (1976) developed a dependency theory of mass media that specified a three-way interaction among audiences, media, and the larger social system. A group's (or audience segment's) dependency on a medium such as television or radio for information increases when (1) that medium supplies information that is central to the needs of that group and (2) when social change, conflict, and social instability increase uncertainty and ambiguity. Increased dependency on mass media for information increases the impact of mass media on knowledge, attitudes, and behavior.

EVALUATING BEHAVIOR CHANGE AS A PROCESS

When communication is recognized as a process that affects different people in different ways at different times, it becomes clear that evaluation of the impact of communication programs also must grow out of this conceptual framework. As the Steps to Behavior Change model indicates, individuals or couples respond to family planning communication in different but related ways depending on where they stand in the process: switching from being undecided to no longer wanting another child; gaining knowledge of modern contraceptives; beginning to talk with other women who support family planning practice; shifting from disagreement to agreement with one's spouse about using a contraceptive; and so forth. They may move one step at a time, or they may take several steps at once. When the intermediate steps of knowledge and attitudes, as well as behavior, change within the time period of the program, this multiple response increases confidence that a communication program has influenced the changes. At the same time, if knowledge and attitudes are observed to change within the period under study, the likelihood that behavior eventually will change, too, is increased.

Statistical analyses of these influences on several hundred or several thousand respondents before and after a communication campaign—including multivariate, regression, and path analysis, for example—can also show how exposure to a campaign is related to the subobjectives or steps to behavioral change, such as an increase in discussion and agreement between spouses or an increase in the belief that modern contraceptives are healthy (see Chapter 7). Such findings suggest that communication not only has a direct impact on behavior in conjunction with other factors, but also that it has an indirect impact because it operates at each step in the process as well. These intermediate steps (intervening variables) can be specified in advance as intended subobjectives of the intervention. Measurement of these intermediate steps (links in the causal chain) greatly increases confidence in attributing outcomes to interventions, because these outcomes are implied by the theories of communication and behavior change used to design the interventions.

A Systematic Process for Developing Strategic Communication Programs

Not only the content and evaluation of communication programs but also the development of these programs is now increasingly systematic and strategic. The design, implementation, monitoring, and evaluation of Johns Hopkins communication projects follow "The Processes and Principles for Health Communication Projects," known as the P Process (see Figure 2.1).

The P Process (in which P can stand for project or program) is valuable because it is (1) systematic and rational, (2) continually responsive to research findings and data, (3) practical for field applications at all levels, and (4) strategic in setting and pursuing long-term objectives. The P Process consists of six s teps that are followed in sequence to develop and implement effective national communication strategies, programs, or, indeed, any organized communication activity:

Figure 2.1
The P Process

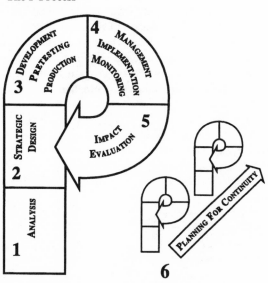

- **Analysis**—Listen to potential audiences; assess existing programs, policies, resources, strengths and weaknesses; and analyze communication resources.
- **Strategic design**—Decide on objectives, identify audience segments, position the concept for the audience, clarify behavior change model, select channels of communication, plan for interpersonal discussion, draw up an action plan, and design evaluation.
- **Development, pretesting and revision, and production**—Develop message concepts, pretest with audience members and gatekeepers, revise and produce messages and materials, retest new and existing materials.
- **Management, implementation, and monitoring**—Mobilize key organizations, create a positive organizational climate, implement the action plan, and monitor the process of dissemination, transmission, and reception of program outputs.
- **Impact evaluation**—Measure impact on audiences and determine how to improve future projects.
- **Planning for continuity**—Adjust to changing conditions; plan for continuity and self-sufficiency.

The P Process was developed in 1983 by the first Population Communication Services project team, which included the Academy for Educational Development; Porter, Novelli and Associates; and the Program for Appropriate Technology in Health. It has continued to provide a solid framework for strategy development, project implementation, technical assistance, institution-building, and training for more than a decade. Somewhat similar processes have been developed by other individuals and organizations to guide their work (Graeff, Elder, & Booth, 1993; L. W. Green & Kreuter, 1991; National Institutes of Health [NIH], 1992). Due to international training programs and technical assistance provided by PCS, many family planning communication programs throughout the developing world have adopted, applied, and institutionalized the P Process over the last decade.

The remainder of the book is organized according to this P Process for program planning and implementation. The experience gained over the last 15 years at each step of a communication program is described in Chapters 3 through 8. The book concludes with a discussion of the challenges facing family planning and health communication in the future. The emphasis throughout is on expanding the role that communication plays in health programs, institutionalizing a systematic approach to developing communication programs, and stimulating the level of creativity needed to make communication effective.

Chapter 3

Preliminary Analysis for Program Planning

PEOPLE

Lesson 1. A communication analysis begins by identifying primary and secondary audiences.

Lesson 2. Analysis should identify what people already know, believe, hope for, and practice.

Lesson 3. Analysis makes it possible to divide large populations into audience segments that will respond to specific appeals.

POLICIES AND PROGRAMS

Lesson 4. Analysis identifies government policies that can impede or assist communication programs.

Lesson 5. Analysis usually indicates that policy-makers are an important secondary audience for family planning communication.

Lesson 6. Analysis identifies strengths and weaknesses so that communication can accentuate the positive and help correct the negative.

ORGANIZATIONS

Lesson 7.   A review of existing organizations shows which
              can best carry out an effective communication
              program and how different organizations can
              collaborate.

COMMUNICATION RESOURCES

Lesson 8.   Analysis identifies the most appropriate and cost-
              effective channels available to reach primary and
              secondary audiences.

VALUE OF RESEARCH AND ANALYSIS

Lesson 9.   A good communication analysis takes both time
              and skill to produce.

Lesson 10.   A good analysis serves many purposes over the life
              of the program.

Communication programs rarely succeed by accident. They succeed as a result of
a systematic planning and implementation process such as the P Process (see Figure
2.1, Chapter 2). The first step in the process is *analysis*. The success of any
communication program depends on an accurate analysis of the problem to be
solved; the people, policies, programs, and organizations needed to resolve it; and
the communication resources that can be mobilized. Various research sources and
methods are used to obtain an accurate account (see Box 3.1).

In most family planning and other health programs, the broad outlines of the
problem have already been defined by high-level policy-makers. For example, the
problem may be too-rapid population growth, high maternal and infant morbidity
and mortality rates, or unacceptable rates of teenage pregnancy or of abortion, or
all of the above. The overall program objectives may also be established—for
example, to reduce fertility or mortality or to increase contraceptive prevalence by
a specified amount.

Whatever the problem and the program objective, the task of the communication analysis is to identify what is needed for communication to help achieve those
objectives. Basically, the initial communication analysis focuses on such strategic
information as the following:

• **People**—Whose behavior must change for program objectives to be reached? How do
  different people perceive the problem? If the problem relates to reproductive health and
  family planning, for example, how much do these people already know about it? What
  are their present attitudes, intentions, and practices? What beliefs and barriers exist that
  impede change? How do society, culture, and religion influence the way people think

and act about the problem? How do people communicate about it, both privately and publicly? Who are the secondary audiences that can influence or reinforce potential users of family planning and other reproductive health services?

- **Policies and programs**—What are the national and local policies, politics, and health care standards and guidelines concerning reproductive health and family planning? Who are the policy-makers and opinion leaders? What programs and services exist, and how good are they? How can they be strengthened?
- **Organizations**—What are the key organizations—government, nongovernmental, and private/commercial—already active in family planning and reproductive health? Which organizations can plan and carry out a communication program? How do public and private organizations work together? What type of collaboration is needed?
- **Communication resources**—What are the best communication channels to reach the primary audiences? Who controls access to these channels? What laws or regulations govern the use of these channels? What technical services are available, such as market research firms, advertising agencies, performers, producers, and distribution services? How knowledgeable are communication professionals about reproductive health and family planning issues?

Box 3.1
Information Sources for Analysis

Analysts must use various research sources and methods to develop a clear and accurate assessment of communication needs and resources.

Quantitative research, notably population-based surveys, permits generalizations about large populations and subgroups. Service and sales statistics help identify where and when people go for family planning advice and supplies.

Qualitative research, such as focus-group discussions and in-depth individual interviews, helps planners understand what people think and how they talk about sensitive topics such as sexual behavior and family planning.

All the following can provide useful information:
- Evaluations of any prior family planning projects;
- Published and unpublished literature, including
  - Demographic and Health Surveys and other household surveys of family planning knowledge, attitudes, and practices;
  - Anthropological, demographic, and sociological studies; and
  - Analyses of the health care and family planning delivery systems;
- Government documents and statistics, including national development plans, legislation, ministry reports, censuses, and official statements;
- Clinic service statistics;
- Inventories of communication materials at service delivery sites;
- Market research such as consumer point-of-purchase or intercept data, inventories of media outlets, and audience profiles for the various outlets;
- In-depth interviews with service providers, clients, and potential clients;
- Observations of counseling sessions, group health talks, and interviews with clients leaving service facilities (includes reports from "mystery clients"—people hired to impersonate clients and visit service providers);
- Focus-group discussions with small groups representative of the audience;
- Interviews with government officials and managers of nongovernmental organizations involved in family planning.

PEOPLE

LESSON 1.

A communication analysis begins by identifying primary and secondary audiences.

Whose behavior must change for program objectives to be achieved? This is the first question that the analysis must address. Married women of reproductive age have always been the major focus of family planning and maternal/child health programs. Thus attention has focused on communicating with those women—in clinics through trained providers, educational lectures, flipcharts, brochures, and increasingly videos, where electricity and VCRs are available; through door-to-door distribution, taking information and supplies directly to women in their homes; through community-based depot-holders, or retail stores where information and supplies can be conveniently obtained; and increasingly through mass media designed to reach women of reproductive age. Because ultimately, if the program is to succeed, these women will have to make an informed personal choice to use family planning or practice other maternal and child health measures in the home, communication programs need to begin with an analysis of their needs and concerns.

Women with unmet need. Demographic and Health Surveys (DHS) in many countries of Asia, Africa, the Near East, and Latin America and the Caribbean show that about 10 to 30 percent of all married women have an unmet need for family planning (Robey, Ross, & Bhushan, 1996; Westoff & Ochoa, 1991; Westoff & Bankole, 1995 & 1996). In other words, they do not want another child, either now or perhaps ever, but they are not currently using family planning. In Nepal, these women—both those who want to delay their next birth and those who want no more births—were identified through a 1993 needs assessment as the key audience for the "Redline Communication Strategy" (Rimon & Lediard, 1993). This analysis made it possible to identify, among the 3.8 million married Nepali women of reproductive age, the subgroup of 1.1 million with unmet need—a group about equally divided between "spacers" (those wanting to space births) and "limiters" (those wanting no more births). These women, both spacers and limiters, became the intended audience who might change their behavior on the basis of a communication campaign designed specifically to address their concerns (see Box 3.4, page 40).

Men. Other audiences also are important. Needs assessments in the late 1980s in Egypt (Rimon & Zimmerman, 1987), Ghana (Ezeh, 1993), Zimbabwe (Kuseka & Silberman, 1990), and elsewhere found that men often made the final decision whether to use family planning. Moreover, these analyses found, communication between spouses about family planning predicted contraceptive use. As a result, later programs in all three countries were designed with specific appeals and information for men as a primary audience and women as a secondary audience. Major objectives were to increase communication between spouses, to stimulate men to use family planning themselves, and to encourage their wives to do so in a shared decision-making process. In Zimbabwe, after two intensive, male-oriented multimedia motivation campaigns, men reported that they became more involved in family planning discussions and decisions and more supportive of family planning (Y. M. Kim, Marangwanda, & Kols, 1996; Piotrow, Kincaid, et al., 1992).

In Chiapas, Mexico, an extensive analysis (Poppe, Rodriguez, & Payne Merritt, 1991) investigated men's and women's roles at four critical points in the process of adopting family planning: (1) initiating discussion with their spouses, (2) seeking information about family planning, (3) obtaining the information, and (4) deciding to adopt a contraceptive method. Male and female respondents agreed that men were responsible for the two most important steps in the process: initiating discussion and deciding to adopt a family planning method. Women, however, were responsible for the two middle steps: seeking and obtaining information. Building on this analysis instead of mere guesswork, the project was then designed to persuade men that family planning was their concern as well as their wives' and called for joint decision-making.

Family and community. Research in some countries shows that the extended family and even male community leaders exert strong influence on the family planning practices of young married couples. Research documenting the influence of the extended family on fertility decisions in Ghana inspired a scene in the film *Dangerous Numbers* (Population Information Project—Ghana, 1987). It featured a mother pressuring her son and daughter-in-law to have more children than the two they already have. The mother is unaware that her daughter-in-law uses family planning. Her son explains that the well-being of his family depends on thinking ahead and knowing how many children he can support. In Bangladesh, baseline research revealed a complex set of influences on a woman's adoption of family planning (Kincaid, Massiah, et al., 1993). While her husband had the dominant voice, the male head of her *bari*, or household compound, usually also had to approve of family planning. Then, even with this approval, to implement the decision, the woman—usually confined by custom to her *bari*—had to spend time with a visiting field worker and with other like-minded women before her desire to use contraception could be legitimated (see Box 3.2).

Other primary or secondary audiences for communication programs might include parents, adolescents, service providers, women whose health might be jeopardized by pregnancy, or any other segments of the population whose behavior or opinion is critical to the achievement of program goals. Representatives of the mass media and policy-makers also can be important audiences because they control access to the public. (For additional discussion of policy-makers as secondary audiences, see Lessons 4 and 5, below).

Thus, long before communication messages are developed and media channels selected, a needs assessment and careful analysis identify who the primary and secondary audiences are, what behaviors they may change, and what information and services they need to make those changes.

Box 3.2

The *Jiggasha* Approach in Bangladesh

In rural Bangladesh, where farming methods have not changed for centuries, a tract of land that two decades ago sustained 2,000 inhabitants today must support 5,000 (Mitra, Lerman, & Islam, 1992)—thanks to rapid population growth. Now, however, things are changing. People increasingly favor family planning, contraceptive use has risen to 45 percent of married women of reproductive age, and the fertility rate is dropping (Cleland, 1994; Mitra, Nawab, Ali, et al., 1994). An energetic family planning program that emphasizes communication has made these changes possible. In a largely rural country where travel is difficult, the population is widely dispersed, and, by Islamic tradition, women do not leave their family compounds. Family planning information and supplies have reached most women through home visits by the government's Family Welfare Assistants. Covering the entire population, however, would require each worker to visit 20 homes per day. In fact, they could reach far fewer.

Challenged to help the Family Welfare Assistants reach more people, communication planners applied modern theory to a familiar approach—group discussions. Theory on the diffusion of innovations points out that new ideas move from person to person through established channels of communication; where and how rapidly ideas spread depend on who talks to whom and how often (Rogers & Kincaid, 1981). The chances that a member of the network will accept a new idea or practice depends partly on how many people in her network already have done so (Valente, 1995).

Communication Network Among Women in Shahidpur Village, Trishal, Bangladesh with Family Planning Users in 1992 Identified.

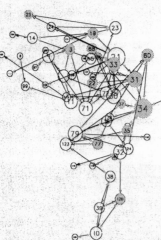

▨ **Users and Perceived Users of FP 24%**
Shahidpur Village, Trishal, 1992

JHU/PCS & MITRA & ASSOC.

Started in 1989, the *jiggasha* approach enables field workers to reach up to a dozen people at a time in groups. In Bangla *jiggasha* means "to inquire." Participants in the *jiggasha* discussion groups convene as guests of influential women in the community. When the most influential women host *jiggashas,* information and attitudes spread most quickly.

Influential women are identified by asking all women about their contacts and who are opinion leaders among women in the community. Then researchers construct a diagram of the social network (see previous page). Each circle represents a woman. A filled circle represents a user of modern contraception. The larger her circle, the more contacts she has. Arrows show who makes contact with whom.

Key women are those with many contacts, such as numbers 34 and 53, and those who link large groups, such as numbers 48 and 49. Field workers ask some of these women to host *jiggashas.*

Research finds that, where highly influential women are active in *jiggashas,* modern contraceptive use among their contacts is generally high.

Women of Shahidpur

"Latifa"

Latifa (number 34) is one of the most influential women in her village. With her husband's approval, Latifa uses a modern family planning method. She welcomes family planning field workers to meet with *jiggasha* groups and is in frequent contact with other women—all of them users of family planning. Most women with whom Latifa talks live in her *bari,* or compound. Of the few outsiders she knows, one is Amina.

"Amina"

Amina (number 48) communicates with relatively few people. Two-thirds of her social contacts do not use family planning. But even without much social support, Amina attends *jiggashas,* has discussed family planning with her husband, and now uses modern contraception.

"Hasina"

Hasina (number 49) neither practices family planning nor attends jiggashas. She interacts with other women slightly more than Amina. One of Hasina's contacts is Sultana, until recently a strong conservative influence in the community; Sultana's influence may help explain why Hasina does not use family planning.

"Sultana"

Sultana (number 53) is one of Trishal's most influential residents. Most of her many contacts, in fact, extend outside her *bari.* Thus she could be an important agent of social change. So far, however, Sultana does not use or discuss family planning; in her social network there is only one user of family planning. Sultana's attitude is changing, however. In 1989 she was firmly opposed to family planning; by 1992 she expressed approval and intention to use family planning. Now, she says, it is her husband's opposition that holds her back.

LESSON 2.

Analysis should identify what people already know, believe, hope for, and practice.

Persuasive communication takes the audience's perspective. Effective messages build on people's current thoughts, feelings, and needs and do not disregard or contradict them. Therefore communication program planners listen to what people say. Through extensive fact-finding, they learn what people really do know, think, and believe. This critically important information, which may be sought from any number of different sources (see Box 3.1, page 31), is essential to design an effective communication program. Perceptual mapping (one of the newer tools for audience analysis) is one way to measure, and also visualize, audience perceptions (see Box 3.3).

In the Philippines, for example, project planners wanted to choose the most appropriate words to describe the benefits of contraceptive methods in television spots. The words "safe," "effective," and "healthy" were being considered to describe important attributes. Then focus-group discussions and in-depth interviews revealed that the Tagalog word *hiyang*, which means "suitable" or "a natural fit" in English, was used repeatedly (Casterline, Perez, & Biddlecom, 1996). The project decided to use that word, which had evolved from the Filipinos' own experience with family planning. So the key message was "visit the health center to find a method that is *hiyang* for you."

A communication project for young people in Brazil provides another example of the critical role of research (Payne Merritt & Raffaelli, 1993). In a 1992 AIDS-prevention project for Brazilian street children, focus-group discussions, interviews, and field observations found that street children of Belo Horizonte did not respond to scare tactics or to the threat of early death. These young people faced death every day. Immediate survival, not future disease, was their concern. Researchers found that street children valued good health only to the extent that it enabled them to survive each day in the streets. So the theme developed for the project was "Street-smart youth can stay strong without AIDS." A video and comic book to convey this message were developed and placed where street children were likely to see them.

LESSON 3.

Analysis makes it possible to divide large populations into audience segments that will respond to specific appeals.

The phrase "the general public" does not belong in any communication plan. Because specific messages are always more powerful than broad, general messages, a communication program should always try, in its initial analysis, to identify specific, fairly homogeneous audiences—that is, audience segments. In other words, once the primary or secondary audience is identified, this audience can be segmented into smaller groupings. Each segment is unified by certain common

Box 3.3
Perceptual Maps: New Tool for Audience Analysis

Perceptual mapping graphically depicts an audience's perceptions. The closer together two concepts, attributes, services, or providers are on the graph, the more closely associated they are in the audience's minds. In particular, the closer something is to the audience itself, the more affinity the audience feels for the product or service, or the more important the attribute is to the audience. Perceptual maps are drawn from survey findings, by computer software called IMAGE, developed by D. L. Kincaid at the Johns Hopkins Center for Communication Programs.

A perceptual map gives communication designers the audience's point of view in one glance. For message design, attributes and benefits that should be emphasized become obvious; the obstacles in people's perceptions that must be surmounted become apparent. Later, "before" and "after" maps can be compared to show how a communication campaign made a difference.

Image of Family Planning Methods, Uttar Pradesh, 1995

In Uttar Pradesh, India, perceptual mapping reveals that people prefer family planning methods that are convenient, effective, and socially acceptable. The Pill, the IUD, and the condom are most associated with these attributes, but the condom is not as popular as the Pill and the IUD.

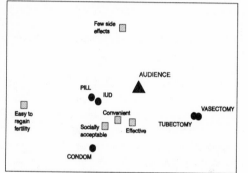

Image of Service Providers, Uttar Pradesh, 1995

In Uttar Pradesh people appreciate health care providers who are effective healers, well-behaved toward clients, and always available. Private doctors and chemists are most strongly associated with these attributes and are preferred by the audience. Now, training is helping health workers develop the traits people want.

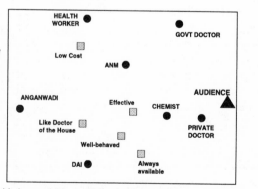

Note: ANMs are auxiliary nurse midwives; a dai is a traditional village midwife; an anganwadi is a traditional healer.

Source: Storey, Chhabra, & Viswanathan, 1995

needs, concerns, or attributes. In selecting which segments to address, good communication analysis looks for audience segments made up of (1) people whose changes in behavior will contribute most to program objectives; (2) people for whom specific messages and materials can be developed; and (3) people who are likely to be exposed to certain channels of communication. With this information, decisions can be made during the strategic design phase about which segments of the audience to concentrate on (see Chapter 4).

Usually overall program priorities determine who the primary audience segment will be. For example, a common program priority is to reach specific geographic areas. But after these primary audiences are established, further audience segmentation can help improve communication. For example, audiences for family planning communication programs can be segmented by:

- demographic characteristics,
- social factors,
- health needs,
- reproductive life stage,
- readiness to change behavior,
- place in the Steps to Behavior Change framework, or
- lifestyle factors.

Conventionally, public health programs have segmented audiences or populations by demographic characteristics such as age, sex, or socioeconomic status, or by various health indicators. These subdivisions can be useful. But now, building on a generation of demographic and market research, family planning communication analyses can use other, more focused ways to segment audiences that will better reflect the different ways that people behave. These often involve thinking about the audience as individuals and looking for relevant motivating or personal characteristics. For example, whether a woman will continue using oral contraceptives may depend more on her fears about health and safety than on her age or socioeconomic status. Whether a man will encourage his wife to use family planning may depend more on his own personality, sense of self-esteem, and openness to new ideas than on his age or place of residence. A woman may experience an unmet need, as discussed in the first lesson, because of lack of knowledge, incorrect knowledge, husband's disapproval, or lack of good services. Based on research within countries, on international data sets, and on recent theories of behavior change, specific population segments that are important to family planning communication programs can be identified. As discussed in Chapter 2, the Steps to Behavior Change framework provides a powerful tool for audience segmentation. Among the various groups identified by the SBC framework, two are often the primary audience for family planning communication: couples who know about family planning but do not plan to practice it, and women who intend to practice family planning.

Couples with high levels of knowledge and even approval of family planning but low rates of practice. Virtually all surveys of health knowledge and behavior find that many people know what is healthy and good for them but do not consistently practice it. This is as true of family planning as of any other health practice. Audience analysis can help to explain this discrepancy in knowledge, attitudes, and practice—the KAP gap—and thus help communication programs address the real concerns that people have. For example, in Pakistan qualitative research investigated why, even though more than 80 percent of married women of reproductive age knew of at least one family planning method, practice of contraception stood at only 15 percent in 1990. The analysis found three main barriers to contraceptive use (Domestic Research Bureau, 1990):

- couples felt that having a son to support them in their old age was essential, and so they would continue having children until they had a son;
- wives raised the topic of adopting family planning but would not act until their husbands approved; and
- both current and potential users of family planning were afraid of contraceptive side effects and mistrusted the quality of available services.

At the same time, all couples had a positive view of spacing births as a way to improve maternal and child health as well as family living conditions. Further analysis, which was carried out by project staff and an anthropologist who had studied sexual practices in several countries, was used to help design a television mini-series, *Aahat*, about a young couple with four daughters spaced too closely and no sons (Lozare, Hess, et al., 1993).

Women who intend to practice family planning. A person's place on the Steps to Behavior Change continuum indicates his or her readiness to change behavior. Thus programs and messages can be designed to meet the unmet communication needs of women (or men) at different stages. When a project objective is to increase overall contraceptive use rapidly, the most appropriate audience segment is often the audience closest to adopting family planning—women who intend to practice family planning but, for one reason or another, are not yet doing so. In Ghana, for example, audience analysis found that almost one-third of women surveyed were at this decision stage—they said they intended to use family planning, and perceived social support for such use (Kumah, Kincaid, et al., 1993; Tweedie et al., 1994). These women, plus current users, became the primary audience for the communication campaign, since theory (Ajzen, 1989) predicted that they would be most likely to adopt or continue using family planning (see Box 3.4, with Figures 3.1 and 3.2).

In the process of audience analysis and segmentation, many different types of data can be used. In the last decade psychographics, a tool used in commercial advertising, has been increasingly applied by health programs. Psychographic profiles create a composite portrait from the statistical findings about the psychological traits of audience members—such as high or low self-esteem, risk-taking tendencies, and fatalism. Psychographic profiles add color and depth to impersonal quantitative socioeconomic data. In effect, psychographic research can create personality profiles of different segments of the audience, allowing project designers to visualize a living person and create messages that would appeal to him

Box 3.4
New Approaches to Audience Segmentation: Examples from Nepal and Ghana

Audience segmentation now goes beyond obvious demographic groups of age, sex, marital status, and socioeconomic status. New approaches to segmentation distinguish potential audiences based on their attitudes and needs and, particularly, where they stand on the Steps to Behavior Change. Segmentation plans in Nepal and Ghana illustrate the new approach.

Nepal
In Nepal the national communication strategy addresses unmet need for family planning—that is, women who say they want to control their fertility but are not using family planning. Among those not now using family planning, the unmet need group is the group most likely to adopt family planning because these women already want to avoid pregnancy (Rimon & Lediard, 1993). In Nepal women with unmet need, who amount to about 1.1 million, outnumber family planning users. The reasons that these women do not use family planning, they report, are lack of access to services and supplies and fear of anticipated side effects (Shrestha, Stoeckel, & Tuladhar, 1988).

Figure 3.1
Unmet Need and Contraceptive Use Among Married Women of Reproductive Age, Nepal, 1991

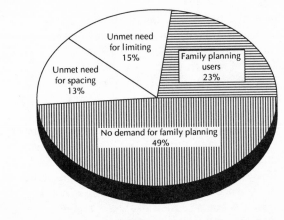

Source: 1991 Nepal Family Planning Survey Preliminary Report.

or her. In the Philippines, for example, researchers used existing studies, focus-group discussion reports, and a nationwide survey to divide low-income Filipinos into seven groups, categorized under the terms Traditionalists, Liberals, Wizened, Tolerants, Strugglers, Rebels, and Go-Getters (Consumer Pulse, 1991). Each category comes to life in a vivid psychographic profile of a composite character,

Ghana

In Ghana women's intentions and perceived social support for contraceptive use shaped the communication strategy. As in Nepal, the strategy focuses on "preaching to the almost converted"—women who intend to practice family planning in the future *and* feel they have social support for doing so. The reasons that these women are not currently practicing family planning suggest the kind of information and encouragement they need—information about methods, information to decrease fear of side effects, and, because research finds that these women are less likely than current users to have talked about family planning, encouragement to obtain more support from partners, friends, and service providers (Ghana Ministry, 1993a; Kumah, Kincaid, et al., 1993).

Figure 3.2
Use, Intention, and Social Support, Ghana, 1993

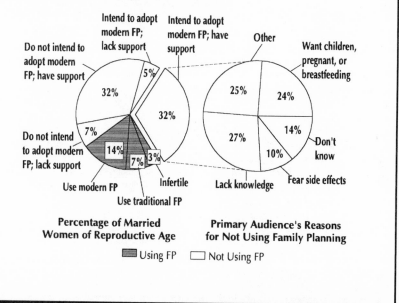

Percentage of Married Women of Reproductive Age

Primary Audience's Reasons for Not Using Family Planning

such as Policarpio, the Traditionalist (see Box 3.5). This type of analysis can bridge the gap between scientific research and creative imagination—both essential in designing an effective communication program.

Box 3.5
A Psychographic Profile from the Philippines: Policarpio, the Traditionalist

Based on findings from both quantitative and qualitative audience research, psychographic profiles of hypothetical personalities evoke vivid pictures of the kinds of people who make up actual audience segments. Researchers in the Philippines discovered the basis for seven distinct personality types in the low-income population. One type, characterized as Traditionalists, is represented by the fictitious character "Policarpio." From what is known of Filipino men like Policarpio, designers can tailor family planning messages to address "Policarpio" and his peers. Messages emphasizing that contraception does not diminish virility would suit Policarpio, as would messages that do not openly challenge conventional gender roles.

Policarpio lives in a barrio in the Visayas. He has been married for seven years now and has four children.

After a day's work in the field, he eats his favorite snack and drinks two glasses of water. He then lies down and sleeps on a bamboo bench near the front door of his hut until his wife wakes him for supper around 6:00. He may spend some time drinking with his neighbors. If they have some cash, they may drink a bottle or two of their favorite local brew. Not drinking would mean effeminacy and weakness.

Occasionally, Policarpio borrows a radio from his brother, who lives just four houses away. Policarpio listens intently to commentaries aired on his favorite AM station.

Policarpio's wife stays at home most of the time. She takes care of the children, prepares the food, washes the clothes, feeds the chickens and the dog. Policarpio likes to tell his friends that a wife should serve the husband because he works hard in the field so that the family will have something to eat. He is content to leave the care of the children to his wife. When it comes to discipline, though, Policarpio takes over, using a bamboo stick. About twice a month, Policarpio goes to town, sometimes with his family, to buy salt, sardines, matches, kerosene, and other essentials. He sticks to essentials and buys little.

Policarpio believes in the old-fashioned values and disapproves of premarital sex and divorce. One of his favorite pronouncements is that the curse of God will strike down those who break His commandments.

Policarpio generally talks only with his closest relatives and a few neighbors. He often prefers to be alone.

POLICIES AND PROGRAMS

LESSON 4.

Analysis identifies government policies that can impede or assist communication programs.

Generally, government policies that impede effective communication about reproductive health include those that:

- restrict the use of specific family planning methods or the eligibility of various providers to offer them,

- discourage services or deny supplies to specific groups,
- limit access to various media, and
- censor communication products.

Analysis can identify what these barriers are, whether they can be surmounted, or whether alternative approaches are possible. In Turkey, for example, when research found that individual contraceptive products could not be advertised in the mass media by brand name, the social marketing project, working with three pharmaceutical firms, promoted three low-dose oral contraceptive brands under one generic logo (Yun & Lewis, 1994). In Kenya, government policies restrict access to family planning services for adolescents and unmarried women. Thus, the Youth Project created an advocacy component to publicize the social consequences of this policy and to spark discussion of policy and program options (Njau, 1994 & 1995). In the Philippines before the 1990s, explicit mention and promotion of contraceptive methods were not allowed on mass media. This policy changed when the Department of Health spearheaded national communication campaigns in 1993 and 1994 informing the public about specific methods. The decision to proceed was based on research documenting that 90 to 95 percent of the population approved of family planning (Social Weather Stations, 1992). Furthermore, other research findings indicated that many different people, including elected local officials, tribal leaders, national and local clergy, major employers, health care providers from doctors to village midwives, broadcast media program directors, journalists, and editors, wanted to learn more about specific contraceptive methods (Consumer Pulse, 1991). This information helped persuade government officials to continue promoting specific contraceptive methods in subsequent mass media campaigns.

LESSON 5.

Analysis usually indicates that policy-makers are an important secondary audience for family planning communication.

Before efforts to reach primary audiences can begin, the preliminary analysis must also identify secondary audiences—namely, the relevant decision-makers in government, religion, business, health care, and the media. Influential people in all these areas control access to primary audiences. Indeed, some would argue that these decision-makers are really the primary audience at the start of a program and become the secondary audience only once the program is under way. Thus the need for high-level support and advocacy starts at the beginning of any program and at the very first step in the P Process of communication program development. It continues throughout the entire process.

Government policy-makers are a crucial audience whose support is especially important for any innovative approach. Thus in Kenya, when family planning leaders wanted to start programs for young people, a first step was to interview national legislators and district health leaders to learn their views (Kumah, Kincaid, et al., 1993). In 1994 in the Philippines, when the Population Commission launched a project to increase awareness of population and environmental issues, one of the first activities was a workshop to orient national legislators, policy-makers, the mass media, the business community, and other influential people to the issues and the purpose of the national campaign (Philippine Legislators' Committee on Population and Development [PLCPD], 1994).

With religious leaders, interviews and discussion before designing communication activities can yield valuable insights. In Peru, for example, project managers met with Roman Catholic leaders before launching an AIDS-prevention campaign (Saba, 1993). To accommodate the clergy's concern for strengthening the institution of marriage, the subsequent campaign mentioned monogamy before promoting condom use. This approach persuaded local clergymen not to oppose TV spots on condom use. Similarly, advance assessment for the Minya Initiative in Egypt prompted project managers to hold workshops on family planning for Muslim and Coptic Christian clerics in the province. As a result, religious leaders of both faiths actively supported the project, collaborating with the government and nongovernmental organizations involved (see Box 3.6).

LESSON 6.

Analysis identifies strengths and weaknesses so that communication can accentuate the positive and help correct the negative.

Service delivery is the bedrock of family planning programs. No matter how motivated people may be, they cannot use most family planning methods without consulting service providers, whether public, private, or commercial. Therefore an effective communication program cannot be designed without an accurate assessment of what services are available at different organizations and locations, how well service-delivery personnel deal with clients, whether facilities complement or duplicate one another, and what the major gaps are. A communication analysis in francophone Africa, for example, found few family planning facilities in rural areas but a number of underutilized clinics in urban centers (Brockerhoff, 1995 & 1996). Since many villagers travel to the city for work or shopping, this pattern creates an opportunity to promote existing urban service sites that could reach some rural populations as well as urban residents. A 1992 analysis of health facilities and outlets in Nigeria found that 40,000 outlets offered family planning information, products, and services in some form (Kiragu, Chapman, & Lewis, 1995). Almost 60 percent were small, privately owned stores offering a limited choice of contraceptive methods. Family planning logos proved useful to help people identify these convenient neighborhood sites, but improved logistics, more training, and better coordination between the public and private sectors were recommended to respond fully to clients' needs.

The tools to analyze service delivery are becoming more sophisticated as USAID's Office of Population and other donors place increasing emphasis on improving the quality of care by maximizing access to and quality of services (the MAQ Initiative). Data from Demographic and Health Surveys are often a first step

**Box 3.6
The Minya Initiative**

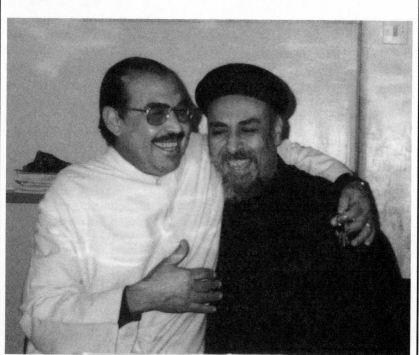

The Minya Initiative, in the rural Minya governorate of Upper Egypt, mobilized the populace in support of family planning with a series of community events in 1992–1993. Some 14 organizations collaborated in the effort, including 3 religious organizations. Leaders of Minya's two major religious groups, Father Sidarous Matta of the Coptic Orthodox Church, and Sheikh Mohammed Abd El Majid, a Muslim cleric, joined the organizing efforts and became friends in the process. Together, they wrote a pamphlet explaining that both Islam and Christianity approve of family planning. Over the 18 months of the initiative, the level of contraceptive use among married women rose from 22 to 30 percent.

in determining who uses which services for which methods, and in tracking trends over time. More recently developed, a research protocol called Situation Analysis, used by the Population Council and combining a number of evaluation methods, assesses the quality of services in individual clinics (Katz, Hardee, & Villinski, 1993; Population Council, 1994). The COPE approach (for Client-Oriented Provider-Efficient), initiated by AVSC International, uses self-evaluation techniques to help providers assess their own facilities and services (Dwyer et al., 1991; Katz, Hardee, & Villinski, 1993).

These and similar methods have helped identify important links—and gaps—between service delivery and communication. For example, a 1994 situation analysis in Turkey found that, to improve the quality of care, it was not enough just to produce more communication materials; indeed, the materials were already there. Rather, providers needed better training in how to use the materials, and clinic supervisors needed upgraded skills to assess their use (Yun & Lewis, 1994). Taking facility-based analysis a step further, a 1995 study in Ghana found that providers delivered services more effectively when they used a variety of communication materials, because more information was exchanged between provider and client, and clients asked more questions during the counseling sessions (Tweedie, 1995). A quality-of-care study in Morocco found that the availability of IEC materials at clinics is significantly associated with contraceptive use (L. Brown, Rice, et al., 1995). Generally, the more types of communication materials used at a facility, the more new family planning acceptors.

A communication analysis needs to consider the viewpoints of both service providers and clients. For a better understanding of the client's perspective, a research project in Nepal used "mystery clients"—that is, impersonators of clients briefed in advance—to visit 16 clinics and ask various questions (Schuler et al., 1985). The research found that at some clinics low-caste clients were treated so rudely that they refused to return—thus identifying a major need for retraining providers in better interpersonal communication. A similar study in Ghana found that providers were especially discouraging to young people—thus identifying the need for special training for those who counseled younger clients (Huntington, Lettenmaier, & Obeng-Quaidoo, 1990; Huntington & Schuler, 1993). In Haiti a needs assessment found that program managers did not recognize the value of counseling or good interpersonal communication and neglected these skills (JHU/PCS, 1993c). Seminars were recommended to sensitize family planning program managers to their importance.

In Chiapas, Mexico, focus groups and in-depth interviews with family planning clients and with the health auxiliaries who served them revealed a different situation (Poppe, Rodriguez, & Payne Merritt, 1991). While the health auxiliaries established good rapport with clients, they gave incomplete or inaccurate information. Because these providers knew about only a few methods and had not been fully trained, they did not offer their clients a full and informed choice. Further, providers did not encourage men to participate and did not offer condoms to men. In addition, the providers themselves believed and spread unfounded rumors about health problems caused by contraceptives. The assessment pointed clearly to a need for more training on technical matters and on serving men.

A good communication analysis that looks closely at access and quality of services not only can identify critical problems but also can suggest constructive solutions. For example, in some Asian and African countries, situation analyses conducted by the Population Council show that most clinics are underutilized and that a high percentage of clinic-based family planning services are provided by only 20 percent of clinics (R. Turner, 1993). Attention-getting signs and logos can spotlight family planning facilities, generate publicity, and thus increase caseloads.

Conversely, when analysis shows that government and nongovernmental facilities are crowded but that people are willing to pay for more attention and better quality services, the solution may lie in communication campaigns to promote private, fee-for-service practitioners as an alternative. In Egypt (Wafai & Associates, 1993), India (Storey, Rimon, et al., 1994), and Indonesia (Rimon, Reed, et al., 1986), analysis showed that private practitioners could serve additional clients, especially in urban areas, and that the professional medical associations would welcome training and promotion to attract more clients for reproductive health services.

A good analysis can lead to more effective marketing of all existing services. For instance, research in the Minya Governorate of Egypt found that several service agencies were competing for the same family planning clients. A 1992 market segmentation study identified the best market position for each agency (Saffitz, 1992). Once each agency began trying to appeal to a different population segment, each attracted more clients, and the whole population was better served.

In short, to correct some of the negative aspects of service-delivery programs, the old adage applies: To change others, we may have to change ourselves first. Rather than blame potential clients for not using services, a needs assessment can look at all the different ways in which providers can offer better service—more supplies and equipment, better training, more attention to quality of care, and more focus on the role of communication in helping clients. Even in assessing service delivery, the primary focus should remain on clients' concerns rather than providers' convenience.

ORGANIZATIONS

LESSON 7.

A review of existing organizations shows which can best carry out an effective communication program and how different organizations can collaborate.

A solid needs assessment reviews all the organizations that can play a role in national communication programs and identifies their strengths and weaknesses for future health communication activities. These organizations vary from country to country and may include both public- and private-sector institutions:

Public-Sector Organizations
- Ministries of Health
- Social Security organizations
- Ministries of Information
- national population councils or commissions
- local government agencies

Private-Sector Organizations
- family planning associations and other nonprofit volunteer organizations

- nongovernmental health organizations
- professional associations, such as organizations of physicians or pharmacists
- other nongovernmental organizations, such as women's groups, environmental agencies, and youth groups
- commercial advertising/marketing and media production firms
- pharmaceutical companies
- large employers
- labor unions

In practice, a good communication analysis or needs assessment applies five criteria to evaluate each major agency: *competence, commitment, political clout, coverage, and continuity* (see Box 3.7). For example, health education units in ministries of health may have continuity and national coverage but may lack commitment to family planning or competence in modern communication skills. Social security organizations have limited coverage, reaching mainly urban employees in large businesses but providing a convenient source of information for them. Ministries of information often exhibit competence, clout, and coverage for communication activities but lack competence in and commitment to family planning. National population councils may appear to have political clout but have sometimes proved disappointing in terms of competence, commitment, and coverage (Indonesia and Mexico are clear exceptions). Family planning associations usually rank high in commitment, continuity, and competence in family planning but may lack national coverage, competence in communication, or political clout. Private nongovernmental agencies—from women's organizations to mission hospitals—vary widely in all the necessary characteristics. Commercial advertising or marketing firms may rank high in communication competence and coverage but are usually low in family planning commitment and competence. A good needs assessment can identify the strengths and weaknesses of all potential players so that the most effective mix of organizations in each specific situation can be identified and can take leadership in the program.

With the current trend toward decentralization, local governments and even communities are developing some of the capacities needed for effective health communication. In Peru, for example, the leaders of Villa el Salvador, a large and well-organized shanty town outside Lima, expressed interest in promoting better reproductive health, using such channels as television spots and talks given by a family planning counselor (Poppe, personal communication, November 13, 1995). Villa el Salvador has its own radio and TV stations, with signals reaching not only the community's 200,000 residents but also neighboring communities. With the cooperation of the Villa el Salvador Communication Center, programming on reproductive health now reaches an audience that extends well beyond the community where it originates.

When, as in most countries, no one organization can undertake a comprehensive national communication program, a good preliminary analysis will identify possible collaborating organizations. A 1990 assessment in Ecuador, for example,

---

Box 3.7
How to Assess Organizations as Strategic Partners: Competence, Commitment, Clout, Coverage, and Continuity

To assess what roles different organizations can play in a communication program and which should be the leaders, preliminary analysis considers the following questions about each organization:

Competence
- ☐ Does the organization have strong technical and management staff?
- ☐ If additional staff are needed, can they be recruited and hired in a timely way?
- ☐ Does the organization have sufficient cash flow and reserves, a financial accounting system, bank accounts, and regular audits?
- ☐ Has it had experience with similar activities?
- ☐ Does it have a positive image and a reputation for high-quality work?

Commitment
- ☐ Does the organization endorse family planning and reproductive health programs?
- ☐ Does it support a strong role for communication?

Clout
- ☐ Does the organization have contacts and access among policy-makers and influential people?
- ☐ Does it have political support for its work?

Coverage
- ☐ Is the organization able to reach intended audiences, including different geographic areas, age groups, or other population segments?

Continuity
- ☐ How long has it been in operation?
- ☐ Has it carried out comparable projects effectively in the past?
- ☐ Has it an institutional base and resources for sustainability in the long run?

---

found that no single institution had the resources and technical expertise to implement a communication strategy directed at hard-to-reach, underserved rural populations (Payne Merritt & Lawrence, 1990). Some organizations had service-delivery networks in place. Others had experience producing broadcast and print materials. Still others offered research capabilities or links with university and health care professionals. The needs assessment identified ways that the different agencies could pool their resources for a common effort.

Collaboration can be largely horizontal, when, for example, a number of service-providing organizations form an informal network or working group to coordinate the development of flipcharts, cue cards, and other clinic-based communication materials. This was the initial pattern in the Bolivia Reproductive Health Project. Or collaboration can be largely vertical, when a single agency, such as the Planned Parenthood Federation of Nigeria, subcontracts with advertising agencies and distribution firms to carry out specific tasks. In most countries, collaboration will be a mix, involving different forms and many levels as communication activities grow from small, separate projects into coordinated components of a national strategy and program.

COMMUNICATION RESOURCES

LESSON 8.

Analysis identifies the most appropriate and cost-effective channels available to reach primary and secondary audiences.

Whether research on communication channels is seen as *audience analysis* (that is, who is reached through what channels?) or *media exposure* (that is, which media reach which audiences?), such research is crucial to designing any communication program. Although channels sometimes are distinguished simply as either interpersonal or mass media communication, channels in fact can be subdivided into many different forms. They can be as varied as the creativity and imaginations of those who use them. Communication channels for health programs can range from individual counseling, group talks, folk dramas, and village festivals to national press, billboards, radio, and television. They can even include key rings, T-shirts and hats, speeches, and cue cards. They can be used singly or, more often with modern campaigns, in various combinations.

To discover which channels have the greatest reach and the highest credibility (which are not necessarily the same), a good communication analysis begins by looking at existing data. Major sources include Demographic and Health Surveys, communication surveys, market research, broadcasters' surveys, and scholarly studies. Drawing on these data, a communication analysis in Uganda, for example, found that only about 30 percent of all Ugandans had access to television, but almost 90 percent listened to radio (Kiragu, 1993a; Kiragu, Galiwango, et al., 1996). Television viewing was largely limited to urban areas; radio predominated in rural areas. In Haiti, a media analysis showed that, with high rates of illiteracy, print media had far less impact on the population than broadcast media (JHU/PCS, 1993c). In both Uganda and Haiti, however, the media with less reach—television in Uganda, newspapers in Haiti—still played valuable secondary roles because their audiences included decision-makers and opinion leaders. By contrast, in both Egypt and Turkey, television reaches almost everyone, making it a high-priority medium for most health messages. Even when levels of radio or television ownership are low, exposure may be much higher because family or friends watch or listen together. To help determine the optimal media mix, a comprehensive communication analysis should obtain the most current data on media costs and coverage, advertising costs, availability of free or discounted public service air time, and possibilities for co-production.

Additional, specific analysis of the habits and preferences of the intended audience can be helpful. Demographic and Health Surveys show, for example, that in contrast to the reluctance of some policy-makers, most married women of reproductive age consider radio and television acceptable sources of family planning information. In Ecuador and Peru, for example, 94 percent of respondents expressed approval of family planning messages on radio or television. Even the lowest levels of approval are substantial; in Pakistan, for example, 49 percent of the women said family planning information on the broadcast media was acceptable (see Table 3.1). In 25 of 33 countries with comparable survey data, at least three-fourths of married women find broadcast media to be acceptable sources of family planning information.

It is important to know not only which media but which days and hours are most popular with the intended audience. For example, audience research for a family planning radio serial drama in 1991 in The Gambia revealed that a 9:30 P.M. time slot on Wednesdays and Sundays would reach far more people than the originally planned 8:30 P.M. slot. The schedule was adjusted accordingly (JHU/PCS, 1992f; Baron et al., 1993).

Research also can determine how community activities and traditional folk media can best reinforce modern health messages and practices. In Ghana, for example, a needs assessment indicated that the traditional late-evening concert parties (*durbars*), where itinerant musical drama troupes perform, would be a fine setting to spread information and stimulate talk among men about family planning (Kumah, 1986). *Durbars* became a popular part of the communication program. In Peru research suggested that street theater actors could create a good opportunity to answer questions about rumors and to correct misinformation for thousands of watchers (Valente, Poppe, et al., 1995). In Morocco, in contrast, a study showed that male street theater players or performers (*helaki*) would not be a credible source of information about modern family planning (Berry, 1991).

VALUE OF RESEARCH AND ANALYSIS

LESSON 9.

A good communication analysis takes both time and skill to produce.

There is always a temptation to skip a comprehensive analysis or needs assessment and instead to begin working directly on specific communication products. Local officials want posters and brochures *now*. Having decided that communication is important, they want attractive products immediately. Sometimes it may even be necessary to produce some material at once or to reprint the best of existing material on a small scale to buy time and ease official impatience until a research-based strategy design and materials can be completed. Officials tend to think that they know what their clients need and that enough research has been done already. But in the long run a comprehensive initial analysis pays off, even though it may require a substantial commitment of time and resources.

Table 3.1
Family Planning Messages in the Broadcast Media:
Access, Exposure, and Acceptability Among Currently Married Women Ages 15–44

Region, Country, & Year	Have Radio	Have Television	Have Heard Family Planning Messages on Radio in Last Month	Have Seen Family Planning Messages on Television in Last Month	Consider Broadcast Family Planning Messages Acceptable
			% of Women Who:		
Africa					
Botswana 1988	NA	NA	40	NA	81
Burkina Faso 1993	54	5	14	3	79
Burundi 1987	81	70	NA	NA	NA
Cameroon 1991	63	20	9	6	60
Ghana 1993	46	16	36	21	88
Kenya 1993	59	7	NA	NA	NA
Madagascar 1992	41	5	7	2	79
Malawi 1992	41	NA	29	NA	86
Mali 1987	53	3	NA	NA	76
Namibia 1992	73	21	NA	NA	73
Niger 1992	39	4	19	4	74
Nigeria 1990	56	17	24	NA	53
Rwanda 1992	35	NA	22	NA	97
Senegal 1993	75	17	19	9	82
Sudan 1990	56	25	NA	NA	74
Togo 1988	49	9	NA	NA	81
Uganda 1988	29	1	NA	NA	68
Zambia 1992	47	10	20	7	75
Zimbabwe 1994	47	18	51	24	92/88[a]
Asia & Pacific					
Bangladesh 1994	29	9	43	17	96
Indonesia 1994	65	40	27	40	NA
Pakistan 1991	37	28	16	16	49
Philippines 1993	NA	44	43	32	88
Sri Lanka 1987	76	19	NA	NA	90
Thailand 1987	75	50	30	NA	89

Table 3.1 cont'd

Region, Country, & Year	Have Radio	Have Television	% of Women Who: Have Heard Family Planning Messages on Radio in Last Month	% of Women Who: Have Seen Family Planning Messages on Television in Last Month	% of Women Who: Consider Broadcast Family Planning Messages Acceptable
Latin America & Caribbean					
Bolivia 1989	85	58	34	30	90/85[a]
Brazil 1991	71	53	17	21	88
Colombia 1995	89	85	43	60	98/98[a]
Dominican Republic 1991	62	62	18	23	95
Ecuador 1987	83	63	75	NA	91
Guatemala 1987	66	30	54	NA	66
Haiti 1994	44	19	16	9	NA
Peru 1991	87	76	38	46	NA
Trinidad & Tobago 1987	93	89	28	NA	96
Near East & North Africa					
Egypt 1992	65	79	22	75	NA
Morocco 1992	88	62	13	11	93
Tunisia 1988	75	73	64	NA	90
Turkey 1993	80	90	NA	NA	NA

Note: [a] The first number is for radio; the second, television.
Source: Demographic and Health Surveys.

There are three major ways of conducting an analysis. First, it can take the form of a comprehensive communication sector analysis focusing on people, policies, programs, organizations, and communication resources. If the information obtained is sufficient, projects and programs can be designed immediately on the basis of the sector analysis. Second, if the program is new and if sufficient information is not available for planning and strategic design, then more data collection or further analysis to fill gaps may be commissioned and undertaken before communication strategies and projects are designed. Third, in countries where timing is a critical factor, an entire project can be designed to include further analysis and formative research as part of the early phase of the project. Then these findings provide the necessary information to develop or refine proposed interventions.

A comprehensive analysis is especially important when an entirely new program is being undertaken. Time and skill are required to produce an analytical report that is both accurate and forward-looking. In Kenya, for example, before a new program to reach young adults was initiated, two full-time staff members and dozens of collaborators spent a full month and almost 10 percent of the project budget in assessing governmental, community, and parental concerns as well as the needs of the young adult audience (Kumah, Odallo, et al., 1992). In addition to personal interviews, the team attended two seminars scheduled over the same period by the Center for the Study of Adolescents and Family Planning Private Sector, a USAID-supported program designed to encourage private-sector programs. The effort proved worthwhile. The program began with a well-informed and concerted effort to win over the policy-makers, local officials, religious leaders, and parents whose support would be essential.

For long-standing programs, a thorough analysis can offer new insights. In Egypt, for instance, in 1987 Population Communication Services was asked to carry out a limited inventory of existing print materials for nonliterates, with the aim of reprinting the best materials or developing new ones. The PCS project director persuaded officials that a broader assessment was needed for the program, which was not expanding as fast as hoped. The rapid assessment concluded that it is not enough for a central government agency (the State Information Service IEC Center) to conduct most of the communication work on behalf of the entire population program (Rimon & Zimmerman, 1987). The assessment team recommended that private-sector agencies be allowed and supported to conduct their own promotions and to market their services, as needed, to particular market niches. This made it possible to create different market niches served by different agencies, giving impetus to what is now a national program focused on improving and promoting the quality of care.

Analysis or a needs assessment is only as good as the people conducting it. The assignment should go to experienced, motivated, and resourceful personnel, most of whom should already be familiar with the local situation. Too often, project managers assemble teams from remote offices, look for consultants with time available, or leave the selection of a needs assessment team to others. Managers are wise to begin well in advance of a planned start-up date to solicit suggestions for research personnel and to recruit experts who can command respect and gain access to relevant sources of information in the community. Members from different backgrounds and countries can bring to the team useful diversity of insights as well. In Kenya, for example, the team included the officers in charge of youth activities from each of three major Kenyan organizations that already sponsored reproductive health programs for youth. Their understanding of local conditions expedited the analysis, while their diverse perspectives, representing both public and private sectors, complemented each other. Two experts from Johns Hopkins University with extensive experience in family planning communication throughout Africa and resident representatives of donor organizations in Kenya rounded out the team (Kumah, Odallo, et al., 1992; Van Hulzen, 1995).

LESSON 10.

A good analysis serves many purposes over the life of the program.

A comprehensive analysis provides strategic guidance, valuable baseline information, a timetable for action, and a basis for future advocacy. It must be seen as the start of an ongoing process and not as an end in itself. The more accurate, insightful, and thorough the initial analysis, the more uses it can serve over the long term in many different ways.

First, a comprehensive analysis should be the guide for strategic project design. To serve this purpose, an assessment must provide more than description and data; it must point toward *a course of action*. When a project manager opens a needs assessment or analysis report, the first question will be, "Where do we go from here?" Unless the assessment provides practical recommendations, it may languish on a shelf.

After summarizing the data collected, a written report must outline the implications for the program, making recommendations for audiences, messages, materials, activities, and communication channels—the basis of a communication program strategy. The Kenya Youth Information, Education, and Communication Needs Assessment provides a good example of taking the research a full step toward program design (Kumah, Odallo, et al., 1992). Rather than merely suggesting that drama might be a good way to reach youth, the report recommended seed funding for youth groups to write and produce their own dramas. It also proposed a series of district, regional, and national contests culminating in a nationally telecast competition and recommended that the best dramas be developed into high-quality videos. Similarly, the 1993 Nepal needs assessment not only called for more use of radio but also specifically proposed (1) a weekly educational radio program on interpersonal communication and contraceptive technology for health care providers and (2) a drama mini-series for couples with an unmet need for family planning (Rimon & Lediard, 1993).

Second, a good needs assessment serves as a convenient reference for project managers, providing relevant data on current communication and service-delivery activities. It can provide a baseline measurement of audience knowledge, attitudes, and behavior as well. This also allows baseline comparisons for future impact evaluation, thus integrating evaluation into the project design from the start. For future consultation, lists of the people who were interviewed and the materials reviewed for background demographic and economic information are helpful. In short, the documentation inherent in the analysis process provides good reference for future analysis, identification of sources of information, and a background for understanding the logic of the strategic design.

Third, a comprehensive analysis can suggest timetables for planning. Depending on the size of the project proposed, the report might cover only the coming year or two. A 1990 Ecuador assessment, for example, was written to bridge a 12- to 18-month gap until a four- to five-year, nationally coordinated communication program could be launched (Payne Merritt & Lawrence, 1990). Alternatively, an analysis might propose a series of activities stretching over a decade, as did the 1991 assessment of family planning and reproductive health activities in Guatemala (Payne Merritt & Poppe, 1991).

Finally, a good analysis can be an advocacy tool. Properly presented, it can help persuade policy-makers and mobilize support. Needs assessments in Bangladesh, Kenya, Nepal, and Nigeria helped win government and donor support for expanded communication programs. Research findings that showed strong public support for family planning helped persuade undecided leaders to move forward in Colombia, Peru, and the Philippines.

Chapter 4

Strategic Design

SETTING OBJECTIVES

Lesson 1. Long-term vision can set bold objectives.

Lesson 2. Setting realistic communication objectives requires knowing and listening to people, not trying to manipulate them.

Lesson 3. Communication objectives reflect the stage and maturity of the overall program.

Lesson 4. Communication objectives are "SMART."

POSITIONING

Lesson 5. Positioning can create a specific image or market niche for a health issue, service, or product that will be memorable and influential to the intended audience.

Lesson 6. Cultural values and national politics influence positioning.

Lesson 7. Positioning is theory-driven and depends on knowing how and why people change their behavior.

DETERMINING HOW TO ACHIEVE OBJECTIVES

Lesson 8.   Communication programs can be implemented in phases, depending on the availability of services, training, and supplies or the readiness of the audience.

Lesson 9.   A multichannel approach can have a synergistic impact.

Lesson 10. Within the multimedia framework, a single medium usually serves as the locomotive or leader to advance the message.

Lesson 11. Mass media are increasingly cost-effective and practical for reaching large numbers.

Lesson 12. The Enter-Educate approach offers many advantages for health communication.

Lesson 13. Communication strategies depend on credible sources who are trusted and respected by the people.

Lesson 14. Satisfied users should be part of communication strategies.

Lesson 15. Communication strategies should be action-oriented and linked to services through recognized symbols.

IDENTIFYING IMPLEMENTING ORGANIZATIONS

Lesson 16. Organizational leadership and cooperation are essential to strategic design.

PLANNING FOR DOCUMENTATION AND EVALUATION

Lesson 17. Plans for monitoring and evaluation, based on the project objectives, should be included in the strategic design, workplans, and budgets.

Every communication program or project, large or small, needs a strategic design. Developing this design is the next step after the initial analysis, and it is a crucial step because all future activities depend upon it. During the strategic design step the basic decisions are made about the key elements in a communication program:

- setting objectives;
- positioning the issue, service, or product to be promoted;
- selecting the means of implementation;
- identifying partner organizations;
- planning for documentation and evaluation.

All five elements are closely interrelated. Program objectives indicate what basic changes are expected in individual behavior in order to achieve positive health impacts. Positioning suggests how these changes can be presented to the intended audience in the most persuasive fashion. The means of implementation constitute the optimal activities, channels, and scheduling to reach intended audiences. The partner organizations develop the messages and means to carry out the activities. Finally, by documenting any changes in individual or community behavior, service and sales statistics, or health indicators, a program can evaluate whether the strategy was appropriate, how well it was implemented, and whether the objectives were achieved. Ideally, each element is spelled out in a national communication strategy that includes an indicative workplan and a budget.

From a communication standpoint, positioning may be the key element because positioning determines the way people will perceive the program, how they will remember the communication activities, and to what extent those activities will prompt action. But every element in a strategic design is important, and every element requires well-informed and creative decision-making.

SETTING OBJECTIVES

Family planning and reproductive health programs may have many different objectives. For example, under the broad national goal of reducing population growth or improving maternal health and child survival, programs will have policy objectives to achieve, for example, high coverage nationwide, selective coverage in specific areas or among specific population groups, a high quality of care, more integrated reproductive health services, or economic sustainability over time. These objectives at the policy level must then be translated into program objectives that can be addressed through various forms of communication.

LESSON 1.

Long-term vision can set bold objectives.

"I have a vision. I want to see an Indonesia twenty years from now in which 80 percent of family planning services are provided by the private sector and 20 percent by the government, with governments serving only those who are poor or cannot afford to pay. Work with us to make this vision a reality." This was the challenge posed by Dr. Haryono Suyono, chairman of the Indonesian National Family Planning Coordinating Board (BKKBN), in late 1986 to a team reviewing the Indonesian IEC program and making recommendations for the next seven years (JHU/PCS, 1986b; Rimon, Reed, et al., 1986).

Out of that vision was born the Blue Circle program. Its primary objective was to shift provision of family planning services from an already successful government program to more self-sustaining private-sector services. In the first three years, private-practice doctors and midwives affiliated with the Indonesian Doctors Association and the Indonesian Midwives Association were trained and given continuing education and materials about family planning. After training, they received the Blue Circle emblem to display at their offices. A major publicity campaign promoted their ability to provide private-sector services at an affordable cost. The project started in 4 cities in the first year and expanded to 10 by the second year and to 300 by the third year. Five months after the 1988 program launch, 32 percent of participating doctors reported some increase, averaging 28 percent, in their weekly family planning caseloads, and 58 percent of midwives reported increases, averaging 36 percent (Haryono, Saffitz, & Rimon, 1990). By the third year, Blue Circle had gained so much recognition that the government launched an array of contraceptive products with the logo as a brand name.

Indonesian leadership was bold in moving an already successful government-funded program toward a less predictable but likely more sustainable future, with more paying clients and expanded private-sector participation. As a result of this partnership of BKKBN with donors, pharmaceutical companies, local governments, doctors, and midwives' associations, as well as other government ministries, the proportion of family planning services provided by the private sector increased from 12 percent in 1987 to 28 percent in 1994 (Indonesia Central Bureau of Statistics [CBS], National Family Planning Coordinating Board [NFPCB], & Institute for Resource Development/Westinghouse [IRD/W], 1989; Indonesia CBS et al., 1995). While the long-term goal of 80 percent private-sector services has not yet been reached, that vision created the innovative Blue Circle strategy, which positioned private-sector providers as an important component of the Indonesian program and stimulated similar campaigns to promote private-sector providers in Egypt, India, and Turkey.

Every program needs a long-term vision. It can empower people because it shows what is important. It can stimulate teamwork because it shows what everyone needs to do. And it can strengthen organizations because it generates new energy.

LESSON 2.

Setting realistic communication objectives requires knowing and listening to people, not trying to manipulate them.

Obviously, objectives that seek to change people's knowledge, attitudes, and especially behavior depend upon those people. Designing an effective strategy requires knowing what people already think and do and finding out what changes they want to make, not trying to manipulate them to make changes they do not want. In fact, the relationship of the audience to the communication objectives is, to quote a Chinese phrase, "like the mouth to the teeth." The Steps to Behavior Change framework (see Chapter 2) provides guidance on where some segments of the audience stand and thus what steps in the change process should receive the most attention in setting program objectives. For example, the audience analysis conducted in Ghana (see Box 3.4, in Chapter 3) revealed that 27 percent of the primary audience who intended to use family planning "lacked knowledge" of contraceptives and that 10 percent feared side effects. Thus improving knowledge by providing accurate information became a major objective because that is what the audience wanted.

This approach reverses the conventional model, which proceeds from source to message to channel to receiver (SMCR) (Berlo, 1960; Laswell, 1948). That model placed the receiver—that is, the audience—last, at the end of a one-way flow of information (see also Chapter 2). Audience feedback was largely omitted. In the 1970s the SMCR model was challenged (Rogers & Kincaid, 1981). Now the experience of the Population Communication Services project and many other communication programs has clearly established that feedback from the audience is essential to designing effective communication. What was once envisioned as one-way communication is now viewed as a two-way dialogue between parties who are both source and receiver. Findings from formative audience research—such as focus-group discussions and in-depth interviews—offer ways to invite audience representatives to participate in strategic communication design. This approach establishes a dialogue between program planners and their audiences. Responding to the hopes, fears, and needs of the audience instead of trying to manipulate the audience is now a crucial part of the strategy.

To design a strategy that is audience-driven and audience-responsive means starting with a sound analysis of the audience, carried out as part of the initial assessment, and then building on it. That analysis makes it possible to segment the audience in different ways. Then, in the design phase the crucial decisions are made on which segments or specific audiences to work with and how to position the program to meet their needs. The audience may be, for example, women with identified unmet need, as in the Redline Strategy for Nepal (see Box 3.4, in Chapter 3), or women who intend to practice family planning and believe they have social support, as in Ghana; or even men, whose support is necessary for their partners' actions, as in Zimbabwe.

LESSON 3.

Communication objectives reflect the stage and maturity of the overall program.

Just as individuals set different reproductive health objectives at different stages of their personal lives, so also national programs set different family planning and reproductive health objectives depending on their stages of maturity and/or success. For the purpose of developing communication strategies, three stages of program development can be identified: (1) early, with a history of 5 to 10 years of organized national effort and a contraceptive prevalence rate (CPR) for modern methods below 20 percent; (2) middle, with a history of 10 to 15 years and a modern method CPR between 20 and 34 percent; and (3) mature, with a history of more than 15 years and a modern method CPR of more than 35 percent (see Destler et al., 1990).

For countries at an early stage of program development, communication objectives focus on influential people and policy-makers to help create a more favorable environment to introduce and fund family planning services. They also focus on creating a basic public awareness of family planning and its benefits. This was certainly the case in the early days of the Asian programs and is currently the case in many African countries. For countries at the middle stage, such as Honduras, Kenya, Nepal, Peru, and the Philippines, often characterized by growth and expansion, communication strategies aim to promote services directly to sectors of the population who are ready to practice, and have access to services, but are still not regular users. For countries at the mature stage, such as Bangladesh, Colombia, Indonesia, and Mexico, communication objectives focus on building institutions, ensuring sustainability, identifying specific audiences that have not yet been reached, promoting quality of care, and reducing dropout rates.

Program maturity can be at different levels within the same country. For example, in Indonesia, program expansion was planned in three strategic places: first, Java and Bali islands; second, the Outer Islands I; and third, the Outer Islands II. Thus, by the time the program was expanding to Outer Islands II, it was already learning from the experience in Java and Bali. By strategically phasing in program expansion, realistic objectives were set in well-defined geographic areas, and program achievements were measured regionally rather than nationally, thus avoiding a common mistake of developing national indicators when programs are actually confined to limited geographic areas.

LESSON 4.

Communication objectives are "SMART."

In management and training jargon, SMART[1] is a well-known acronym that defines good objectives and helps in setting them. It stands for the following:

S **Specific**—defining what is to be accomplished in terms of specific steps to behavioral change among specific, well-defined audiences

M **Measurable**—quantifying the objectives by indicating a numerical or percentage change expected

A **Appropriate**—defining intended changes that are culturally and locally acceptable

R **Realistic**—avoiding objectives that are beyond the scope of available resources, contrary to relevant experience, or unrelated to communication efforts

T **Timebound**—identifying the time frame in which changes should be achieved

The 1993 Family Planning and Health Project campaign in Ghana offers an example of SMART communication objectives. The strategy was *specific* because it sought to increase the use of modern contraceptive methods among the primary audience of women ages 15 to 45 who approved of and intended to use family planning, and who had social support to do so—about 32 percent of all Ghanaian women; it was *measurable* because it set four percentage points as the expected numerical increase in modern contraceptive use; it was *appropriate* because the local health staff participated actively in drawing up plans that were based on local conditions; it was *realistic* because the intended audience was women who were "ready" and had already expressed their intention to limit or space pregnancies; and it was *timebound* because the behavior change was expected to take place in a 24-month period (Ghana Ministry of Health/Health Education Unit [Ghana MOH/HEU] & Johns Hopkins University/Population Communication Services [JHU/PCS], 1993a & b).

Setting realistic objectives is a special concern in public health programs because public health officials or political leaders often want to achieve 100 percent audience coverage or to reach the hardest-to-reach population very quickly with limited resources. In setting objectives, public health communication programs can learn from the commercial sector. Private businesses are pleased when they can increase market share by a few percentage points. Private businesses also expect to continue their promotions or repeat campaigns many times instead of expecting that a onetime effort will be sufficient. When objectives are out of reach, a program is doomed to disappointment and criticism, no matter what it actually achieves. By setting realistic objectives, communication programs can change the indicators by which success is gauged and set a climate of positive reinforcement for real accomplishments. When programs can document and achieve their realistic objectives, the individuals and organizations involved develop a culture and expectation of achievement that boosts their chances for further success.

POSITIONING

Positioning is a concept from the commercial world of advertising and marketing that can play a key role in modern health communication. In the context of strategic design, positioning means presenting an issue, service, or product in such a way that it stands out from other comparable or competing issues, services, or products and is appealing and persuasive. Positioning creates a distinctive and attractive image, a perpetual foothold in the minds of the intended audience. Also, positioning provides a framework within which a consistent appeal can be developed and publicized (Ogilvy, 1963; D. E. Schultz, Martin, & Brown, 1987; Trout & Ries, 1972a, b, & c).

In the commercial world, positioning creates terminology and images that can be positive and can last long after specific campaigns have been completed. Advertising is largely based on positioning that makes a brand name a household word and creates a clear and distinguishing image that the brand name carries with it. For example, Levi's jeans are positioned as durable and "cool." Hewlett-Packard computer printers are positioned as state-of-the-art and reliable. A Rolls-Royce is positioned as top-of-the-line—a flawless, elegant status symbol available only to someone with impeccable taste and substantial wealth.

Positioning can also be applied to promote different forms of health care, including family planning and reproductive health services. A communication program that positions family planning well can become a steering wheel for the whole program instead of just a spare wheel, used only when the program is not going well. Strategic positioning helps to ensure that all stakeholders and participants in the communication program, from the top to the bottom, from the planners to the field workers and volunteers, understand what the central thrust of the strategy is. It makes possible a consistent understanding at all levels of what is "on strategy" and what is "off strategy" in terms of message development. Strategic positioning also helps to ensure that the communication component is taken seriously; it would be next to impossible strategically to position a product, service, or idea without using communication skills as a steering wheel.

LESSON 5.

Positioning can create a specific image or market niche for a health issue, service, or product that will be memorable and influential to the intended audience.

Just as commercial producers and advertisers need to position their products to meet customer needs or preferences, so also health communication programs can position health services to find their niche and attract appropriate clients. The Gold Star campaign in Egypt is a good example of strategic positioning. The overall program objective is to provide high-quality reproductive health services in Egypt through Ministry of Health and Population clinics. The Gold Star becomes the symbol for quality improvement. The Gold Star campaign links overall program objectives and communication strategies in a marketing approach that serves both clients (customers) and providers.

How was this strategy and positioning developed? The Egyptian Ministry of Health and Population, spurred on by nongovernmental agencies who promote "distinguished service at an affordable price," was already working on quality improvement. It formally adopted the objective of improving the quality of government family planning clinics because it did not want to be perceived as providing a lower quality of care than the private sector. Because improved quality will not attract clients if no one knows about it, achieving the objective depends on the communication strategy of publicizing the improved-quality, gold-star service. It is the first nationwide family planning communication strategy in a developing country focused on promoting quality of care and positioning government clinics as a source of high-quality care. Clinics that can pass a 101-item checklist of quality improvement indicators in two consecutive quarters will receive the mark of quality, the Gold Star symbol, identified and developed through extensive pretesting. The Gold Star is posted on the doors of qualifying clinics and in high traffic areas to direct clients to service locations. Within the clinic, the Gold Star is used to personalize service, to highlight upgraded quality, and to help identify specially trained service providers. Gold Star pins are given to health care providers to remind both them and their clients of the need for high-quality service. Television spots feature the Gold Star by a clinic door and remind viewers that "behind every door, there are friends whose main concern is to help you."

In phase one, the campaign focuses on training and promoting individual providers in different aspects of reproductive health. In the second phase, as an increasing number of high-quality clinics are identified and marked, the strategy focuses on promoting certified Gold Star locations for family planning and other reproductive health services. These facilities are positioned as a high-quality service to meet reproductive health needs. Training will continue as the quality improvement program extends nationally so that better quality becomes a reality, not just a promise. At the same time, because quality is being publicized and promoted in the media and the concept of quality is being legitimated, clients will come to expect more, and providers will be pressured by client expectations to provide better care. The strategy is another example of the way communication can become a steering wheel that guides both the supply and the demand sides of quality improvement. As a USAID official put it, "Egypt is the 'Gold Star' of the worldwide family planning program in improving quality of care" (JHU/PCS, 1996a).

The Johns Hopkins Population Communication Services project especially encourages marketing strategies that position and promote special types of providers rather than individual products or specific methods of family planning. The PRO Approach (*Pro*moting *Pro*fessional *Pro*viders) was used in Ghana. Since family planning is a complex and sometimes sensitive subject, and since most couples benefit from counseling and medical advice, the role of service providers is crucial. Also, promoting providers is often a more acceptable and more credible way to position a national program than promoting specific products or methods. The approach addresses a larger audience and at the same time puts a human face on the issue. In Ghana one major reason that the program was not moving forward, according to qualitative research done in 1988, was the perception among potential clients that Ministry of Health service providers were rude, uncaring, and incompetent. The service providers themselves reported that they were uninformed, poorly motivated, and too busy. These research findings provided the basis for designing a strategy to give family planning a human face, to raise the performance and morale of service providers, and to build trust among potential clients.

Borrowing from experience in the commercial sector that it is possible and sometimes preferable to promote the *provider* of complex or controversial products rather than the products themselves, the planners developed their strategic positioning: "Talk to your family planning advisors. They care." More than 5,000 family planning providers were trained in counseling and primed for the campaign in three regions of Ghana (Y. M. Kim, Amissah, et al., 1994). Clinic data collected by the Ministry of Health showed that couple-years of protection (CYP) increased by nearly 90 percent during the one-year campaign period (Ghana MOH/HEU & JHU/PCS, 1992). A postcampaign survey of more than 2,000 respondents found that, among those most exposed to campaign messages, 58 percent talked to their spouses about family planning, 48 percent talked to friends, 36 percent talked to providers, and 12 percent began using contraception. Men's use of modern methods increased from 19 percent to 25 percent over the course of the 1990–1991 campaign (Kincaid, Hindin, & Foreman, 1993). Moreover, a different and independent social marketing survey conducted later showed that government providers were rated higher on quality of service than any other family planning providers, including nongovernmental organizations, pharmacies, private midwives, and even private doctors (Marketing & Social Research Institute, 1993) (see Figure 4.1). This is the opposite of findings in most countries, where government service providers are rated lower than other providers.

An added benefit of positioning providers, also learned from marketplace experience, is that promoting the skills of service providers helps them set for themselves a higher standard of service and at the same time boosts their morale. Thus health care clients, providers, and even their supervisors all come to expect a higher quality of service as a result of the well-publicized claims. In this way the Gold Star strategy in Egypt and "I Care" in Ghana resemble the well-known slogan of United Airlines: "Fly the Friendly Skies of United." Through this often-repeated slogan, the employees of United are constantly reminded to treat their customers as friends.

LESSON 6.

Cultural values and national politics influence positioning.

Positioning issues or services is never value-neutral. Therefore the positioning of a health program as personal and sensitive as family planning must reflect the basic values of each society. It must offer a benefit that is important to the members

Figure 4.1
Quality Ratings of Selected Family Planning Service Providers in Ghana, 1993

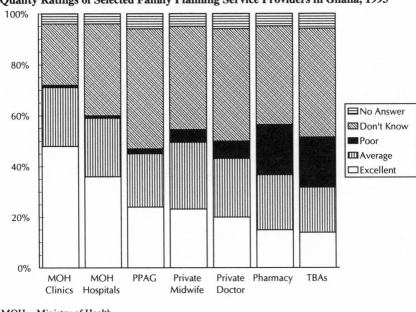

MOH = Ministry of Health.
PPAG = Planned Parenthood Association of Ghana.
TBAs = traditional birth attendants.
N = 1,049 women ages 15–49.
Source: Ghana Family Planning and Health Project, Marketing and Social Research Institute, 1993.

of that society. For many Western nations, individual human rights are highly valued; thus the absence of coercion and the presence of respect for individual religious beliefs are reflected in such positioning as emphasis on informed individual choice, meeting existing but still unmet need, and supporting a cafeteria approach to family planning in which the client chooses his or her preferred method. In many African and Asian countries, the family may be valued more than the individual, especially individual women. Thus the approval of the husband, mother-in-law, or family leader is also essential. Family planning can be positioned in the context of benefitting family life. In China, political leaders have subordinated individual and family values to the perceived national demographic and economic benefits of reducing population growth; consequently, they have positioned family planning as a patriotic duty.

Thus, while three United Nations conferences on population, from Bucharest in 1974 to Mexico City in 1984 to Cairo in 1994, have affirmed "the basic human right of couples and individuals to determine the number and spacing of their children," in each country the way that family planning can be positioned in communication strategies will reflect this value in different ways. More specifically, a family planning program can be positioned exclusively in health terms, that is, to reduce high-risk births; or in demographic terms, that is, to reduce population growth; or in terms of human rights, that is, to foster informed individual choices; or in terms of personal financial well-being and security. Value judgments and political decisions will determine whether the appropriate primary goal is to increase contraceptive prevalence overall or to satisfy the needs of particular groups perceived to be in greatest need or hardest to reach. For example, in the predominantly Catholic Philippines, the population program set as its primary objective reducing the number of high-risk births rather than slowing the population growth rate or reducing the total fertility rate. This positioned family planning as a health issue, a means of contributing to the reduction of maternal and infant mortality (USAID, 1993a). At the same time, reflecting the strong Philippine love of children, the campaign adopted a logo with a little girl and boy skipping gaily above the slogan, "If you love them, plan for them." This approach positions family planning as a manifestation of parents' love for their children—an appealing concept in Philippine society.

In Nigeria, the terminology of the new family planning national logo was changed from "family planning" to "child spacing" because the President was expected to inaugurate the logo. High officials believed that positioning the program to space births was more consistent with Nigerian family values and more politically acceptable in the conservative northern part of the country than positioning to limit births or promote small families.

Political considerations must always be taken into account in positioning health services. The larger the constituency and the more organizations that participate in developing a communication strategy and then agree to support it, the greater the likelihood of achieving the ultimate objectives. In Bangladesh, more than 40 government agencies, nongovernmental organizations, and donor agencies participated in a two-year process of developing a national communication strategy for family planning and maternal and child health for 1993 through 2000. The strategy emphasizes an integrated program that will promote a wide range of reproductive and child health services available at multipurpose centers. This approach was confirmed through an audience or customer appraisal, conducted by Bangladeshi staff of the USAID Mission, which indicated that most women were willing to pay a small fee to secure adequate supplies and high-quality services at integrated reproductive health centers (USAID, 1995). These facilities are being promoted as convenient, one-stop service centers under the Green Umbrella logo, a colorful image that positions the health centers as a source of protection and help with many health problems.

LESSON 7.

Positioning is theory-driven and depends on knowing how and why people change their behavior.

Positioning an issue, a service, or a product depends, like the whole process of strategic design, on knowing why people behave as they do. In the field of health communication, this means not only knowing and listening to the immediate audience but also building on a whole body of knowledge about health behavior that can help to inform decisions. Strategic design and positioning benefit when they are based on theories of behavior change that have been empirically tested and can be adapted to meet the needs of specific audiences.

As discussed in Chapter 2, there are many different theories of behavior change, but most confirm that sustained behavior change is a process through steps or stages—a process that can be accelerated by purposeful communication. Using the Steps to Behavior Change model, communication strategies can be designed to move individuals from one stage to another in sequence over time—for example, from ignorance to knowledge, from knowledge to approval, from approval to intention, and from intention to action.

Other behavior change models focus less on the individual and more on community norms or existing communication networks (Festinger, 1954; Rogers & Kincaid, 1981). In rural Bangladesh, for example, where women's roles are defined by family and community networks, the *jiggasha* strategy was designed to position the program as a way of mobilizing women in groups so that they could reinforce one another's behavior. Building on network analysis and diffusion theory, the *jiggasha* strategy empowered women to confer about health needs while encouraging men to see family planning as a community norm rather than a purely individual decision (Kincaid, Das Gupta, et al., 1993; Kincaid, Kapadia-Kundu, et al., 1994; Massiah et al., 1992; Rogers & Kincaid, 1981).

Another important theoretical guide that Johns Hopkins programs have used to help position desired behavior change is social learning theory (Bandura, 1977). Based on Bandura's thesis that people learn by observing others—in person or by means of mass media—and then adapt similar practices to their own lives, communication strategies use popular role models to position responsible sexual behavior as appropriate, modern, and above all, popular. The Enter-Educate approach (see below, Lesson 12) offers unique opportunities to put a powerful theory into practice, presenting an issue, a service, a product, or even a behavior vividly and with strong emotional impact.

Understanding how and why people behave as they do rather than simply producing a high volume of print or other materials is the key to effective communication. In fact, any time a communication project is designed, some assumption about behavior change is implicit in the design, whether it was adopted consciously or not. The more explicit this model is, however, the more systematic the development, execution, and evaluation of the project can be.

DETERMINING HOW TO ACHIEVE OBJECTIVES

Once objectives, audiences, and positioning are established, the strategic design must provide a guide to what actions to take. The design must indicate the activities, channels, and scheduling that will be most likely to lead to the desired destination. In other words, strategic design is like a road map, showing precisely how to get from here to there.

In communication, as in geography, the best maps are designed by those who know the territory. Therefore, good strategies are rarely designed by short-term consultants or under the time and page limitations of competitive procurements. Good strategies need to be developed from good research, comprehensive analysis, and extensive consultation with local experts and decision-makers. Listening to the audience and knowing the basic terrain are essential.

LESSON 8.

Communication programs can be implmented in phases, depending on the availability of services, training, and supplies or the readiness of the audience.

Communication programs are usually designed to increase demand for services. That means that the facilities, the providers, and the supplies must be ready for an influx of new clients or customers. Potential family planning clients can become discouraged and cynical if they respond to a promotion only to find that service providers are not ready and no supplies are available. After such an experience, some may never return. From another point of view, service providers who are not informed about upcoming campaigns may be ignorant or misinformed about the services clients want. They may be annoyed when a flood of clients arrives. They may even turn people away.

Figure 4.2
The Ghana Health and Family Planning Information Project Timeline, 1987–1993

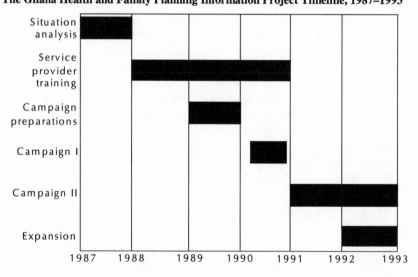

Source: Y. M. Kim, Kumah, et al., 1992.

A well-designed strategy will recognize that any public campaign requires months and sometimes years of preparation before it can be launched. In fact, the public launch of a communication program usually occurs about halfway through the entire P Process, as shown in the timeline in Figure 4.2.

During the five-year communication project in Ghana, the first two years were devoted to training, development of print and audiovisual materials, working with opinion leaders and religious leaders, preparing a health bulletin for service providers, and producing radio and television programs. Only in the third year was the "I Care" campaign launched, with a coordinated array of mass media productions, rallies, and sporting events. Even then coordination of logistics was not complete (Ghana MOH/HEU & JHU/PCS, 1992; Y. M. Kim, Kumah, et al., 1992). Similarly, in Bolivia planning for the Reproductive Health Program began in 1989, but the official launch with television spots and a speech by the Minister of Health did not take place until April 1994.

For those who are designing a health promotion campaign, it is important to know (1) what facilities are available that really can offer the services being promoted; (2) what facilities people actually use; (3) whether providers are trained in the necessary technical and interpersonal communication/counseling skills; and (4) how supplies will be increased to meet the greater demand. Knowing what facilities are available to promote is crucial in developing a strategic design. When programs are just beginning, as for family planning in Kwara State, Nigeria, in 1984 and for reproductive health in Bolivia in the 1990s, campaigns had to promote specific model clinics, since other facilities were not ready to provide services (Piotrow, Rimon, et al., 1990; JHU/PCS, 1990a & 1992d). In francophone Africa today, since there are few clinics providing reproductive health services in rural areas, the promotion strategy focuses on urban clinics. As the number of urban users increases, they will be encouraged to recruit friends and relatives from rural areas (Brockerhoff, 1995 & 1996).

Training health care providers is not usually the task of a communication program. Yet in the field of family planning/reproductive health, counseling and good interpersonal communication are increasingly recognized as essential to informed choice and satisfied, continuing clients. Therefore, health communication units or training teams have played important roles in training providers to communicate better with their clients. In addition to providing useful client-oriented materials, some family planning communication programs have helped train providers in interpersonal communication and counseling before undertaking major service promotion campaigns. Not only in Ghana but also in the Minya Initiative in Egypt and the Bolivian National Reproductive Health Program, for example, refresher courses in counseling skills and client-friendly materials for counseling were developed to accompany the promotion campaigns. In Nepal the first volume of the National Medical Standard for Reproductive Health covers contraceptive services, including interpersonal communication and counseling and the GATHER

Box 4.1
GATHER: Counseling in Many Tongues
The acronym GATHER helps family planning providers remember six crucial elements in the counseling process:

G – Greet clients
A – Ask clients about themselves
T – Tell clients about family planning methods
H – Help clients choose a method
E – Explain how to use the chosen method
R – Refer or return for follow-up

GATHER in Other Languages:
Arabic—*mustakhdim* (user)
French—*bercer* (to rock [a cradle])
Portuguese—*afiado* (sharp)
Russian—*pomogi* (help)
Spanish—*acceda* (access)
Turkish—*kaynak* (the source)
Urdu—*khuda awal* (God is first)

GATHER was introduced in 1987 in *Population Reports*, published by Johns Hopkins Population Information Program. Since then, training programs around the world have developed acronyms in languages ranging from Arabic to Urdu. When combined with training in how to develop interactive, emphatic relationships with clients and how to adapt counseling to clients' individual needs, situations, and wishes, this step-by-step process has proved to be a powerful tool for improving family planning counseling.

In Nepal, the Ministry of Health (MOH) has incorporated the Nepali equivalent of GATHER, *abhibadan* ("to greet"), into the National Medical Standards for Reproductive Health and added a new acronym, *namaskaar* (a respectful greeting). *Namaskaar* reminds providers and clients that clients, too, have an active role in the counseling process. The two—*namaskaar* and *abhibadan*—go together like two hands in respectful greeting.

Namaskaar

Na   LEARN. You have the right to know and to value your needs.
Ma   ASK the provider to clarify.
S   SEEK services from health workers and lead the conversation.
Kaa DISCUSS and UNDERSTAND benefits for you and your family.
Ra   ENCOURAGE others and ESTABLISH action plan for your well-planned family.

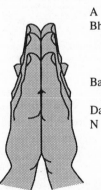

Abhibadan

A   GREET the client.
Bhi ASK questions without discrimination. ASSESS the individual needs of clients or couples.
Ba   SOLVE problems or remove obstacles.
Da   HELP wholeheartedly.
N   BID goodby and ask clients to come again.

approach to counseling in Nepali (Nepal Ministry of Health/Family Health Division, 1995) (see Box 4.1).

Training providers in communication skills can be planned in various ways, including training of all providers directly, as in the community-based distribution program in Kenya (JHU/PCS, 1989b), training of senior providers who in turn will train others; training of trainers, as in El Salvador, where three workshops prepared

86 trainers to train almost 4,000 rural outreach workers (JHU/PCS, 1992e); or, as is becoming the preferred approach, training of selected master trainers/practitioners, who have the professional and personal skills both to practice and to teach effectively (Bromham et al., 1995). However it is designed, training in technical clinical skills and also in interpersonal communication skills and counseling, including appropriate use of print and audiovisual materials and other resources, is an important first phase in any promotion campaign that expects to highlight these skills in providers.

Finally, health communication strategies must be based on a realistic appraisal of supply systems, to be sure that contraceptives and other commodities will flow in sufficient quantity to meet the increased demand. In Ghana, unfortunately, despite extensive preparations for the "I Care" campaign, demand for oral contraceptives increased so much that many clinics ran out of pills and others had to ration supplies, thus diminishing the impact of the campaign and disappointing clients (Y. M. Kim & Olsen, 1992).

LESSON 9.

A multichannel approach can have a synergistic impact.

A good strategy always employs a multichannel, mutually reinforcing approach appropriate to the audience and prevailing conditions. Communication can be divided into three broad channels: *interpersonal*, including family, friends, and health care providers; *group*, including mobilization of community organizations; and *mass media*, including print and broadcast.

The conventional wisdom, based on U.S. research in the 1930s and 1940s, was that mass media create awareness, group activities stimulate approval, but only interpersonal communication can influence behavior (Lazarsfeld, Berelson, & Gaudet, 1948; Rogers, 1962). The last three decades of research have demonstrated that such generalizations are unwarranted and have often led to circular arguments whether interpersonal communication is better than mass media or vice versa. As in the case of a carpenter who knows when to use a hammer as opposed to a screwdriver, a communication planner knows when to use radio, print materials, or counseling, depending on what the objectives are.

Much experience in family planning communication shows that a multimedia approach works best, that no one medium or channel is sufficient, and that, when properly developed, mass media can certainly influence behavior, just as interpersonal communication can spread awareness and knowledge (Chaffee, 1982; Hornik, 1989; Rogers, 1995). A combination of appropriate media and activities can produce synergy, achieving more than each medium alone.

A good communication strategy will combine different media to repeat and reinforce key messages. Not everyone is reached by the same channels of communication, so a multimedia approach is the only way to reach a substantial proportion of the audience. A recent example is the *Haki Yako* (It's Your Right) campaign in Kenya. Designed to emphasize the basic human right of women and men to control their own fertility, the campaign used radio spots and a radio serial drama to publicize the slogan; community visits by field workers to reach rural areas; posters and billboards to create a visual image of men and women talking together; and T-shirts to stimulate more interpersonal communication and to encourage advocacy by satisfied users. A 1994 national sample survey of men conducted in Kenya found that 68 percent had heard family planning messages on the radio, 54 percent had seen family planning posters, 46 percent had heard about family planning in newspapers and magazines, 38 percent had seen family planning pamphlets, and 26 percent had seen family planning billboards. Thus, except for radio and posters, no one channel reached more than half the population. Exposure to any one of the five channels was 83 percent, however (Kekevole et al., 1996). In Kenya, radio should continue to be used as the "lead" channel in the media mix. Reach is only one aspect of channel synergy, however. Hearing about family planning on the radio can reinforce what is seen on posters or in pamphlets; both print and radio can enhance the credibility and acceptance of local community-based volunteer distributors.

In Kenya, radio and print reinforced services at clinics. New family planning users interviewed at clinics said they had heard about family planning through a variety of mass media: 38 percent cited the radio drama *Kuelewana ni Kuzungumza* (*Understanding Comes Through Discussion*); 27 percent cited other radio sources; 22 percent mentioned group talks; and 42 percent cited print media such as posters, leaflets, and newspapers as their source of referral (Y. M. Kim, Lettenmaier, et al., 1996). Before the *Haki Yako* campaign in 1991, only one-fifth of new family planning clients could describe either the advantages of their chosen method or how to use it. One year later, more than four-fifths of new clients could describe both. This is a clear example of how communication outside the clinic can support counseling in the clinic.

Bolivia's Reproductive Health Campaign, under the slogan *La Salud Reproductiva Esta en Tus Manos* (Reproductive Health Is in Your Hands), used a similar approach. It was designed to reach 500,000 men and women through a media mix that included television and radio spots; audiocassettes for buses; in-clinic videos that focused on communication among women, with husbands, and with health care providers; print materials; and signs to identify clinics. All were linked by the lilac-colored logo of *Las Manitos*, the little hand of an infant clinging to a mother's finger. Surveys undertaken in El Alto, La Paz, Cochabamba, and Santa Cruz before and after the campaign showed an increase of 8.7 percentage points in the number of new users of family planning during the eight-month campaign, compared with an increase of 5.4 percentage points in the eight months before the campaign period (Valente, Poppe, & Payne Merritt, 1996).

A radio soap opera and distance-learning series in Nepal exemplify an innovative application of the multimedia approach. While the soap opera, intended for couples of reproductive age, seeks to spur discussion between spouses and to prompt clinic visits, the radio distance-learning series is designed to train district health workers in technical matters and in interpersonal communication and counseling. These radio broadcasts are being used in combination with face-to-face counseling training and print materials to promote interpersonal communication in the home and in the health centers.

LESSON 10.

Within the multimedia framework, a single medium usually serves as the locomotive or leader to advance the message.

Since resources are always limited, communication strategies should identify a leading medium to carry the message and focus major efforts there. This decision should be made primarily on the basis of the initial audience analysis. Whatever medium best reaches the intended audience deserves the most attention. Thus, for example, market research showed that television was the medium of choice in Egypt and several Latin American countries, radio in Nepal and much of Africa, and community-based *jiggasha* meetings with field workers in rural Bangladesh.

In each case, however, the major medium was reinforced by other forms of communication that repeated some of the same themes, logos, or messages. In Egypt television soap operas and spots were reinforced by local community mobilization campaigns, similar to the Minya Initiative, and by training providers in interpersonal communication and counseling. In Latin America television spots and drama are reinforced by counseling training for providers, videos for use in clinics, street theater presentations, and print materials for clients and providers. In Nepal the radio shows will be reinforced by classroom training for health care providers, local radio listening groups, audiocassettes for buses, convenient cloth kits in which field workers can carry brochures and contraceptives, and local newspaper stories. In Bangladesh the *jiggasha* community meetings are reinforced by Enter-Educate audiotapes, portable flipcharts, and regular national radio broadcasts. Everywhere, posters and client materials help providers to explain what family planning means and how to use specific methods.

LESSON 11.

Mass media are increasingly cost-effective and practical for reaching large numbers.

Mass media, despite the initial costs of production and the ongoing complexities of coverage, content, and control, usually reach a large audience at a relatively low cost per person when they are used strategically. The Turkish multimedia campaign and the first Zimbabwe male motivation campaigns are good examples. The Turkish multimedia campaign relied heavily on television and incurred direct costs of slightly less than US$232,000. Turkish Television and Radio donated an additional US$2 million worth of prime air time. Projections from the findings of a representative sample survey suggest that within six months the campaign had reached more than 6.5 million married women of reproductive age at a direct project cost of US$0.04 per woman reached (Kincaid, Yun, Piotrow, & Yaser,

1993). After the campaign, an estimated 345,000 more women were using modern contraceptive methods, about a 3 percentage point increase. If this increase is attributed to the campaign, the cost amounts to about US$0.67 for each new modern-method user (see Table 4.1). In Zimbabwe, the radio drama *Akarumwa Nechekuchera* (You Reap What You Sow) reached over half a million men. It cost $0.16 to reach each man and $2.41 to gain each new user (see Table 4.1). Before the male motivation campaign in Zimbabwe, the average annual increase of modern contraceptive use between 1984 and 1988 was 2.25 percentage points. During the 16-month campaign period in 1988 and 1989, the average increase of modern methods rose to 2.7 percentage points—20 percent greater than the previous trend (Piotrow, Kincaid, et al., 1992).

Radio and television are probably more cost-effective in reaching people than field workers are. A 1985 health campaign in Swaziland, supported by the HEALTHCOM Project, used both mass media and interpersonal channels to promote oral rehydration therapy. Evaluation comparing the effectiveness of mass media and interpersonal communication found that people exposed to radio were just as likely to take action as those exposed to various interpersonal or group channels. Radio, however, reached 60 percent of the population, whereas the health volunteers reached only 16 percent, and the clinic nurses only 22 percent (Hornik, 1989). In any case, it would be virtually impossible as well as prohibitively expensive to recruit, train, deploy, and pay the legions of field workers that would be needed to reach as many people as the mass media can, and as often. In addition, the mass media can depict scenes and bring up subjects that field workers may be unable or reluctant to discuss with people face to face (see Lesson 12).

LESSON 12.

The enter-educate approach offers many advantages for health communication.

Entertainment has been used for educational purposes since the beginning of human history. Greek tragedies, parables in the Bible, songs and stories in every religion and culture present the conflicts and values of different societies in vivid, dramatic, and, above all, entertaining terms. Modern mass media carries on this tradition, reaching millions with popular radio and television shows that entertain and educate simultaneously.

Johns Hopkins has used what is called the Enter-Educate approach for more than a decade to make health messages more appealing. Songs encouraging young people not to rush into sexual relationships were the first effort. Although the message contradicted the themes of most popular music, the songs were big hits in Latin America, the Philippines, and Nigeria. In Latin America, Tatiana and Johnny urged young people to wait until they were ready—for sexual relations, marriage, or pregnancy. The messages were well and correctly remembered years later (Kincaid, Jara, et al., 1988), and the songs were played long after the peak of their popularity.

Table 4.1
Cost-Effectiveness of Multimedia Communication Campaigns
in Kenya, Nigeria, the Philippines, Turkey, and Zimbabwe

Country, Campaign, & Year	Total Cost ($US)	Measure of Effect	Estimated Number of People Affected	Cost Per Person Affected ($US)
Kenya—Youth Variety Show	97,170	• To reach one person	3,354,439*	.03
		• To take some action	838,610	.12
		• To call show, write to producers, or visit a clinic	60,000	1.63
Nigeria—Benue State Mobile Drama, 1992	6,400	• To reach one person through the dramas	26,000	.25
Philippines Campaign for Young People, 1987	355,500	• To reach one person	1,196,000	.30
		• To motivate one person to seek more information	325,000	1.09
Turkey—Mass Media Family Planning Campaign, 1988	231,637	• To reach one woman	6,566,400	.04
		• To increase one woman's awareness of family planning	1,723,700	.13
		• To motivate one woman to visit a clinic	426,800	.54
		• To motivate one person to use family planning	344,700	.67
Zimbabwe—Male Motivation Campaign Phase 1, 1989	92,948**	• To reach one person	576,074	.16
		• To increase one person's knowledge of family planning	434,936	.21
		• To motivate one person to discuss family planning with his/her partner	305,895	.30
		• To motivate one person to use family planning	38,597	2.41

*Refers to young people age 15–24 of which about three-fourths were already sexually active.
**Based on the reach and total cost of the radio drama *Akarumwa Nechekuchera* (You Reap What You Sow).

Sources: Kincaid, Yun, et al.,1993; Kiragu, 1997; Piotrow, 1992; Piotrow, Kincaid, et al., 1992.

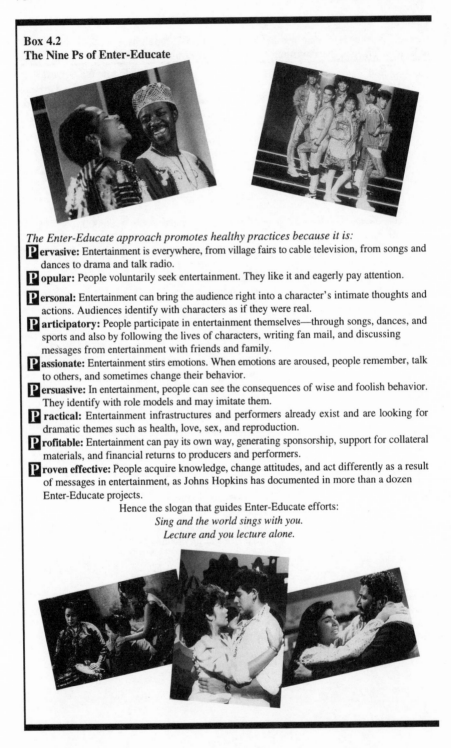

Box 4.2
The Nine Ps of Enter-Educate

The Enter-Educate approach promotes healthy practices because it is:

Pervasive: Entertainment is everywhere, from village fairs to cable television, from songs and dances to drama and talk radio.

Popular: People voluntarily seek entertainment. They like it and eagerly pay attention.

Personal: Entertainment can bring the audience right into a character's intimate thoughts and actions. Audiences identify with characters as if they were real.

Participatory: People participate in entertainment themselves—through songs, dances, and sports and also by following the lives of characters, writing fan mail, and discussing messages from entertainment with friends and family.

Passionate: Entertainment stirs emotions. When emotions are aroused, people remember, talk to others, and sometimes change their behavior.

Persuasive: In entertainment, people can see the consequences of wise and foolish behavior. They identify with role models and may imitate them.

Practical: Entertainment infrastructures and performers already exist and are looking for dramatic themes such as health, love, sex, and reproduction.

Profitable: Entertainment can pay its own way, generating sponsorship, support for collateral materials, and financial returns to producers and performers.

Proven effective: People acquire knowledge, change attitudes, and act differently as a result of messages in entertainment, as Johns Hopkins has documented in more than a dozen Enter-Educate projects.

Hence the slogan that guides Enter-Educate efforts:
Sing and the world sings with you.
Lecture and you lecture alone.

Nigeria:
Choices
Performed by Onyeka Onwenu and King Sunny Ade
Written by Onyeka Onwenu

Chorus: Choices,
(together twice) Choices,
               Choices,
               We can make the choice.

Onyeka: This is the time
               When we have to make a choice.
               Take a stand
               On the kind of world we want.
               Is it love with peace of mind
               Or children we are not prepared for?
               We can make that choice.

King Sunny: I want you,
               And I know you want me, too.
               That's a natural way to be
               for you and me.

Onyeka: But love has its rewards
               and responsibility.
               Let us love with care.

(Repeat chorus twice together)

Onyeka (spoken): You know,
               Making love is beautiful.
               But don't forget,
               You can make children sometimes
               When you don't want to.

King Sunny: Yes, we shouldn't make children
(spoken)   We cannot take care of.
               There are ways of making love
               Without making children.

Onyeka: That's Family Planning.

(Repeat chorus together twice, then repeat first v

Onyeka: I love you
               And I know you love me, t
               I know you'll understand
               When I make my choice.

King Sunny: Let's work it out togeth
               I know we can.

Together: Let us love with care.

Repeat Chorus

Philippines:
That Situation
Performed by Lea Salonga and Menudo
Written by Manny Aquino

Together: There's so much in life
               That we would like to do.
               We can wait for love
               Until we know it's true.
               It's up to us
               Not to jump into "that situation."

First male: I'm too young, not ready yet.
               I've got so much to do
               Got to take it step by step.
               It's best for me and you.
               It's up to us
               Not to jump into "that situation."

Second male: Let's take it easy.
               One step at a time.
               Why should we risk it?
               Our future's on the line.
               It's up to us
               Not to get into "that situation."

a: Is this what we want?
               Is it worth risking
               All we have ahead to do?
               t make that mistake.

Mexico:
Detenté ("Wait")
Performed by Tatiana Palacios
and Johnny Lozada
Written by Prisma

Tatiana: Hear how our heart beats,
               Hear how fast it beats.

Johnny: Wait.

Tatiana: Feel how this great love grows,
               Feel how everything is shaken up.

Tatiana: Understand.

Johnny: I no longer can, I no longer can.
               I want you in my arms,
               I want to love you.

Tatiana: Let's take love step by step.
               Let's go step by step. Wait.

Johnny: I can't (Tatiana: I understand)

Tatiana: Try it bit by bit, it will be better.
               Try it bit by bit so that it can grow.
               There's no need to run.
               Love that is rushed
               Is love that is lost.

Together: Understand,
               Let's not love at the wrong time.
               Wait. Later it will be a shame.
               Understand
               That love on the run creates
               Bread and water children,
               Bread and water children.
               Creates children without love,
               Without anything.

In the Philippines, Lea Salonga urged young people not to get into "that situation," that is, pregnant before they were ready. (See Box 4.2.) She warned young people not to make the wrong decisions—"Why should we risk it? Our future's on the line." Benefitting from more advance preparation and from the successful experience with Tatiana, the Lea Salonga songs were promoted on T-shirts and posters, through contests, and in radio and television spots, and were linked with a telephone hotline. All repeated the message that young girls should avoid premarital sex.

Evaluation in Metropolitan Manila showed that more than 90 percent of the young people surveyed remembered the message, about half said they were influenced by it and talked to others about it, and 25 percent sought more information. The Dial-A-Friend Telephone Hotline promoted in radio and television spots was overwhelmed by calls (Rimon, Treiman, et al., 1994).

In Nigeria, King Sunny Adé and Onyeka Onwenu sang "Choices" and "Wait for Me" to carry the message that "you can make love without making children—that's family planning." The Nigeria songs were part of a three-phase campaign to attract public attention, promote family planning, and stimulate clients to visit the clinics of the Planned Parenthood Federation of Nigeria.

Serial dramas or soap operas have carried Enter-Educate messages about reproductive health on radio or television in countries as varied as Egypt, Ghana, India, Indonesia, Kenya, Mexico, Nepal, Nigeria, Pakistan, the Philippines, Tanzania, Turkey, Zambia, and Zimbabwe. Ever since the 1950s, when *The Archers,* a serial about a farm family in England, was used to promote modern farming practices, and the 1970s, when Miguel Sabido's television soap operas in Mexico stimulated adult literacy and family planning, soap operas have proved an effective way to present social messages (Fraser, 1987; Noel-Nariman, 1993). The Nine Ps of the Enter-Educate approach help to explain why entertainment is being used more and more by Johns Hopkins and other organizations to present, promote, and popularize health practices worldwide (S. I. Cohen, 1993; Gao, 1995; Piotrow, 1994; Ramlow, 1994; Ranganath, 1980; Ryerson, 1994; Senanayake, 1992) (see Box 4.2).

Even on a small scale, an entertainment approach can be effective. Short radio or television spots that tell a story or involve popular characters are more compelling than those that preach at people or simply tell them to take action. Both humor and tragedy can move an audience. In Turkey, the best remembered component of a family planning campaign was a tragic but totally wordless spot that showed a young couple having more and more children until the debilitated mother disappears from the scene, presumably dead. Paradoxically, during the same campaign, a series of humorous spots starring Turkey's leading comedian, Uger Yucel, was almost equally well remembered (Kincaid, Yun, et al., 1993). On an even smaller scale, village-based entertainment that reaches only a few hundred people can carry important health messages. Puppet shows, street theater, school dramas, video vans traveling to rural areas—all can bring valuable health information to people who might not pay attention to or understand a formal lecture.

The Johns Hopkins experience illustrates, however, that Enter-Educate programs must be carefully planned, following all the steps of the P Process. A successful Enter-Educate effort requires research on audience preferences; strategic decisions on top-quality talent, scripting, and positioning of the issues to be covered; pretesting; media promotion; personal appearances; monitoring; and evaluation (de Fossard, 1997; Rimon, Treiman, et al., 1994).

LESSON 13.

Communication strategies depend on credible sources who are trusted and respected by the people.

Persuasive communication depends on trust as well as expertise. People will not follow advisors they do not trust. Thus a communication strategy needs to identify and mobilize leaders and institutions that people trust. In 1973 Rogers identified the most credible sources as those who were similar to the intended audience (homophily) but had enough expertise to convey new and accurate information (Rogers, 1973, p. 59).

Who are these sources today? In traditional societies, such as rural Bangladesh, they are husbands, village heads, religious leaders, and opinion leaders in women's social networks (see Box 3.2, in Chapter 3). In many countries such as Bangladesh, village health workers also play this role. In some cases national leaders are highly credible. A Tunisian woman told an interviewer: "Men are much better these days than they were before. They respect women more. Now they learn things, they are more understanding, they understand the rights of men and of women, too. And now a man can no longer divorce a wife he tires of. Before, a woman could be divorced, beaten, and poorly treated. That kind of thing doesn't exist anymore, thanks to President Bourguiba. Thanks to him and the laws, women are much better off today" (Huston, 1979, p. 28).

Celebrities can command attention and build trust—but only if they are credible spokespersons. In the Philippines, for example, teenage singer Lea Salonga was a credible and effective source of advice on sexual responsibility for young people because her own life was disciplined and consistent with her message. Moreover, by taking the time to make personal appearances in high schools, she demonstrated a real concern about the issue of sexual responsibility. In Latin America, the teenage star singer Tatiana Palacios was a credible source in urging young people to wait before becoming sexually active because, even though she was flirtatious, she insisted that "you can say 'no' " (Kincaid, Jara, et al., 1988). Two other young singers, Karina and Charlie, were less successful in Latin America, however, because they were not seen as credible or committed sources. Karina's private life was not perceived as exemplifying abstinence and sexual responsibility, and she did not go to schools and youth centers to reinforce those messages (JHU/PCS, 1994a).

Messengers need to match the message. For men in Cameroon, Roger Milla, the soccer star, proved a highly credible source. His television spots with his wife, son, and daughter urged couples to plan their families and to have only the number of children they could afford. The spots were seen by millions and evoked much favorable comment. Evaluation before and after the multimedia campaign found a large increase in clinic visits after the television spots had aired. The number of visits in five selected clinics rose from 50 in January 1991 to nearly 500 in December 1993 (Serlemitsos, 1994). In Nigeria King Sunny Adé is well known not only as one of Africa's top juju singers but also as a man with many women and children. Coming from him, the message "You should not have children you cannot take care of" was more credible than a plea for sexual abstinence would have been. In visits to maternity hospitals and in news media interviews, he admitted that, even though he was well off, it was difficult to take care of many children. He advised others not to follow his example but to plan their own families carefully.

Well-produced broadcast spots or dramas can position actors and actresses as convincing spokespersons and create a higher level of credibility. In Egypt, the beloved actress Kareema Moukhtar played the role of a doctor in *Memoirs of a Female Doctor*. In these television spots, she advised mothers not to let their daughters marry too young or begin childbearing too early. She recommended family planning for child-spacing and limiting. People later came to clinics and asked to consult "Doctora Kareema" (El-Bakly & Hess, 1994). When Moukhtar visited a clinic with USAID officials, women flocked to her to ask for advice on family planning (Maguire, personal communication, 1996). Others tried to find her house in Cairo to get contraceptives.

LESSON 14.

Satisfied users should be part of communication strategies.

Advocacy by satisfied users is not only the final step in individual behavior change but also a powerful force in any communication strategy to establish a community norm and encourage others to adopt new practices. Satisfied users include men and women who have used specific family planning methods successfully or found good service at local facilities. Because family planning has been perceived as a taboo subject, too sensitive for public or even much private discussion, satisfied users often remain silent. They need encouragement to speak out and to encourage others who may still be uninformed, uncertain, or reluctant to act.

One of the objectives of communication strategies, although often unstated, is to legitimate family planning and reproductive health issues as appropriate subjects for family and media discussion. Satisfied users can play a major role in this effort. At interpersonal and community levels, discussion about personal experiences plays an important role. In the *jiggasha* approach in Bangladesh, where women meet in groups and discuss their own problems, family planning users give advice on side effects and encourage women who, without such advice and reinforcement, might discontinue use of contraception. Mothers' clubs in South Korea and Indonesia have long performed the same role (Rogers & Kincaid, 1981).

On the mass media level, testimonials and role models of satisfied users can be extremely influential, as Roger Milla demonstrated in Cameroon. In Kenya, a male motivation project, supported by AVSC International and Johns Hopkins, recruited men who had had vasectomies and were willing first to meet with one another, then to talk with other men, and finally to appear in television spots. In Peru, the *Las Tromes* (female) and *Los Tromes* (male) television spots depicted typical couples who were satisfied users of modern methods. Two sets of spots were needed because, after the first *Las Tromes* spots for women, men wanted an opportunity to appear as smart, modern role models, too (Poppe & Leon, 1993).

LESSON 15.

Communication strategies should be action-oriented and linked to services through recognized symbols.

To change their own behavior, people need to know exactly where to go and what to do. Thirty years ago the typical family planning communication product might have been a poster contrasting a rich, smiling, small family with a poor, unhappy-looking, large family, and showing, in small type at the bottom, the address of a family planning association open one or two days a week. Today communication about reproductive health needs to be much more focused and to call for some specific action: talk to one's spouse, visit a service site for counseling, choose and begin using a family planning method. Recognizing that most people have heard about family planning and that many say they intend to use it, health communication programs are looking for new ways to be sure people know where to find services, supplies, and further information and to be sure they do not postpone their visits.

An innovative approach now being applied in communication strategies worldwide is the use of distinctive family planning or reproductive health logos to identify service sites. Borrowing from the commercial sector, Johns Hopkins encourages every national program to develop and use an attractive logo to identify sites where people can obtain services. The ideal logo is attention-getting, attractive, easy to describe orally (as on the radio), durable, and recognizable regardless of size.

In the largest logo project to date, family planning logos were distributed to more than 40,000 information and service sites in Nigeria (JHU/PCS, 1993f). The logo took two years to develop and launch in a country that had never had a family planning program before. It was reproduced on posters, brochures, mobiles, billboards, and television spots but especially on durable signs, and was distributed to all locations, including pharmacies and clinics, where services, information or products were available. "Nigeria's New Baby," the logo was called. Nine months after distribution more than 60 percent of the population in Enugu, Kano, and Lagos had seen the logo and knew what it meant (Kiragu, Krenn, et al., 1996). Similar national logos have been developed, with government and nongovernmental organizations deeply involved, elsewhere, including the Green Star in Tanzania, the

Yellow Flower in Uganda, the lively children in the Philippines, the Green Umbrella in Bangladesh, the Happy Couple in Peru, and *Las Manitas* in Bolivia (see Box 4.3).

Developing and distributing a national logo can be an important element in bringing different groups together, focusing attention on the strengths and weaknesses of existing services, and developing an overall national strategy. The process of bringing audience research, organizational resources, and service providers together in a coordinated effort focused on national program objectives can be a key component in strategic design.

Logos can also be used as part of the positioning process, to designate distinctive organizations or services or to highlight distinctive features—such as high quality—in existing services. In Indonesia, for example, where a national family planning logo already existed, the Blue Circle was used to identify private practitioners and to position them as well-trained, knowledgeable, fee-for-service providers (see Lesson 1). In India, the Indian Medical Association developed a logo to help recruit new members for the organization, to promote training courses in reproductive health, and to attract more clients for its members (Storey, Rimon, et al., 1994). In Egypt, as noted, the Gold Star helps to highlight public-sector clinics as a source of high-quality service and thus to position the entire program in the eyes of the public as a program of distinction and excellence.

IDENTIFYING IMPLEMENTING ORGANIZATIONS

LESSON 16.

Organizational leadership and cooperation are essential to strategic design.

The major criteria for implementing organizations are competence, commitment, coverage, clout, and continuity, as noted in Chapter 3, Lesson 7. Sometimes organizational leadership does not require strategic decisions because it is obvious to all where leadership resides. In Indonesia, for example, the Ministry of Population/BKKBN is a clear voice of authority in all aspects of family planning and is strong in all five attributes. Minister Haryono Suyono is the only head of a national program with a doctorate in communication and sociology. He helps to ensure that communication is a major element in the program and that all efforts convey a consistent message. The National Population Council (CONAPO) in Mexico plays a similar role. The Zimbabwe National Family Planning Council plays a comparable role in that country, although on a different level as a quasi-governmental agency.

Box 4.3
The Images of Strategic Positioning

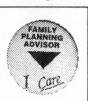

Ghana

We Care

After special training in communicating with clients, the Ghana Ministry of Health family planning advisors proudly told the public, "We care." This positioning improved morale, performance, and public perceptions.

Bolivia

Las Manitos

"Reproductive health is in your hands." The logo empowers and encourages people to act for their own benefit.

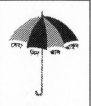

Kenya

Haki Yako

"It's your right." The Haki Yako emblem tells people that they are entitled to plan their families with high-quality services.

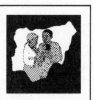

Nigeria

Nigeria's New Baby

The logo of a couple cradling their baby suggests that child-spacing will ensure the baby's health. The logo links a wide variety of providers together under one symbol—clinics, hospitals, pharmacies, and others.

By focusing on a unique characteristic, strategic positioning gives a family planning/reproductive health program a memorable identity, occupying a niche in the minds of the public and providers. A well-designed symbol can help position a service, product, idea, or program.

Bangladesh

Green Umbrella

A range of protective family health services—family planning, maternal, and child health care—are offered under the symbol of the green umbrella.

Indonesia

Blue Circle

The logo stands for family planning services by private doctors and midwives. "KB" stands for "family planning."

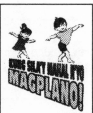

Philippines

"If you love them, plan for them!"

The logo and slogan link family planning with caring about your children.

Egypt

Gold Star

A symbol of quality, the gold star on display tells the public that this clinic meets high standards. Clients expect good service, and providers expect to offer it.

In other countries, however, different institutions play different roles, and, for specific communication programs or activities, some agencies are better qualified than others. In those circumstances, determining the lead organization or deciding what roles different groups will play is an important strategic decision. Whether the decision is made by the government, by various donors, or by an active organization that simply takes the lead, it is a decision crucial to program design. In Nigeria and Kenya, for example, on the basis of initial needs assessments, the Planned Parenthood Federation of Nigeria and the Family Planning Association of Kenya, respectively, stood out as the strongest agencies to implement communication programs. In Ghana, the Health Education Division of the Ministry of Health developed the necessary commitment, competence, continuity, and coverage to run regional campaigns when funded directly by donors. Unfortunately, it lacked the political clout to ensure adequate support when ministry officials made the key funding allocations. In both Egypt and Pakistan, subunits of the Ministry of Information showed the competence, clout, and commitment to produce high-quality mass media products with wide coverage. In Turkey an early needs assessment identified the Turkish Family Health and Planning Foundation, a nongovernmental organization formed by leading businessmen, as a competent group. This was a major strategic decision. The foundation carried out a successful mass media project and, in part as a result, was selected to carry out a national social marketing and clinical service promotion effort. As a result of these efforts, its president, Vebhi Koç, won the prestigious United Nations Population Award in 1994 (Turkish Family Health and Planning Foundation [TFHPF] Annual Report, 1995–1996).

PLANNING FOR DOCUMENTATION AND EVALUATION

LESSON 17.

Plans for monitoring and evaluation, based on the project objectives, should be included in the strategic design, workplans, and budgets.

One of the most common misconceptions about evaluation is that it is something that is done after a project is finished to find out whether the project was successful. Yet one of the first principles of evaluation is that, if evaluation is not planned at the start of a program, it is too late to be informative or useful any time (see Chapter 7). Planning for evaluation is therefore an integral part of strategic design. In fact, in setting program objectives and subobjectives, planners should simultaneously be asking themselves, "How will we find out whether these objectives have been achieved?" While many of the decisions to be made about evaluation methodology and major lessons learned from Johns Hopkins' experiences are discussed in Chapter 7, in fact evaluation itself calls for a step-by-step process, comparable to the P Process, that begins before any activity is implemented and continues after all activities are concluded.

During the strategic design phase, it is especially important to plan adequate time and funds for monitoring and evaluation. Whatever type of evaluation design is selected—whether randomized or quasi-experimental and control groups, one-group before-after design with sample surveys, comparison of exposed or unexposed individuals or communities, longitudinal panel surveys, service statistics, or referral data—some type of baseline or trend information is essential to establish change over time. Even where the initial response is expected to be low or nonexistent, as in measuring exposure to materials before they are distributed, a baseline to gauge other audience characteristics is useful. It can also show how many people reply incorrectly or misidentify messages. The decision on which data to collect for baseline measurements is closely related to the findings of the initial analysis, to the theory of behavior change that underlies the basic strategy, and to the audience, participating organizations, timeline, and budget for the entire program.

For campaigns with large-scale activities, the most common type of program evaluation depends on survey data from representative samples of the population. To collect data in surveys of 1,000 to 2,000 persons can take from a minimum of three months—if questions are already prepared, interviewers trained, and sampling frames established—to a maximum of a year or more if no preparatory work has been done. Data entry, editing, and analysis can take even longer, depending on available people and resources. Where new surveys are an essential part of formative research or analysis, they will precede strategic design. Where data already exist that permit strategic design, baseline surveys for evaluation purposes usually take place after the design and just before implementation begins. This is often a rushed period, but incomplete questions, poorly trained interviewers, poorly documented sampling frames, and data entry errors can complicate later analysis and muddy conclusions. To ensure good data and good analysis, budgets for pre- and post-survey research should be realistic. The minimal cost of fielding a sample survey is about US$35,000, compared with the cost of a major Demographic and Health Survey with 10,000 respondents, which can run as high as $300,000 for field costs alone. At least six months to a year should be allocated from start to finish of the baseline survey. Slightly less funding and time can be allocated for follow-up surveys. For projects of one year or less, two surveys are usually sufficient. The number and timing of additional survey rounds depend on the duration of the project, the extent of change that the program expects to cause, and, of course, available resources.

In Ghana, for example, the second Family Health Project called for a baseline survey and one follow-up survey. With support from the Futures Group, the baseline survey was carried out in April 1993, and the follow-up two years later, in November 1995. In Mali, surveys to measure the impact of a onetime campaign were conducted in December 1992 and six months later in July 1993. In contrast, the more extensive Peruvian program called for six rounds of a subnational survey at six-month intervals for three years. Feedback from the initial rounds made it possible to improve and simplify the questionnaires, but evaluators concluded that fewer rounds and a smaller number of simpler, more method-specific questions would have been even more useful (Valente, Sabar, et al., 1996).

To evaluate training, training materials, or print materials that can be distributed selectively, experimental designs with comparable control groups are feasible but must be planned well in advance. Since it is not possible to train everyone at once, nor is it always necessary to distribute brochures, posters, or similar material to all areas or clinics at the same time, it is theoretically possible to assign individuals or units to experimental or control groups. Nevertheless, to be sure that those individuals or areas selected for training or receipt of materials are comparable, they must be assigned either randomly or on a matched basis. This assignment process will require background information, current data, and an eye for political concerns as well—a time-consuming process that needs to be planned in the design phase.

All too often, plans are not made to evaluate print materials further after pretesting. For example, illustrated booklets on contraceptive methods prepared for early Population Communication Services projects in Nepal and Nigeria could not be adequately evaluated since no funds had been allocated and prevailing distribution methods did not establish separate experimental and control areas. Subsequent evaluations in both countries have focused less on evaluating individual items or materials—which usually have a limited impact that is hard to mea-sure—and more on evaluating campaigns or large-scale activities which can have a larger or synergistic impact that is more easily measured. In both countries questions have also been included on surveys conducted by other organizations—an efficient way to save both time and money but an approach that needs to be included in the strategic design from the start (see Chapter 7, Lesson 12).

NOTE

1. SMART is a commonly used acronym in training and management. An exhaustive search did not find the source for the acronym; however, the concepts underlying SMART can be found in educational psychology literature. Specifically, see Robert F. Mager, *Preparing Instructional Objectives* (rev. 2nd ed.), Belmont, CA: Lake Publishing Co., 1984.

Chapter 5

Development, Pretesting and Revision, Production

PROFESSIONAL QUALITY AND CREATIVITY

Lesson 1.   The approaches that work in developing messages and materials for professional marketing and advertising can be applied to health communication.

Lesson 2.   Communication professionals know best how to develop communication products, but finding the right professionals takes time and care.

Lesson 3.   Communication professionals need close supervision in developing appropriate health and family planning materials.

HEALTH EXPERTISE

Lesson 4.   Health professionals need to provide input and to review materials for technical accuracy.

AUDIENCE PARTICIPATION AND FEEDBACK

Lesson 5.   Message development is a collaborative and participatory process.

Lesson 6.   The participation of representatives of intended audiences in pretesting helps ensure that the materials will speak effectively to actual audiences.

Lesson 7.   Pretesting and revision take time and money but help to avoid the even greater costs of ineffective materials.

Lesson 8.   Pretesting can inform and reassure government officials and other gatekeepers about communication strategies.

VALUE

Lesson 9.   Producing high-quality materials in large volume is cost-effective.

Lesson 10.   High-quality materials hold up over time and encourage reuse.

Once the strategic design for a communication program is established, work begins on developing specific messages and materials to support that strategy. Developing messages and materials that can increase knowledge, change attitudes, and, especially, encourage new behavior is no easy task. It combines art and science. It calls for a creative process that applies imagination and talent within the framework of an agreed-upon strategic design.

Every communication project can offer its own lessons in how to develop specific messages and materials. From the experience of the Population Communication Services project in more than 50 countries, an overriding principle for message and materials development has emerged. It is the need to combine:

- professional quality and creativity in communication,
- health expertise,
- audience participation and feedback, and
- value for money spent.

This combination is important, of course, to every aspect of health communication from the first assessment to the final evaluation, but it is especially important in designing the products and materials that will be the most conspicuous and costly part of any communication program. Whether the products developed are brochures, posters, television spots, radio serial dramas, or live performances and events, the same principle applies.

Only with such a combined effort can messages and materials achieve the high quality that is crucial to effectiveness. In practice, high quality means health communication products that are:

- comparable to the best commercial communication products,
- accurate in addressing health issues, and
- appealing to the intended audience.

Thus the specific lessons that follow on materials and message development, pretesting, and production link creativity and skill in communication, professionalism in health care, and the participation of audiences in developing high-quality products. Such products can be used widely and repeatedly—thus making their production cost-effective and their impact durable.

PROFESSIONAL QUALITY AND CREATIVITY

LESSON 1.

The approaches that work in developing messages and materials for professional marketing and advertising can be applied to health communication.

Family planning messages compete for attention with professionally developed commercial marketing messages crafted by creative and skillful message-makers with ample resources. In the United States, for example, the average person is potentially exposed to hundreds of commercial appeals every day (Media Dynamics, 1995). For family planning messages to be noticed, remembered, understood, and acted on, they must compete in quality (if not in quantity) with other messages.

To be effective, staff of Population Communication Services and their colleagues around the world have learned to play the game the way the competition plays it. Therefore family planning messages are now developed according to many of the principles and techniques that successful commercial advertisers apply. The Seven Cs of Effective Communication, adopted from standard advertising practices, offer a convenient guide to the key attributes of effective communication (J. R. Williams, 1992) (see Chapter 2). Whether promoting consumer products or encouraging healthful behavior, persuasive communication follows these seven basic rules:

- Command attention,
- Cater to the heart and head,
- Clarify the message,
- Communicate a benefit,
- Create trust,
- Call for action, and
- Consistency counts.

Command attention. Only messages that are noticed and remembered can be effective. An unnoticed message might as well not have been sent. Messages will not be noticed if they are dull or nondescript. Effective messages should be daring enough to attract attention and elicit comment while at the same time remaining sensitive to cultural context, social values, and political priorities. Slogans such as *Haki Yako* (It's Your Right) in Kenya or the two skipping children in the Philippine logo with the slogan *Kung sila'y mahal n'yo, magplano* (If you love them, plan for them) meet that test. Sometimes it is the medium even more than the message that is the attention-getter. For example, using the Goodyear blimp or the sides of elephants as billboards to promote condoms, as was done by the founding Secretary-General of Thailand's Population and Community Development Association, Mechai Viravaidya, always commands attention.

Cater to the heart and head. Most people are moved at least as much by emotions as by reason. A message that arouses emotion is effective because people learn better when their emotions are aroused (see Chapter 2). Emotional appeals usually involve storytelling—reflecting, however briefly, the situation and feelings of an individual. Thus emotional messages are often best delivered in an entertainment format, as a song, a drama, or even a comic sequence. Appeals to reason at the same time add staying power to a message. After emotion has cooled, the message still makes sense. For example, in an Egyptian television spot, the wise and caring "Doctora" (Kareema Mouhktar) loses her temper at the mother who wants to lie about her young daughter's age so that she can be married to a rich man. The Doctora's emotional outburst reinforces her sensible message against early marriage.

Clarify the message. Focus and freedom from clutter are crucial. A message should convey a single, important point. Ancillary information and multiple themes can distract the audience, and some people will miss the point. The technical information and complex qualifications used by epidemiologists and many health care providers confuse many audiences. Such detailed information, put in terms that are meaningful and understandable to clients, is best communicated in counseling or other interpersonal communication. Above all, the audience must understand what the message means. Hence the motto Focus Demands Sacrifice. A single, clear, and comprehensible message is best. For example, in Ghana the simple message, "Trust your family planning advisor. She cares," proved more powerful on a billboard than attempts to depict the wide range of contraceptive methods.

Communicate a benefit. People need a strong motive to change their behavior. The best motivator is the expectation of a personal benefit; people rarely buy a new product or take up a new practice unless they see some direct personal benefit in it. In the commercial field, advertisers know that consumers do not merely buy products; they buy expectations of benefits. As Charles Revson, a major cosmetics company magnate, put it, "In the factory, we make cosmetics; in the store, we sell hope" (Tobias, 1976).

The benefits that family planning promises must reflect the positioning of the product, which in turn will reflect the values, expectations, and hopes of the intended audience. Depending on the audience's concerns (learned from the analysis of formative research described in Chapter 3), a message might promise such benefits as good health, beauty, sex appeal, financial security, or a happier marriage. The *Las Tromes* campaign in Peru, for example, suggested that contraceptive users could join the ranks of "with-it" young women (*tromes*) who enjoy modern lifestyles and supportive husbands. In Nepal, in contrast, attractive posters suggested that young men and women who use family planning will be strong and healthy for the necessary work on their farms.

Create trust. A message that people will act on of their own accord must come from sources that they trust (see Chapter 4, Lesson 13). If the promise of a future benefit does not come from a credible source, people will not believe it. Many family planning messages are expressed by the character of a benevolent, trustworthy local nurse or a doctor, such as Egyptian television's "Doctora Kareema," to show that the message can be trusted. Also, sources can inspire trust if they are people similar to the intended audience or to what the audience aspires to be. To reinforce trust, messages often are phrased informally, the way one person speaks to another—that is, "you" in the familiar second-person singular, rather than "they." For example, the Bolivian *Salud Reproductiva* (Reproductive Health) campaign used as its tag line, *Salud Reproductiva—Está en Tus manos* (Reproductive health is in your hands) (Valente, Saba, et al., 1996).

Call for action. After seeing or hearing a persuasive message, the audience should know exactly *what to do*. Once convinced that the promised benefit is worth pursuing, people need to know how to act on this belief—where to go, whom to call, what to buy. Directives should be clearly stated. Without a specific cue to action, people may hear, understand, and even approve of a message but still take no action. For example, in promoting sexual responsibility among young people in the Philippines, television spots showed the telephone numbers of the Dial-A-Friend hotline while singing star Lea Salonga urged, "If you want to talk it over, just Dial-A-Friend" (Rimon, Treiman, et al., 1994).

Consistency counts. Repetition is essential. A message that is repeated many times, perhaps with variations but always with basic consistency, becomes familiar, and people come to recognize and understand it without having to stop to think. As it gains recognition, it also reaches wider and more diverse audiences. A good logo, slogan, or central message theme therefore should be used and reused until, like the dynamic white ribbon on a red background in the Coca-Cola logo, or the American Express slogan "Don't leave home without it," people know what it stands for even without seeing the name of the product. In family planning communication, the use of logos to identify service providers' posts, contraceptive distribution sources, informational materials, and contraceptive products is an example of consistency and repetition to make an idea more familiar (see Chapter 4, Lesson 15 and Box 4.3). Of course, where technical information is involved, as in flipcharts, client brochures, and training material, consistency is especially important to prevent misunderstandings.

The Seven Cs correspond to some degree to the different Steps to Behavior Change (see Chapter 2). They help to indicate which type of information is most needed at each stage of change (see Figure 5.1). In the initial, or knowledge, stage,

Figure 5.1
**Meeting Communication Needs at Each Step to Behavior Change Through the
Seven Cs of Effective Communication**

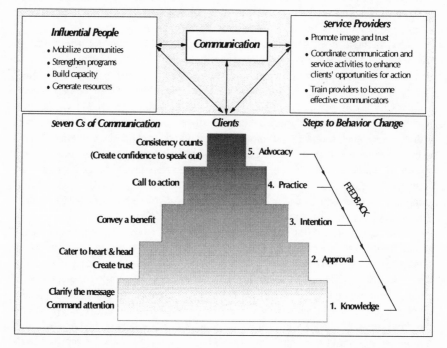

education is a primary need. Thus commanding attention, clarity, and consistency
are important. During the approval stage, persuasion becomes more important.
Therefore it is crucial to create trust and to cater to the heart and to the head. In the
intention stage, people are trying to decide whether to change their behavior. This
is when communication needs to convey plausible personal benefits. In the practice
stage, when behavior change occurs, a call to a specific action is needed. This is the
time when providing information about service locations and hours, for example,
can provide the incentive to practice. In terms of behavior change, beyond the
Seven Cs of message development, another characteristic of effective messages and
activities is that they can create confidence to speak out. In this way they can
empower people to serve as advocates for programs and services.

Of course, good communication needs to combine these elements, as much as
possible. For example, the Pro-Pater campaign that promoted vasectomy in three
cities in Brazil in 1990 exemplified nearly all of the Seven Cs (see Box 5.1).

The campaign's animated television spot won a Bronze Lion Award at the
1990 Cannes International Advertising Festival, a recognition of high quality. More
important, Brazilian men implicitly endorsed the campaign by showing up for
vasectomies in greater numbers (Kincaid, Payne Merritt, et al., 1996) (see Chapter
7, Lesson 4).

Box 5.1
Brazil Vasectomy Spot: Navigating the Seven Cs

In just 30 seconds a Brazilian television spot promoting Pro-Pater vasectomy clinics embodies all of the Seven Cs of Effective Communication:

1. Command attention. A few measures of a wedding march attract the viewer's attention to two cartoon hearts standing side-by-side as bride and groom.

2. Cater to the heart and head. The viewer has a moment to puzzle over these creatures before amusement takes over: The male figure has obviously—although abstractly—become sexually aroused, and the two nudge amid giggling and kissing sounds. The consequence is the appearance of a little third heart.

3. Clarify the message. The male heart becomes sexually aroused again, and more nudging and kissing follow. This time the result is two more bouncing little hearts.

4. Create trust. The male is aroused again but this time the female pushes him away, objecting noisily—a familiar situation that suggests these cartoon characters have a trustworthy message.

5. Communicate a benefit. Voice-over suggests a visit to a Pro-Pater clinic, and two small black lines on the male heart suggest a vasectomy. When the male becomes aroused again, his mate happily accepts him.

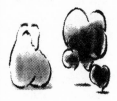

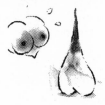

6. Call to action. On-screen type shows the telephone number and address of a Pro-Pater clinic, and a voice-over urges viewers to call. The spot concludes with a clever tag line positioning vasectomy in the viewer's mind: "Vasectomy—an act of love."

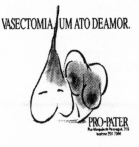

VASECTOMIA, UM ATO DE AMOR.

PRO-PATER

7. Consistency counts. The loving hearts also appeared in newspapers and magazines, even on an electronic billboard above a busy Rio de Janeiro intersection. Over the years, a constant theme of Pro-Pater promotion has been that vasectomy is an act of caring and responsibility.

LESSON 2.

Communication professionals know best how to develop communication products, but finding the right professionals takes time and care.

However expert in their own fields, few health officials have the artistic or technical skills needed to develop high-quality communication products on their own. Whether a program is developing posters and brochures or organizing sophisticated multimedia communication campaigns, professionals from the media, advertising, or entertainment industries can almost always add quality and creativity.

The motto to follow is Buy It, Don't Build It—in other words, use professionals. This approach has been vital to the development of major Enter-Educate campaigns in Africa, Latin America, Egypt, Indonesia, and the Philippines, to the logo distribution campaign in Nigeria, and to many other multimedia efforts. Recruiting first-class writers, actors, singers, and producers—who often are willing to work at a considerable discount—has led to prize-winning products in many countries. Over more than a decade, Johns Hopkins has recruited and worked effectively with numerous professionals (see Appendix).

Identifying and then recruiting the right professionals takes time and care. In the Philippines, for example, the 1980s Music for Young People project starring Lea Salonga began with audience research—a survey of high school students to identify singers who were popular with young people. Next came interviews with each singer and reviews of performance videotapes. Final selection was based on the performers' popularity, image with young people, willingness to be involved in a controversial project encouraging sexual responsibility, availability to promote the project, and personal commitment to the campaign objectives (Rimon, Treiman, et al., 1994). This effort led to the choice of Lea Salonga, the young Filipina singer who later achieved international fame playing the title role in London and New York in the musical *Miss Saigon.*

Equal effort went into developing the songs themselves. A contest elicited 13 songs from professional Filipino composers. The seven best submissions were pretested with students, entertainers, and health professionals. As a result of the care given to selecting the right talent at every step, the winning songs, "That Situation" and "I Still Believe," sung by Lea Salonga and the group Menudo, became big hits on radio and in the record stores (see Box 4.2, in Chapter 4).

Finding the right advertising agency to design messages or manage a campaign also requires care. A combination of independent research and competitive bidding helps to ensure a broad choice, high quality, and a fair price (Greenberg et al., 1996). For example, project managers in Bolivia reviewed more than 40 advertising agencies and media production houses in 1992 and conducted in-depth interviews before selecting Grey Advertising to design a multimedia campaign (JHU/PCS, 1993g). In Indonesia the National Family Planning Coordinating Board (BKKBN) identified eight advertising agencies with the capability to develop what later became the Blue Circle campaign for private-sector providers. The BKKBN invited each agency to submit a design strategy and develop initial materials for the campaign, reimbursing each US$1,000 for its efforts. Then a review committee selected the firm of PT Fortune as the best (Saffitz & Rimon, 1992). The manual *How to Select and Work with an Advertising Agency*, a collaboration between Prospect Associates and Johns Hopkins Population Communication Services, provides detailed guidance for the process (Greenberg et al., 1996).

Government approval to use commercial vendors is sometimes difficult to obtain. In countries where the ministries of health have their own donor-funded production studios or where government-operated broadcasting agencies want additional business, there may be strong resistance to the use of private-sector professionals. Both donors and communication experts need to emphasize the quality and skills that trained and experienced communication professionals from the private sector can bring to health campaigns. Generally, while in-house government facilities may be able to produce excellent training materials, brochures, or posters for clinic use, private-sector professionals have the experience needed to develop creative messages for the public. These professionals are best for producing multimedia campaigns, broadcast-quality radio and video productions, and commercial-quality billboards, posters, point-of-purchase promotion, and other materials for the public.

LESSON 3.

Communication professionals need close supervision in developing appropriate health and family planning materials.

Obtaining good products from media professionals demands considerable time and energy—not only to find the best available skills but also to oversee the work. Communication project managers and health experts must make clear from the start that they expect to work closely with creative and production personnel. Spelling out the degree of oversight at the beginning is important. It is essential that advertising agencies, which are hired and fully compensated for their work, recognize the need to accept guidance from their clients, the program managers. Otherwise some firms or individuals may object to what they regard as interference. In fact, the initial working agreement should stipulate that project managers will check production work at every stage. Such close monitoring can avoid the need to reprint a poster or reshoot a film—costly steps that can throw a project off budget and off schedule. Even more important, close monitoring can prevent products that do not convey clear or accurate messages. Furthermore, the agreement should hold the production team responsible for the quality of its work. This means, for example, that printers should be required to redo poor print jobs at their own expense (de Fossard, 1997).

Similarly, unless the nature of the collaboration is established in advance, a director filming a television spot, for example, may refuse suggestions from project staff during shooting and accept comments only after rough editing. At that stage, of course, if scenes have to be reshot, actors must be called back and scenes reconstructed. By alerting a director that ongoing supervision is normal and in the long run economical, project managers can reduce such delays and needless costs.

Even experienced communication professionals can benefit from guidance and close supervision in promoting family planning and other health issues. In Peru, for example, the advertising agency responsible for campaigns designed to reach young couples initially directed the television spots toward upper socioeconomic classes. That was the audience the agency knew and usually addressed in consumer product advertising. To refocus the advertising agency on the intended audience of mid- to low-level socioeconomic status, project managers had to supervise every step, including casting and selecting locations, sets, and even props (Poppe, personal communication, June 5, 1996a). In Indonesia, a production company that had not received sufficient guidance cast a stylish actress in full makeup to depict a typical rural midwife. Substantial changes were necessary before the video could be used. Had a script been prepared, reviewed by program managers in advance, and discussed with the production company, time and expense could have been saved.

Where entertainment rather than advertisements is being prepared, the program manager's idea of necessary supervision may be the creative personnel's idea of unwelcome interference. In a Turkish film, for example, officials expressed the desire to see references to specific family planning methods early and prominently. An episode in which women listened to a lecture about family planning was included, but it interrupted the narrative and was one of the least interesting scenes. In the Philippines, in contrast, commercial co-producers of an Enter-Educate film refused to incorporate many of the suggestions provided by Johns Hopkins on the grounds that conspicuous promotion of family planning would detract from the dramatic, action-filled plot and reduce the commercial appeal of the films. As a result, both Johns Hopkins and the donor agency were dissatisfied with the final production, even though it won numerous cinema awards.

To try to clarify the line between professional creativity and social messages, Esta de Fossard, an actress and producer, has developed a manual for radio social drama scriptwriters: *How To Write a Radio Serial Drama for Social Development: A Script Writer's Manual.* A key element she recommends is the design document, prepared at the start of the project. It spells out all the key messages to be presented and identifies in detail how the characters, plot, and setting will be developed to present those messages clearly (de Fossard, 1997). International workshops have been held in Zimbabwe (1994) and Nepal (1996), and national workshops in Bangladesh and Indonesia (1996), to help scriptwriters and directors practice the science and the art of producing high-quality artistic work that is both convincing in its health messages and commercially successful.

HEALTH EXPERTISE

LESSON 4.

Health professionals need to provide input and to review materials for technical accuracy.

The input of health professionals is essential throughout the process, not only in the selection of appropriate broad objectives and accurate messages but also in the design of specific materials. Expert input is, of course, most essential in preparing training materials or materials designed primarily for health professionals. For example, when the Family Planning Association of Kenya and AVSC International decided to develop a training film for use in Africa on counseling for voluntary female sterilization by means of minilaparotomy, they invited groups of 20 to 50 health care providers in three countries to participate in focus-group discussions. The health professionals first assessed various scripts for the film and later previewed early versions. The first round of discussions revealed that minilaparotomy was in fact performed in various ways throughout Africa, with different anesthesia and operative techniques and with patients in different positions. The script for the training films therefore had to be adapted for each audience to reflect these differences. Although the involvement of and repeated pretesting with health personnel increased the time and cost by about one-fourth, the knowledge gained was invaluable (Harper, Schneider, & Mworia, 1990; Harper, 1991).

AUDIENCE PARTICIPATION AND FEEDBACK

LESSON 5.

Message development is a collaborative and participatory process.

Communication is a dialogue, not a monologue (see Chapter 2). Participation by the intended audience as well as by program management, health care providers, researchers, advertising agencies, scriptwriters, and even performers helps to ensure high quality. Ideally, creative personnel should talk directly with the kind of people they want to depict and reach. In fact, an effective way to design messages is to ask audience members to talk about family planning in their own words and then to design program messages accordingly. Many men and women have already engaged in a dialogue with their spouses and friends about the advantages and disadvantages of family planning. They have already passed through an extensive "feedback" process and have discovered what kind of messages are effective, what expressions are ambiguous, and what words are understood or misinterpreted. For example, in Turkey, Bilge Olgaç, scriptwriter of the drama *Hope Was Always There*, about rural midwives, visited rural centers to talk directly with midwives and their clients. In Indonesia, Teguh Karya, the distinguished writer and director of the television drama *Alang, Alang,* participated in focus-group discussions with the trash scavengers who were featured in the drama. At the press conference when the video was released, he acknowledged the value of this personal involvement and dialogue.

When direct personal contact is not possible, the creative team should review the initial audience analysis or market research as the first step to creative message development. Workshops offer a practical way to share the results of audience research. In Indonesia, for example, before developing the three population and environment dramas in the *Equatorial Trilogy,* film directors, scriptwriters, and producers attended a two-day orientation workshop to review what the public perceived as the links between population and environmental problems. They watched videotapes of focus-group discussions to learn what potential audiences said (JHU/PCS, 1992j). Seeing and hearing members of the audience talk about their personal problems brought the research findings to life. Creative personnel later commented on how helpful the videotapes had been to writing dialogue.

In Tanzania a 1993 workshop to develop a radio soap opera not only presented the results of audience research but also provided guidance on the Enter-Educate approach. Kenyan actor/producer Tom Kazungu, who had developed a popular soap opera in Kenya featuring health messages, was invited to show Tanzanian scriptwriters how to combine education and entertainment through effective plots, setting them in familiar places and creating characters that the audience could identify with (Kazungu, 1993).

Psychographic profiles, such as that of "Policarpio" (see Box 3.5, in Chapter 3), also can help creative personnel speak effectively to their audiences—not as an anonymous mass of people but as distinct individuals. Giving scriptwriters a name and a face, or even a photograph, can help them identify with listeners or viewers. In Uganda, for example, project managers vividly evoked the intended audience for the scriptwriters of a radio drama. Married men were represented by "Musa Kitayimbwa," a hypothetical 30-year-old Muslim shop assistant living with his wife and six children in two rented rooms; Musa dreams of owning his own business and wants his children to be more educated than he is (Glass & Smith, 1993). Scriptwriters were encouraged to write their scripts specifically for listeners like Musa.

LESSON 6.

The participation of representatives of intended audiences in pretesting helps ensure that the materials will speak effectively to actual audiences.

Even the most careful preparation cannot guarantee that the intended audience will understand messages and materials or find them appropriate, relevant, and persuasive. Pretesting—that is, asking selected members of the intended audience what they think about the messages and materials—is an excellent way to make sure that the audience is involved and the best way to ensure that materials do indeed evoke the intended response. When behind schedule and over budget, project managers may be tempted to skip pretesting altogether or take the shortcut of having colleagues review the materials. But no colleagues—whether government officials, project personnel, foreign experts, or next-door neighbors—can serve as a proxy audience to predict real audience reactions. Even the best trained health communicators and the most creative designers must test their messages to make sure they are meaningful to the people that they hope to persuade. When the audience does not respond positively to a message, the only course, however painful, is to revise and test again until something that does work is developed. In health communication, as in retail sales, the customer is always right.

Pretesting not only checks how well project managers, artists, and writers have interpreted audience analysis, but it also uncovers matters that researchers and officials may have overlooked. Even when pretest participants generally like an overall concept, they usually can suggest significant changes that will make materials easier to understand and more appealing. For example, Bolivian project managers were surprised to learn from pretesting that indigenous men and women, although bilingual, differed in the languages they preferred for radio messages. Men, because they were accustomed to working in Spanish-speaking environments, preferred hearing family planning radio spots in Spanish. Messages in Spanish sounded more authoritative, the men said. Women, in contrast, preferred the indigenous languages of Quechua and Aymara, which they heard at home. Messages in Quechua and Aymara sounded more personal. With this information, the managers revised their broadcast plans and aired spots on appropriate stations and at times to reach men and women separately, each in their preferred language (Payne Merritt, 1992).

Pretesting can shed light on subtle aspects of materials being created—pictures, colors, music, choice of actors, even facial expressions. Drawings in a Bolivian flipchart for reproductive health counseling underwent numerous changes—some conspicuous, some subtle—as a result of points raised in pretesting. Before pretesting, the family featured in the drawings was pale and nondescript; after pretesting, they were redrawn with pronounced ethnic characteristics and facial expressions. Before pretesting, the mother wore a look of apprehension as she received an injection; after pretesting, she was shown with a relaxed smile. The doctor, meanwhile, was transformed into an entirely different character (see Box 5.2).

Ideally, a pretest elicits comments on every feature that might limit or enhance effectiveness. At a minimum, pretesting seeks answers to these basic questions:

- Is the message clear to the intended audiences? Do different audiences interpret the message differently (for example, men and women, people of different ages, rural and urban residents)?
- Is the message trustworthy and believable? In particular, does the message make a credible promise of personal benefits to be gained?

Box 5.2
Listening to the Audience

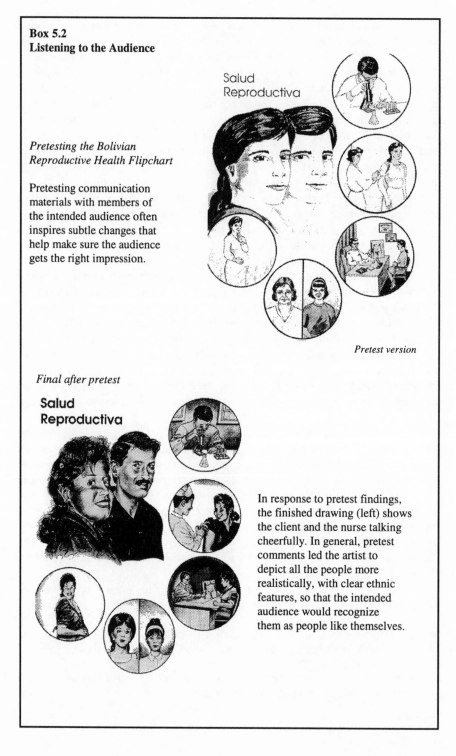

Salud
Reproductiva

*Pretesting the Bolivian
Reproductive Health Flipchart*

Pretesting communication
materials with members of
the intended audience often
inspires subtle changes that
help make sure the audience
gets the right impression.

Pretest version

Final after pretest

**Salud
Reproductiva**

In response to pretest findings,
the finished drawing (left) shows
the client and the nurse talking
cheerfully. In general, pretest
comments led the artist to
depict all the people more
realistically, with clear ethnic
features, so that the intended
audience would recognize
them as people like themselves.

- Does the audience like the material? Why or why not? Do they like it for the right reasons?
- Are the images culturally appropriate?
- Are there too many messages? Must some information be sacrificed for better focus?
- Is there anything offensive in the material?
- Would people talk to their friends and relatives about the message?
- Does it make the audience want to take appropriate action?

In short, pretesting should help determine how well the message meets the criteria of the Seven Cs and the Steps to Behavior Change model for its specific audience.

Pretesting can yield very specific solutions to problems identified. When Johns Hopkins staff members were working in 1989 with the Planned Parenthood Federation of Nigeria to develop songs promoting sexual responsibility, focus-group participants with whom the song "Wait for Me" was pretested revealed a possible serious misunderstanding. As first written, the lyrics repeated the phrase "wait for me." To some listeners in the focus group, the phrase mainly connoted patience in love relationships and the need to plan one's whole life; the message about family planning was not coming through clearly. Finally, on the focus group's advice, the phrase "plan with me" was incorporated into the lyrics, clarifying the family planning message that the song was intended to deliver (Baron et al., 1993).

Sometimes pretesting reveals that an author's favorite ideas or clever creative slogans simply do not work with the intended audience. In a U.S. campaign to encourage childhood immunization before age two, Johns Hopkins staff came up with the slogan "Up to two—it's up to you," meaning "You should have your child immunized before the age of two." At pretesting, the slogan had no impact on its intended audience of low-income mothers using public health facilities. For them, the best message was simply "Immunize on time. Your baby's counting on you" (Henderson, 1994b; Warner & Associates, 1994). A simple, straightforward slogan that emphasized the mother's responsibility to care for her trusting baby was more persuasive, both rationally and emotionally, than a catchy slogan that was hard to understand.

LESSON 7.

Pretesting and revision take time and money but help to avoid the even greater costs of ineffective materials.

The cost and effort required for pretesting and revising communication materials vary greatly. Generally, pretesting print materials with an intended audience can be done rapidly and at low cost, although drawings may need to be revised and pretested several times (Zimmerman & Steckel, 1985). The more complex and technical the subject matter or the intended product, the more costly—but also the more important—pretesting becomes. Several rounds of pretesting may be necessary before creative staff can depict complex health matters clearly and accurately. In Cameroon, for example, an artist made initial drawings for a flipchart about Norplant® implants based on illustrations from another booklet. During pretests, service providers commented that the drawings did not accurately show either where the syringe was positioned during insertion or how the capsules were inserted. To correct the problem, a service provider sat with the artist while he revised the pictures. Even then, a second round of pretesting revealed further inaccuracies. A new artist was hired and required to observe a Norplant insertion before starting to draw. Finally, the second artist was able to draw accurate pictures for a flipchart that project managers could produce and distribute to clinics with confidence (Vondrasek, personal communication, May 1994).

Pretesting need not always be expensive or time-consuming, however. In developing Enter-Educate materials, the key is early and direct contact with members of the intended audience. For example, from informal pretests during a materials development workshop in Uganda, scriptwriters obtained rapid feedback on the first two episodes of *Konoweka* (A Stitch in Time). The drama was designed to promote family planning use among women, engender more positive family planning attitudes among men, tell listeners where to find family planning services, and encourage communication with partners. This simple pretest found that the drama did not appeal to its intended audience, married women ages 20 to 35. The younger women complained that it sounded like something their parents would listen to. The scriptwriters thus learned early on that they would need to use themes, characters, and vocabulary more appropriate to younger listeners (Glass & Smith, 1993).

Sometimes pretesting results can be rejected or modified—if there are good reasons for doing so. In Morocco, for example, project managers developing television spots promoting family planning found from focus-group research that women preferred a male narrator. The women thought a man's voice sounded more authoritative—"like a doctor's," they said. Nevertheless, the Ministry of Public Health wanted the spots to convey intimacy, a sense that one woman was speaking to another privately about family planning. They decided, therefore, to use a woman's voice despite the pretest results. The ministry wanted viewers to think about family planning as a subject for friends and relatives to discuss rather than as a message from someone in authority.

LESSON 8.

Pretesting can inform and reassure government officials and other gatekeepers about communication strategies.

While the view of government officials does not necessarily reflect the views of primary audiences—especially audiences very different from them, such as adolescents or nonliterate villagers—the endorsement of these officials is usually essential to ensure media placement. In Kazahkstan, for example, two television spots for young adults were successfully pretested with the intended audiences, but a too-tight schedule prevented pretesting with health officials and other community influentials. As soon as the television spots were aired, complaints from officials about any family planning messages on television forced them off the air. The accompanying posters and brochures remained in the youth facilities, however, and were in great demand among young people (Gushin, Hooper, & Saffitz, 1994).

In general, messages to be shown on television require more pretesting at all levels than other material. Because television reaches such a large and undifferentiated audience with vivid images, material that would be acceptable in posters or brochures or even in clinic or community videos may be offensive to some television viewers. Also, television comes right into the home, where parents, grandparents, and young children may be watching together. In that setting, intimate conversation, rude behavior, or unaccustomed candor may be personally embarrassing. A member of Parliament in Kenya objected to a television program supported by the Ministry of Health and the World Bank, *Usiniharakishe* (Don't Rush Me), in which a teenage boy attempted to seduce a schoolgirl in his bedroom and was slapped in the face. Pretesting had indicated that some people—a small minority—might be offended by the scene, but complaints multiplied when it appeared on prime-time national television ("Usiniharakishe," 1986).

By demonstrating that materials will be acceptable and effective for the intended audience once they are made public, pretesting can help win the support of apprehensive officials. Clear documentation is important, as is solid research. In Colombia, high-level officials delayed a broadcast condom-promotion campaign for two weeks. Only when they were able to review the favorable pretest results did they agree that the material could be aired (JHU/PCS, 1986a). Good documentation of pretest results is especially important in selecting national logos and slogans, since officials often have their own ideas about what is attractive or effective—ideas that may differ substantially from the ideas of the intended audience.

Setting up committees of influential people to review materials in advance can help prevent delays or cancellations. For example, for the Nigerian family planning drama broadcast as part of the television variety program *In a Lighter Mood*, advisory councils consisting of representatives from University Teaching Hospital, the Nigerian Television Association, and the State Ministry of Health reviewed the script for each episode. This allowed the committee to attest to the medical accuracy, cultural appropriateness, and clarity of the production (Piotrow, Rimon, et al., 1990; JHU/PCS, 1990d).

In the rush to implement programs and to meet the never-ending demand for more communication materials in the field, the temptation to omit audience research and pretesting is always strong. Yet a communication campaign, like a house, is only as strong as its foundation. A health communication program built on a rock-solid foundation of competent analysis, appropriate strategy, and high-quality professional production that is pretested with the intended audience will be easier to implement and far more effective than a program built in haste on the shifting sands of improvisation and ad hoc materials.

VALUE

LESSON 9.

Producing high-quality materials in large volume is cost-effective.

Almost too obvious to require proof, this lesson has been a basic principle underlying Johns Hopkins family planning communication work for two decades. For example, the publication *Population Reports*, an authoritative review of research findings and program experience published by the Population Information Program in the Johns Hopkins Center for Communication Programs, is the most widely distributed publication in the population field. The publication has been cited in parliamentary debates in Peru and the Philippines to settle questions relating to family planning methods and programs. With more than 130,000 copies distributed in English, French, and Spanish, each 32-page copy costs only about US$2.60, including mailing.

Another example is the 1991 flipchart entitled *Planning Your Family*, a collaborative effort between Population Communication Services and the International Planned Parenthood Federation (IPPF). The flipchart was pretested extensively in English- and French-speaking countries throughout Africa and then printed in five basic colors on durable stock with thick, laminated covers. The quality of the handsome flipchart is obviously very high. In the short run, it was expensive, including the initial development, pretesting, and print run of 10,000 copies in two sizes, a large version for clinics and a smaller one for community-based workers.

In the long run, however, the high quality proved cost-effective because the product is credible, durable, and salable. The flipchart was first presented at the November 1991 Annual Meeting of the American Public Health Association (APHA). The presenters reported, "The Africa flipchart received such a positive response at APHA that we are already being asked for costs on bulk orders" (Church & Bashin, 1991). Between 1992 and 1995 most of the first printing was sold or distributed to programs. Reprinting 1,000 copies of the smaller-size flipchart in 1995 cost US$23.28 per unit. By comparison, printing 2,000 copies initially would have cost only US$16.82 per unit, but in this case limited funding prompted a decision that was penny-wise and pound-foolish.

LESSON 10.

High-quality materials hold up over time and encourage reuse.

Reuse extends the life of communication materials and saves resources. Entertainment, especially, can be repeated many times to reach new and wider audiences. In fact, songs, plays, and films are created to be performed or shown over and over again. Popular radio and television dramas also can be broadcast many times—in fact, as long as characters, plot, messages, and, above all, production quality meet prevailing standards. Some materials may have to be revised to suit different audiences or different media. *Umut Hep Vardi* (Hope Was Always There) was a two-episode Turkish television drama about the problems that a young rural midwife faced at her first posting in a small, rural community. The drama was designed to appeal to viewers in eastern Anatolia, where contraceptive prevalence rates were the lowest in the country, although the drama was broadcast nationwide. Called by some the "*Dr. Zhivago* of Turkey," the drama proved so popular that within three years it was aired twice more and seen by 57 percent of the population—approximately 32 million people nationwide (TFHPF Annual Report, 1992–1993; ZET-Medya Research, 1992). A panel study conducted in six regions of eastern Anatolia found that 29 percent of the men and women who saw the drama said that they intended to visit a midwife (Kincaid, 1992).

Berdel (Barter), a feature film directed by Atif Yilmaz and produced by the Turkish Family Health and Planning Foundation, told the tragic story of a woman who could not produce a son for her husband. He then bartered away his oldest daughter to obtain a new young wife. This drama, which emphasized the need for family planning and more respect for women, was shown in theaters throughout Turkey and won seven international film awards. Because of its popularity, *Berdel* was also aired seven times within five years on television, where it was seen by an estimated 35 million people. In audience surveys after the second showing, 41 percent of viewers said that, as a result of watching the film, they would try to stop discrimination against daughters, and 25 percent said that they would give family planning more attention (TFHPF Annual Report, 1992–1993; ZET-Medya Research, 1992).

Sometimes parts of materials have multiple uses. In Nigeria several versions of two different television spots promoting child-spacing were made in 1994 to suit audiences in the three regions of the country. One music bed provided background for all versions of the spots, while scripts and casting changed from one version to the next (Kiragu, Krenn, et al., 1996).

Repackaged materials can reach new and different audiences. In Burkina Faso, for example, folk dramas first performed live in towns and villages were later videotaped for television broadcast to audiences many times larger. In contrast, the Indonesian drama *Alang, Alang* was edited down from three hour-long television episodes to a single 100-minute version to show from mobile video vans that reach rural areas lacking access to television broadcasts.

With still more effort, high-quality materials can be recycled into totally new products. Thus, segments of footage from the documentary *Living Stories of Yemeni Families* and from popular Nigerian and Philippine music videos have been incorporated into television spots used over long periods. Such reuse not only saves money but also links campaigns. The new campaigns call to mind the earlier messages.

Sometimes materials with a proven record in one country can be exported successfully to other countries. For example, popular songs produced in Mexico to promote sexual responsibility among young people were played all over Latin America in other Spanish-speaking countries. In Africa family planning materials frequently travel across national boundaries. In one case, *It's Not Easy*, a feature film about AIDS produced in Uganda for the AIDSCOM project, has been distributed to more than 60 television stations throughout the continent, in both English and French versions. Surveys in Kenya and Zimbabwe have confirmed that the Ugandan production is effective elsewhere. *It's Not Easy* attracted substantial audiences in both countries and inspired many viewers to take some action—discussing the video with friends, practicing monogamy, or using condoms (McCombie & Hornik, 1992). In Africa, the Union of National Radio and Television Organizations of Africa (URTNA) encourages the exchange of radio and television programming through its Program Exchange Center, even dubbing films and videotapes into different languages when necessary. Currently, these include films and videos on family planning, sexually transmitted diseases (STDs), HIV/AIDS prevention, child survival, and other health interventions.

Illegal pirating of popular songs and videos is another way that many people are reached, even though it deprives producers and performers of legitimate income. Johns Hopkins staff found the popular Pakistani TV series *Aahat* available at Baltimore video centers. Tapes of King Sunny Adé and Onyeka Onwenu's family planning songs were on sale in the markets of Ghana within a month after their release in Nigeria.

Although some widespread distribution occurs spontaneously, prompted by the very success of good materials, it can be efficient to plan from the start to produce and distribute materials regionally. The Zimbabwe film *More Time*, directed by John Riber and produced by Media Development for Trust to alert adolescents to the dangers of early, unprotected sex, was designed for use throughout Africa. Distributed and promoted by Johns Hopkins in Kenya, the film was an immediate hit. Project managers must make certain, however, that materials are appropriate for audiences in different countries.

Additional pretests and revisions may be needed before a film, flipchart, or other material produced in one country can be distributed elsewhere. For example, a series of training videos on family planning counseling produced in Peru in 1995 was pretested for use in Bolivia, Brazil, Mexico, and Nicaragua in 1996. After pretesting showed that the videos do cross cultural borders, they were distributed throughout Latin America (Poppe, personal communication, November 13, 1995). These videos were conceived for regional use because experience had shown that counseling strengths and weaknesses, as well as training approaches, are similar throughout the region.

In short, while service delivery takes place exclusively within a local or national infrastructure, communication products often can travel wherever a regional language, such as Arabic, English, French, or Spanish, is understood. In fact, many popular commercial film dramas and television serials are dubbed into different languages and distributed around the world. The more the world moves into an electronic age, the more opportunities arise for wider international use of modern communication products. The most effective programs in the long run may be those that combine appropriate community-based activities with top professional-quality national or international broadcast materials.

Chapter 6

Management, Implementation, and Monitoring

MANAGEMENT

Lesson 1. Identification of the lead agency and clear lines of responsibility for each phase of the program enable everyone to focus on achieving communication objectives.

Lesson 2. Training can build a critical mass of communication experts in each country who share the same conceptual framework, pursue the same strategic goals, and apply relevant technical skills.

Lesson 3. Activities at the community level depend on strong local support and decentralized initiatives.

Lesson 4. The funding for communication activities, materials production, and technical assistance needs to be closely coordinated.

Lesson 5. All parties need to understand and follow established consultation and clearance requirements.

IMPLEMENTATION

Lesson 6.   Dissemination of materials is a separate activity, requiring a specific plan and budget.

Lesson 7.   A campaign launch is an opportunity for maximum public, press, and political attention.

Lesson 8.   Compensation or appropriate recognition for the people who work on a communication program improves morale and performance.

MONITORING

Lesson 9.   Regular and accurate monitoring helps ensure that outputs are produced and distributed as planned.

Lesson 10.   Rapid feedback allows managers to fine-tune program operations and improves the organizational climate.

Lesson 11.   Too much information can clog a monitoring system.

Lesson 12.   When monitoring reveals unexpected problems or opportunities, a flexible and rapid response is necessary.

Implementation—Step Four in the P Process—is where everything comes together. After months of analysis, design, materials development, pretesting, revision, and production, the public campaign begins. It may be only the tip of a massive iceberg of effort, but this is what the public sees and will respond to. Even the most revealing research and a brilliant strategic design will not produce results unless they are well implemented.

Implementing a campaign, a project, or a program is a complex, challenging task. Managers and their staffs must keep dozens of interrelated and overlapping activities moving forward on schedule (see Chapter 4, Lesson 8). The relatively small 1993 MotherCare program to reduce maternal mortality in Bauchi State, Nigeria, provides a good example. This campaign lasted only six months and was limited to a single state—albeit one with a population of 4.2 million (JHU/PCS, 1993b; Ajiboye et al., 1995). For this campaign, program managers had to coordinate:

- distribution of 40,000 posters, 40,000 pamphlets, counseling materials for midwives, 500 pieces of promotional dress fabric, and 500 T-shirts;
- a rally to launch the project;
- mobilization activities (group talks, drama performances, and distribution of print materials) in 15 communities; and

- broadcast of 446 radio spots, 26 episodes of a radio drama, 13 radio discussion programs, 13 episodes of a radio talk show, 13 episodes of a television drama, and 8 television discussion programs.

Just before the launch, managers also were responsible for:

- an orientation workshop for representatives from nongovernmental organizations and the mass media;
- a seminar to introduce village leaders to the project; and
- the training of 92 midwives, 240 birth attendants, 30 community health education workers, and 30 health educators.

As communication programs grow in size and duration, the need for careful preparation, good management, and close monitoring multiplies. Responsibility for managing different activities must be assigned from the start. Then, to spot problems—such as lack of trained providers, inadequate supplies, incomplete distribution of materials, or poor turnouts for community events—managers must monitor activities closely, reviewing reports from site visits, service statistics, and other tracking systems. When problems arise, managers must resolve them quickly. In fact, managers must stimulate an organizational style or culture that welcomes feedback and encourages all involved to identify problems and make suggestions to correct them as rapidly as possible.

MANAGEMENT

LESSON 1.

Identification of the lead agency and clear lines of responsibility for each phase of the program enable everyone to focus on achieving communication objectives.

As noted in Chapter 4, it is important for all involved to identify and support a lead agency among the many possible agencies involved in a complex health communication program. Without a lead agency, accountability for results may become so diffused that the program will suffer. Who selects the lead agency? In a well-established program such as Indonesia's, there is little doubt that the Ministry of Health/BKKBN is the responsible government agency. In other cases, the Ministry of Health or a national commission may be the lead agency. Elsewhere, or for small projects, a nongovernmental agency such as a family planning association may simply assume that role. In some cases, donor agencies will select a public or private organization to direct a specific project or program. In any case, the strategic design for any program, large or small, should clearly identify the lead organization based on preliminary analysis and with the agreement of the governmental and nongovernmental organizations involved (see Chapter 3, Lesson 7).

The lead organization will, of course, have to work cooperatively with many others to achieve maximum impact. At this point, organizational communication, both within an agency and with the other partners, becomes an important skill. Co-workers need to share their findings and concerns politely with one another so that all involved have the information and encouragement they need to perform well. In Ghana, for example, the Health Education Unit in the Ministry of Health has been the lead agency, but it has developed many partnerships with other ministries and organizations to work at the local level (Ghana MOH/HEU & JHU/PCS, 1992). In Bolivia, the IEC Technical Committee took initial leadership, and various agencies worked to develop materials until the Ministry of Health formally launched the program and became the national leader (Valente, Saba, et al., 1996).

Whether the health communication program is run in a hierarchical fashion by one agency or is a team effort, specific individuals or groups need to be responsible for specified activities. These activities usually include preparation of print materials, radio or television spots or programs, community outreach and meetings, distribution of materials, training, regular publicity, monitoring, and evaluation. Responsibility is usually divided by type of activity and by geographic area, with materials production and evaluation usually handled centrally, while community activities and monitoring are handled locally. Many variations are possible, but all the organizations and individuals involved should have a clear understanding of their own responsibilities. These are best spelled out in a workplan (see Figure 6.1).

To implement large programs, additional personnel may be needed. This can involve recruiting more staff or consultants, as was done by the Health Education Division in Ghana, or by temporarily releasing current staff from other duties. For larger tasks, subcontractors, task forces, or reallocations of workloads should be considered. Commercial advertising or distribution agencies may be needed. Special and demanding communication programs rarely succeed if new duties are simply loaded onto already-overworked staff.

An increasingly common management problem can occur when many donor agencies are working in the same country. One agency, often a multilateral donor, may provide multiyear program support for staff salaries, while other donors support specific projects. Thus job security is not linked to achieving project results. Health communication projects, which are more conspicuous and often face closer scrutiny than training or service delivery, need to produce results. Thus, however funded, they need to emphasize management by results, and all donors need to look for those results. This means clearly identifying what final results are expected, what intermediate results may occur, and how to proceed step by step to achieve those results. It also means seeking the active endorsements of all relevant donor agencies so that it is clear that all donors expect results.

In the long run, the best way to protect individual positions and ensure institutional survival is to demonstrate results. A valid theory, such as the Steps to Behavior Change model on the individual level (see Chapter 2), clear processes such as the P Process at the project level (see Chapter 2), and useful guidelines such as SMART for the objectives within the strategic design (see Chapter 4, Lesson 4), all help to define what results can be expected and how to achieve them.

Figure 6.1
The Minya Initiative Project Workplan, Egypt, 1990–1993

Activity	1990			1991												1992					Responsibility
	O	N	D	J	F	M	A	M	J	J	A	S	O	N	D	J	F	M	A	M	
1. Initial Data Gathering	█																				NPC/Minya
2. Translation/ Analysis		█																			JHU/PCS
3. Draft Project Design			█																		JHU/PCS
4. Orientation of LPCs & Review of Draft Design				█																	JHU/PCS, NPC/ Minya, Local Population Council
5. Baseline Research						█															JHU/PCS Local Affiliate
6. Message Development, Implementation, Design, Pretesting, and Production							█	█	█				█	█							Local Population Council
7. Training of Supervisors and Trainers*								█	█												Training Specialists
8. Training of Service Providers												█	█								Trained Staff*
9. Launch "Centers of Excellence" Campaign										█	█	█	█	█	█						Local Population Council
10. Management & Monitoring					█	█	█	█	█	█	█	█	█	█	█						NPC/Minya
11. Impact Evaluation				█	█	█	█	█	█	█	█	█	█	█	█						JHU/PCS Local Affiliate
12. Review and Replanning Workshop															█	█	█				NPC Minya

Ultimately, institutions that produce results can create an institutional climate of achievement that is the best guarantee of long-term success in a changing environment.

LESSON 2.

Training can build a critical mass of communication experts in each country who share the same conceptual framework, pursue the same strategic goals, and apply relevant technical skills.

As communication becomes a recognized discipline with a specific body of knowledge and skills, people who carry out large-scale communication programs require training in the field. Working together on national programs, communication experts need to speak the same language, understand the strategic nature of a communication program, and apply their skills in a consistent, step-by-step process. They can then become a critical mass, stimulating and reinforcing one another and articulating their role persuasively to others. Training can create this critical mass.

To develop a critical mass of competent communication practitioners calls for training at all levels. Policy-level personnel need to know how to develop a strategic design and manage public- and private-sector collaborators. Mid-level personnel usually need skills in community organization and/or materials development. Health care providers need special training in interpersonal communication and counseling. Grassroots workers need to know how to stimulate community participation, from local people with influence to families who need help. And all those who work in the field of communication need to know how to communicate a can-do institutional climate that will inspire others (see Box 6.1).

A single workshop or a variety of long-term degree programs is not enough. The best approach is a continuing series of highly participatory workshops followed by on-the-job experience implementing a program. All those involved in a country program can learn a basic conceptual framework and a step-by-step model that they can then elaborate and pursue together as they carry out their program. Workshops for high-level staff and national, regional, and district workshops should all use the same basic concepts and terminology.

In a number of countries, including Bangladesh, Bolivia, Egypt, Ghana, Indonesia, Nigeria, and Zimbabwe, a critical mass of health communication practitioners has been trained in the P Process of project development. The interactive computerized training program SCOPE (strategic communication planning and evaluation) helps participants work through the entire P Process from analysis to evaluation, often with data on their own country.

A key lesson in SCOPE training is how to improve the institutional climate within an organization so that the program and products also can improve. Good organizational communication helps address "product problems" and not just "selling problems." SCOPE training emphasizes that good communication within an organization is an "upstream" activity that can stimulate innovation, improve morale, and energize workers. Materials production is a "downstream" activity that can often be best managed by improving quality upstream (Latzko & Saunders, 1995). In other words,it pays to build in quality upstream rather than to rely on "quality control" to remove poor quality downstream. (See Box 6.2.)

Box 6.1

How to Make an Effective Presentation

Lessons from the Johns Hopkins Center for Communication Programs Advances in Family Health Communication workshops:

1. "How Does This Help Me?"

Most participants especially appreciate presentations that will be useful to them in their jobs (and lives). So present what the audience wants to learn. Don't try to overwhelm them with data or dazzle them.

2. Know the Audience

Have respect for your audience. Avoid talking down to them. Some resource persons ask participants in advance about their knowledge and experience. It is usually better to err on the side of sophistication.

3. Present New Insights

Participants expect state-of-the-art communication information. If you have been giving the same presentation each year, it is time for an update.

4. Identify a Single Most Important Concept

Present it early, keep focusing on it as your presentation unfolds, return to it often, and reiterate it during your wrap-up.

5. Plan a Wrap-Up

The wrap-up is the most important part of your presentation. Know how you want to finish, and plan everything to lead to or support the conclusion.

6. Manage Your Time Well

Nothing loses an audience faster than complaining about lack of time. They feel that the presenter is cramming and that their brains are full.

7. Less Is More

Allow at least one-third of your time for questions and discussion throughout the session. Also, about 20 minutes is the most you can expect participants to follow your train of thought. Then they need a break, a change of pace or style, or a participatory exercise.

8. Do Exercises Early

Use exercises right away to build excitement. Bring in the main points after participants have struggled firsthand with the concepts in the exercise.

9. Rehearse and Prepare

Cue videos before sessions begin. Make sure that slides are in order and will not show up upside down or backward. Make sure overheads are ready; detach the printer backing paper before the session, not during.

10. Keep Support Materials Simple

No more than six lines of large type (36 point) plus title (42 point) per slide or overhead.

Box 6.2

SCOPE—Training Communicators with the Virtual P Process

The computer software SCOPE, for Strategic COmmunication Planning and Evaluation, teaches the P Process of communication project development. Developed at Johns Hopkins Center for Communication Programs for its Advances in Family Health Communication workshops, SCOPE has grown increasingly sophisticated since its introduction in 1992. The software is on the verge of becoming a real-world analysis and planning tool in addition to a flexible interactive training tool.

Working with SCOPE, trainees come to appreciate the value of carefully analyzed data as a basis for strategic planning and the systematic, step-by-step approach of the P Process. From its start in 1992, SCOPE has used real country data. Working with a hypothetical budget of US$1 million, SCOPE trainees work through the steps in the P Process. They invest in research, analyze the real data, develop a strategic design, and even prepare messages and mock-ups of products, and plan evaluation for an 18-month communication campaign for their country. The SCOPE exercise is a decision-making process. With each choice the users make, the software leads in a particular direction. As explained by Benjamin Lozare, chief of the Center's Training Division and leader of SCOPE development, SCOPE teaches that decisions have consequences.

Continuously upgraded, SCOPE had been produced for 14 countries and in four languages by the end of 1996. The latest enhancements include district-level maps of health and socioeconomic indicators or of program impact as well as a function that reads national trend data from a periodically updated World Bank database. Under discussion are a SCOPE version for AIDS prevention programs, an edition for youth organizations, and a SCOPE-based software to help communities record and analyze their own data and develop their own development and health plans.

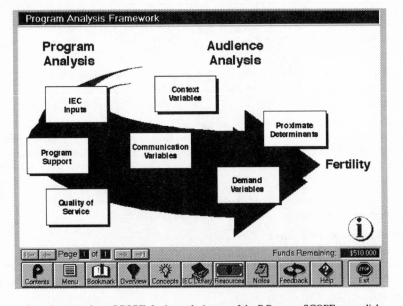

Sample screen from SCOPE: In the analysis step of the P Process, SCOPE users click the computer mouse on one of these boxes to choose the data they want to analyze.

LESSON 3.

**Activities at the community level depend on strong local support
and decentralized initiatives.**

Complementing the power and reach of mass media, community-based field
activities are important, especially for rural areas, for their participatory, normative
role. Community activities should be an integral part in the overall strategic design.
They may range from folk song festivals and group sessions with field workers, as
in Bangladesh, to lectures and discussion groups, as in Bolivia, to puppet shows, as
in India and francophone Africa, to street theater, as in Latin America and North
Africa, to football games, as in Zimbabwe, to concert parties and parades, as in
Ghana, to poetry readings and plays, as in Egypt. These and other Enter-Educate
approaches are especially effective. Further examples include mobile cinema vans
in India and Indonesia and Hits for Hope song contests, carried out by itinerant
troops traveling in vans with their equipment, and bicycle races in Uganda.

Whatever the event, community activities require local support and activism
to succeed. In Egypt, Ghana, and Zimbabwe, for example, Ministry of Health
officials at the district level, nongovernmental agencies, and local leaders combined
forces to put on local events that attracted large audiences and popular participation.
To draw in local organizations and individuals for appropriate entertainment,
education, and family planning promotion, local committees were formed in each
case—in Minya governorate, Egypt, around the National Population Council
representative, the governor, and state family planning services; in Ghana around
the district health education officers; and in Zimbabwe around the Zimbabwe
National Family Planning Council field representatives (Ghana MOH/HEU &
JHU/PCS, 1992; Piotrow, Kincaid, et al., 1992; Kemprecos et al., 1994). As more
countries decentralize responsibility for health services, health communication
programs will depend increasingly on grassroots leadership—through local advisory
and implementing committees that include and can mobilize local governments and
local private organizations, including women's organizations and other civic
groups.

LESSON 4.

**The funding for communication activities, materials production,
and technical assistance needs to be closely coordinated.**

As international development programs move into their fourth decade of
operations, funding patterns are changing. Small projects funded by a single donor
and managed by a single government agency or nongovernmental organization are
increasingly giving way to larger programs with multiple donors and implementing
agencies. Major cost items, such as in-country training, commodities, and
production costs, are more likely to be directly funded either by or through host-

country institutions, while expert technical assistance may still be funded separately, through international organizations. This is true in communication programs as well as in training, service delivery, research, and evaluation.

As a result, coordination, to make sure all the required inputs are available at the same time, is becoming a major task, and in a health communication project or campaign, timing can be crucial. Examples of poor coordination abound. In India, for example, technical assistance to train district-level health educators was organized and ready for a full year while the local agency selected and funded separately to carry out the training failed to produce a satisfactory curriculum. In Ghana, regional-level health educators were trained and ready to manage multimedia regional family planning campaigns, but the funding for campaign supplies, transport, and local activities was diverted to other programs, including the construction of an AIDS laboratory and health education office building and resource center in the capital. In Ethiopia, technical assistance teams arrived on site only to find their government counterparts not ready to put them to work because of conflicts over funding. By contrast, in Indonesia, funding for Johns Hopkins technical assistance to the Ministry of Health/BKKBN's International Training Program has been well coordinated with planned workshops and observation tours to train family planning workers from other countries. As a result, training facilitators have become more proficient, training materials and curricula have improved, and the reputation of the program has grown.

Generally, coordination improves with time and experience, especially when programs have stable leadership. But coordination depends in fact on a strong host-country institution or donor support that channels adequate communication resources in a timely manner through a coordinating unit. Also, to be sure that centrally produced materials are ready when local-level activities begin calls for a comprehensive plan of events at each level, regular meetings to share information, and a schedule for all technical assistance requested.

LESSON 5.

All parties need to understand and follow established consultation and clearance requirements.

Because communication programs are designed to be conspicuous and far-reaching, reviews at all levels are unavoidable. No donors or other responsible agencies want to be surprised by a poster, billboard, television or radio spot or drama, or even a flipchart or packet of materials that they have never seen or heard of before. In fact, the more a communication program commands attention and caters to the emotions (see Chapter 4), the more important it is that local gatekeepers and appropriate officials have opportunities to review and approve the basic themes and materials in advance. Ensuring that organizations implementing health communication programs understand clearance procedures is part of good management.

This means not only that advertising agencies need clearances from host-country agencies and possibly international donors, but also that the creative talent—scriptwriters and directors—recognize that they need these clearances. The objective of clearances should not be to censor or second-guess cultural sensitivities or expenditures but rather to prevent surprises and to enable officials to explain programs and their messages fully and accurately if any criticisms arise. In Egypt, donors and government agencies were embarrassed when the scriptwriter for a population/environment film submitted his draft manuscript to the censor's office before it had been reviewed by the donor and the sponsoring agency. To avoid this, not only should pretesting results be documented, but project advisory committees representing local gatekeepers should also be set up to provide advice, especially before mass media productions. The Planned Parenthood Federation of Nigeria established an advisory panel composed of religious leaders and other respected individuals to review the two music videos of King Sunny Adé and Onyeka Onwenu promoting sexual responsibility and family planning before they were released.

IMPLEMENTATION

LESSON 6.

Dissemination of materials is a separate activity, requiring a specific plan and budget.

Distribution is often a neglected task because it is not perceived as glamorous or challenging. Yet print, broadcast, and other materials must be in place before the launch of a communication campaign. Materials for health care providers, such as flipcharts, posters, leaflets, anatomical models, reference manuals and, where feasible, videos for client education, need to be delivered to the appropriate site. When print or video materials designed to be used by various providers do not reach those providers, the effect is the same as taping a radio or television show and never broadcasting it. Billboards and posters must be mounted in conspicuous public places. Relevant articles and advertisements must be in the hands of newspapers and magazines. Radio and television programs must be scheduled in advance, and tapes distributed.

Disseminating and distributing this wide array of material poses a major logistical challenge to any communication program. Each item must reach the correct destination intact and on time. If a billboard goes up late or in an obscure spot, fewer people will see it. For example, during the Blue Circle campaign in Indonesia, only two of the five billboards supplied to the city of Semarang were posted, and neither of those was appropriately placed. Although the intended audience for the campaign was couples who could afford to pay private practitioners for family planning services, the billboards were placed in low-income areas, where clients had to rely on government-supported services (Saffitz & Rimon, 1992).

Print materials require specific distribution plans. Simply determining how many items to deliver, and where, is the first challenge. For the logo promotion campaign in Nigeria, for example, estimates of the number of family planning outlets varied so widely—anywhere from 10,000 to 150,000—that a special inventory was conducted in 10 local government areas just to make the rough projection of 40,000 outlets nationwide on which to base print orders and distribution plans (Kiragu, Krenn, et al., 1996).

Distribution also posed problems during the Blue Circle campaign in Indonesia. At first, complete and accurate names and addresses for all participating physicians and midwives were hard to gather. The spot checks conducted during the campaign uncovered another problem: Equal amounts of materials were delivered to each location, even though some service providers saw many more family planning clients than others. Not surprisingly, the busiest practices ran out of leaflets very quickly. The sheer volume and weight of print materials and the large number of destinations involved also complicated distribution. In just the first year of the campaign, for example, nearly 2 million items had to be received, stored, sorted, grouped by city, shipped, collated, and delivered to the offices of more than 3,000 physicians and midwives in four cities on two islands (Saffitz & Rimon, 1992). A job of this size is often too large for project staff or for existing distribution systems run by a government ministry to undertake in a short time.

There are alternatives, some low-cost, some expensive. For example, when large-scale training held in central locations accompanies a communication project, trainees can carry materials home and distribute them in their local areas. This approach means free transport and special handling. Kenyan providers trained in a workshop on interpersonal counseling skills, for example, were so enthusiastic about their new materials that they took them home, and many took the initiative of setting up displays in their clinics (Rudy, personal communication, June 1996). Another possibility is to ship communication materials together with contraceptive supplies so that only one delivery is necessary for each facility. In the Philippines, arrangements are made with the printing companies to package and send materials directly to the provinces together with contraceptive supplies, thus avoiding expensive repackaging or warehousing. The Family Planning Association of Uganda (FPAU) used another low-cost approach in preparation for a local project launch: They hired unemployed students to hang posters and clinic signboards and to distribute leaflets (Kiragu, Galiwango, et al., 1996).

The surest way to distribute print materials, but also the most costly, is to hire a commercial firm that specializes in materials distribution. In Nigeria, for example, the Family Health Services Project contracted with an outside firm to distribute materials promoting the new family planning logo to every family planning service and supply outlet in the nation. The firm hired 3,000 census workers to carry the materials to the approximately 40,000 destinations that had been identified in the preliminary inventory. Despite fuel shortages, ethnic hostilities, political crises, and rough terrain, almost all of the materials reached their destination (Kiragu, Krenn, et al., 1996).

Storage is an ongoing problem. To achieve economies of scale and have print materials always available, large print orders make sense. But the costs and logistics problems involved in warehousing and reshipping print materials need to be considered, too. For each country and even for different types of material, special plans should be made and adequate funds should be set aside in the budget for storage as well as distribution.

When counseling materials such as flipcharts or cue cards are to be developed, service providers must be prepared for their arrival. Distributing counseling materials is more than a matter of quantities and transportation. Collaborating organizations and service providers must be prepared to receive and use the materials. Project personnel must tell recipients what materials will be coming and when, so that the boxes do not sit unopened in warehouses or on loading docks.

A passive system of distribution—where clinics receive an initial supply of materials and have to reorder when more are needed—does not work. Distribution systems for contraceptives and communication materials, like the distribution systems for Coca-Cola and other consumer products, need to be proactive, estimating needs in advance, monitoring the use of those materials, and arranging for regular and automatic resupply (Descouens & Dow, 1986; World Health Organization [WHO], 1995).

Training in how to use the materials also is vital. Without training, even enthusiastic providers may be unable to use new materials effectively. In Brazil, thorough training helped to build providers' demand for an integrated package of posters, pamphlets, flipcharts, and other family planning materials developed by the Brazilian Association of Family Planning Agencies (ABEPF) in 1986. ABEPF produced training guides for part of the package and trained 391 health workers from 89 organizations throughout the country on how to use the materials. These health workers, in turn, used the training guides to teach their co-workers about the materials (JHU/PCS, 1988).

While print materials are not usually the most effective part of a health promotion campaign, their distribution is the easiest for an ad hoc or outside evaluation team to monitor—and criticize. Outside evaluation teams usually cannot listen to local radio shows, and rarely do they interview a representative sample of the audience. But they can easily look into clinic cupboards and see what print materials are available. Thus almost every communication evaluation in every country comments on insufficient distribution of supporting print materials to clinics and other health facilities. For this reason alone, an astute communication director should make a special effort to be sure that print materials are delivered in ample quantity to all health facilities. This may require designating a specific individual to arrange and report regularly on distribution of print materials. With respect to radio and television, program schedules and costs must be negotiated and agreed upon before the campaign launch. The dissemination of broadcast materials poses its own unique challenges. Project managers need to draw up a media plan, specifying broadcast schedules for each station. This may require a lot of groundwork. For example, in 1992, when the Planned Parenthood Federation of Nigeria (PPFN) broadcast a series of public service announcements encouraging couples to visit family planning clinics, the federation selected and negotiated contracts with 17 radio and 18 television stations throughout the country for more than 8,000 broadcasts. Negotiating teams, consisting of project managers and local PPFN staff, arranged the placements, at the same time negotiating discounts of up to 35 percent including agency, volume, block-booking, and prompt-payment discounts (PPFN, 1992).

LESSON 7.

A campaign launch is an opportunity for maximum public, press, and political attention.

The launch of a campaign is a critical moment. After months of behind-the-scenes preparation, this is the first time a program reaches the public. At this point, the program launch can be a news event with a better chance than ever again for major media coverage. As one advertising slogan goes, you never get a second chance to make a first impression. A good launch can generate momentum for the whole campaign.

Preparation for launch entails myriad decisions both small and large, from the colors of ushers' uniforms to which dignitaries and celebrities to invite and how to be sure that they attend. Project managers orchestrating a launch must draw up a set of objectives for the launch itself, a timetable, a detailed checklist of what needs to be done, and a clear statement of who is responsible for what.

The 1993 *Haki Yako* (It's Your Right) campaign in Kenya, which used a variety of print and broadcast media, provides a good illustration. Nine weeks of intense preparation, carefully laid out in a separate workplan, preceded the launch. A meeting was held to inform all family planning organizations about the launch and to enlist their support. Radio and television spots, newspaper ads, flyers, and public address system announcements were arranged to herald the upcoming launch and invite the public to attend. Bumper stickers, T-shirts, visors, and flags were designed and produced for distribution during the launch ceremonies. A press conference was held. Activities for the day of the actual launch were all carefully arranged—a parade, speeches by dignitaries, display stands for family planning organizations, a mobile family planning clinic, a full day of entertainment by musical groups, comedians, acrobats, poets, and drama troupes, and more (Kim, Lettenmaier, et al., 1996).

To heighten the initial impact, large-scale projects may sponsor regional- or district-level launch events as well as a national ceremony. This gives managers an opportunity to involve influential local politicians and opinion leaders. Local ceremonies also carry the excitement of the launch to other areas. In Kenya, *Haki Yako* managers conducted a workshop to help regional managers develop local launch activities. District launch ceremonies in Kakamega, Mombasa, and Nyeri, featuring speeches by regional leaders and local entertainment, took place at the same time as the national launch of the campaign in Nairobi (Kim, Lettenmaier, et al., 1996).

Cultivating the interest of the news media requires special attention and creativity (Robey & Stauffer, 1995). Part of good preparation is having the right people present at the launch. When celebrities and political leaders are involved in the launch, members of the press are likely to be there, too. The combination can generate far-reaching, long-lasting momentum. In Pakistan, the launch of the film *Aahat* was a major social event, with sports heroes, movie stars, and government leaders vying for invitations to the gala affair. Helping everybody celebrate the occasion and giving awards was Imran Khan, national hero and captain of the world-champion cricket team. World-famous Pakistani musician Nusrat Fateh Ali gave a concert. In Mali, plays and songs that had won awards at a recent festival drew public and news media attention to the launch of the family planning logo (JHU/PCS, 1993d). In Indonesia, a helicopter deposited a truck carrying Blue Circle signboards in the middle of a Jakarta stadium while journalists, photographers, and thousands of other guests looked on (Saffitz & Rimon, 1992). In Nepal, the launch of a radio soap opera and distance-learning program included a live performance by the actors and a speech by the U.S. ambassador. The launch received front-page press coverage. (See Box 6.3.)

LESSON 8.

Compensation or appropriate recognition for the people who work on a communication program improves morale and performance.

In all development programs, there is a tendency to pay for the services of professionals who work at the highest levels while expecting community-level workers to serve as volunteers. Communication programs and campaigns depend heavily on the time and commitment of community leaders and activists. While advertising agencies, production houses, the media, and, of course, most medical personnel expect compensation, grassroots workers often receive only token wages, small commissions, or nothing. Thus it is especially important that the contributions of grassroots workers and volunteers be recognized in some way.

Compensation can take many forms. The International Planned Parenthood Federation, whose member associations depend on high-level volunteers for many advocacy, public relations, and program responsibilities, recognizes this service through honorary positions, titles, and travel to international meetings. For mid- and lower-level professionals, the best form of recognition is often training opportunities—workshops, observation tours to other sites, or even international training or study tours. Such activities, which can include attendance at the Johns Hopkins–sponsored series of national and regional workshops Advances in Family Health Communication, the Centre for African Family Studies workshops in Nairobi, or travel as observer-participants to the Indonesian International Training Program, not only reward good performance but also provide stimulus and newideas for even better performance in the future. Participants must be chosen according to fair and objective criteria so that those who deserve recognition and will stay on the job are rewarded.

Box 6.3

Campaign Launch—Getting Off to a Good Start

Getting a communication campaign off to a good start is crucial. An impressive ceremony to launch a campaign attracts attention from the press, the public, and political leaders. A good launch ceremony requires advance publicity, dignitaries and celebrities on hand, well-organized press coverage, pageantry emphasizing the symbols or logo of the campaign, detailed planning and coordination to make sure everything goes as planned—and the flexibility to respond creatively if it does not.

At the 1996 launch of the Green Umbrella logo in Bangladesh, nearly 3,000 family planning field workers paraded in the streets of Dhaka carrying their own green umbrellas, emblems of their key role as providers of protective family health services.

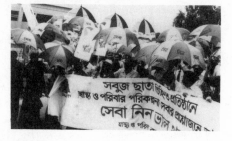

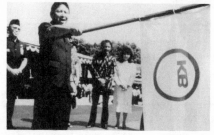

The 1989 launch of Indonesia's Blue Circle campaign in Jakarta emphasized ceremony, with government officials attending, flags flying, and a typical couple, representing satisfied users, among the guests of honor.

A traditional dance troupe, wearing campaign T-shirts, entertained the crowd at opening ceremonies for Kenya's *Haki Yako* (It's Your Right) campaign in 1993.

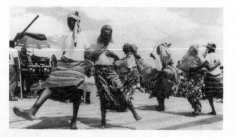

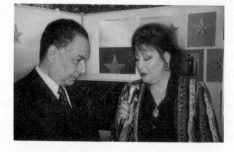

Egypt's Minister of Health and Population being interviewed after addressing the 1996 ceremonies launching the Gold Star Quality Improvement Program, a major initiative to improve and to publicize the quality of services in family planning clinics.

At the community level, support for campaigns and community programs can be rewarded by higher status in the village, recognized through seating on a dais with honored guests, attendance at district-level trainings, and travel to the capital city, for example. Sometimes bicycles, special supply kits, or commodities that can be sold for a small profit are also given to community workers in recognition for their work. In Ghana, nurses who had been trained and participated in the "I Care" campaign were given diplomas and special badges that said, "I Care" at a public ceremony pledging high-quality services (Ghana MOH/HEU & JHU/PCS, 1992).

At all levels, contributing organizations, materials, and individuals can be given full public credit for their work—orally, in print, and in video or audio credits. Outstanding performers can be nominated for national and international awards, such as the Media Awards presented annually by the Population Institute or the annual United Nations Population Fund Awards to individuals and organizations.

MONITORING

LESSON 9.

Regular and accurate monitoring helps ensure that outputs are produced and distributed as planned.

Both monitoring and impact evaluation are essential to any communication project, but they serve different functions and operate in different ways. *Monitoring* is part of project implementation. It focuses on outputs—processes and products. It tells project managers whether activities are taking place as planned or whether there are significant deviations. Were print materials prepared and distributed to the appropriate destinations? Were billboards put up in the designated locations? Were radio and television announcements or dramas aired at the appropriate times and places? Did community events take place, with widespread participation? And, important but often neglected, were suppliers and subcontractors paid promptly so that they will continue to work for the program? In short, project monitoring measures the nuts and bolts of project activities as they take place to determine whether they are being carried out as specified in the workplan.

Impact evaluation, also referred to as "evaluation" or "assessment," determines whether the original project objectives were met—that is, whether the intended audience changed its knowledge, attitudes, or behavior. Impact evaluation usually is completed after implementation is finished, but, where feasible, some rapid impact evaluation can be undertaken while the program is under way (see Chapter 7).

Monitoring project outputs should be simple and routine, so that project managers will know immediately if activities are not carried out properly. Typical monitoring techniques include verification of print runs, review of delivery invoices for print material, site visits to delivery points, checks of warehouse inventories, monitoring of radio and television broadcasts, and regular reporting on community activities. These tasks should be assigned to project staff before campaign launch. Since project managers must react immediately if a particular job is not being done, monitoring reports should be submitted regularly and often—that is, monthly, weekly, or sometimes even daily.

Monitoring techniques need to be appropriate to the media involved. For example, radio and television broadcasts must be carefully followed to check whether public service announcements and especially paid advertisements are aired on schedule and that broadcast quality is acceptable. The Planned Parenthood Federation of Nigeria initially used volunteers to monitor public service announcements daily. There was little incentive, however, for them to complete a task they perceived as very demanding (PPFN, 1992). As a result, paid staff at the state level were assigned the task. They proved to be more effective monitors. Carrying out this function also gave them a sense of ownership in the nationally organized project and increased their sense of responsibility for promoting the local services. Once monthly broadcast monitoring reports were compiled from daily logs, project managers could immediately ask radio and TV stations to make up for any broadcasts that had been missed. At the same time, some stations ran announcements more frequently than they agreed to, and they could be specially recognized. The very knowledge that broadcasts and spots are being closely monitored may motivate station managers to follow the agreed-upon schedules and thus may prevent omissions (JHU/PCS, 1994c).

Similarly, in monitoring radio spots to promote community-based workers in Honduras, the workers themselves proved the most effective monitors because they lived in the same area as the intended audience and had direct and personal interest in the success of the campaign. As in Nigeria, asking the local providers and other staff in Honduras to monitor broadcast spots gave them a bigger stake in the promotion and helped ensure accuracy in monitoring (Payne Merritt, personal communication, April 1, 1996).

Monitoring the distribution of print materials may call for other approaches. At the Family Planning Association of Kenya, staff members regularly check to see whether print materials arrive as scheduled. They found that clinic-based providers were far more likely than community-based workers to have received the print materials. They also found that clinics run by nongovernmental organizations were receiving materials more consistently than the Ministry of Health clinics. As a result, the distribution system was strengthened to give higher priority to Ministry of Health clinics and community-based workers. In Indonesia, Blue Circle supervisors visited service providers' offices regularly to see whether project materials had been delivered and were correctly displayed inside and outside the offices (Saffitz & Rimon, 1992).

Community mobilization campaigns also need close monitoring to be sure local events take place as planned. In Brazil, for example, the monitoring system built into the AIDS-prevention project for street children in the city of Belo Horizonte collected data on the number of outreach sessions held, attendance at the sessions, topics covered, and the materials distributed. With this information the project managers could be sure that enough sessions were held in each area, could track attendance and the number of materials distributed, and could provide complementary data for impact evaluation. During the first three months of campaign implementation, monitoring showed that over 600 youth had participated in 55 sessions and that over 68 percent of the youth had attended several outreach sessions and other community activities (Payne Merritt & Raffaelli, 1993). In the first Zimbabwe male motivation campaign, managers needed to know if and when the scheduled motivational talks took place. Speakers were required to fill out a form listing the date, location, and time of each talk, as well as the topics covered and how many people attended. In-depth interviews were also conducted with community leaders and participants to evaluate the effect of the talks (Kuseka & Silberman, 1990). In the Minya Initiative in Egypt, staff used an observation checklist to monitor a sample of the activities held during each Health Week. With this checklist, staff confirmed which activities were carried out and recorded how many people attended (Jabre et al., 1993).

LESSON 10.

Rapid feedback allows managers to fine-tune program operations and improves the organizational climate.

Although the objectives of any communication project are to influence family planning knowledge, attitudes, and behavior over the long run, the immediate reactions of the audience should also be tracked continually to provide as much feedback as quickly as possible. Monitoring audience impact is more difficult than monitoring program outputs, but it should be attempted wherever possible. In the Minya Initiative, for example, project managers established a media-event tracking system to try to relate increases in client attendance to various meetings (Jabre et al., 1993; Kemprecos et al., 1994).

Feedback about radio and television materials can sometimes combine monitoring of the broadcasts with assessment of the impact on intended audiences and can even generate suggestions for future activities. In Kenya, for example, radio programs and print materials produced by the Provider and Client Project invited listeners and readers to write in for more information. More than 3,000 letters poured in over nine months, providing information about the relative reach and impact of different media. Project staff analyzed the letters by district, the gender of senders, the nature of the information requested, and the programs and articles that prompted the request. As a result, the ongoing radio programs could include the kind of information listeners asked for. In The Gambia and Tanzania, project staff members led regular discussions of radio soap operas with groups of listeners and then passed their suggestions on to scriptwriters for inclusion in later episodes (Jato, personal communication, November 11, 1996). Likewise, in Uganda managers used feedback from the men and women monitoring a weekly radio drama series to help direct the course of future episodes. Listeners made note of their reactions after each episode and then met monthly to discuss their observations. The producers responded to these comments by building future episodes around a popular character who was drawing a strong following, by toning down characters perceived to laugh too much or to be too boastful, by simplifying the language used by the nurse, and by paying more attention to continuity between episodes. Regular monitoring also found that one episode incorrectly suggested that men could use injectable contraceptives for family planning. The error was corrected in a subsequent program. Thereafter the Family Planning Association of Uganda (FPAU) became more vigilant about reviewing scripts before recording episodes (JHU/PCS, 1994d).

LESSON 11.

Too much information can clog a monitoring system.

The basic purpose of monitoring is to permit rapid changes if they are needed to make the program more effective. Thus, busy project managers need feedback quickly so that they can react while there is still time to make improvements. Excessive information can slow down analysis and obscure conclusions. Ideally, local project staff should collect only as much information as they can analyze and apply immediately.

An overambitious sentinel site system designed to monitor the "I Care" campaign in Ghana illustrates the pitfalls of collecting too much information. The initial plan was to collect data from household interviews and focus-group discussions conducted every three months at 25 sentinel sites and to analyze the data at the University of Ghana in Accra. Since it took months and sometimes years for busy researchers in Accra to analyze even a portion of these data, the results did not reach the local project managers in time. A project review recommended that future monitoring systems be far simpler and that on-site data collectors and regional managers be trained to analyze and interpret their own essential data promptly (Ghana MOH/HEU & JHU/PCS, 1992).

Similar problems occurred in Peru, where a total of eight waves of surveys were conducted to evaluate reproductive health campaigns. When the data proved too extensive and complex for rapid analysis, the survey was streamlined between rounds five and six and a new firm was contracted for on a competitive basis. Thereafter results were available faster, and the impact of the campaign became clear (Valente, Saba, et al., 1996; Valente, personal communication, November 21, 1996a).

LESSON 12.

When monitoring reveals unexpected problems or opportunities, a flexible and rapid response is necessary.

Good managers are quick to recognize and take advantage of any unexpected opportunities that show up during project monitoring. In Egypt, for example, managers of the Minya Initiative discovered that after motivational meetings people did not want to set up a clinic appointment for a later date. They wanted information and supplies right away. As a result, two of the implementing organizations—the Ministry of Health and Population and the Ministry of Information/State Information Service—began conducting joint meetings in rural areas with a physician present to provide services at the end of the talk (JHU/PCS, 1993e).

A similar approach was applied in Peru, where family planning counselors doubling as field monitors attended close to 200 performances of the street theater drama *Ms. Rumors*. The counselors from Advocacy for Population Programs (APROPO), the family planning association in charge of the presentations, were on hand to answer any questions sparked by the drama's family planning themes. In total, counselors conducted face-to-face sessions with approximately 4,500 audience members. At the same time, they monitored the quality of performances and recorded the number of people in attendance. It is estimated that in 1994 and 1995 over 61,000 people saw the dramas. *Ms. Rumors* was also performed outside clinics and hospitals to entertain and educate people waiting for services (Valente, Poppe, et al., 1995). In each case, bringing services directly to the people proved more effective than trying to persuade the people to go to the services.

Also in Peru, monitoring the *Las (Los) Tromes* television spots provided feedback that permitted immediate improvement. Many viewers found 30-second public service announcements too short and too general to convey specific information or to increase knowledge. As a result, longer spots were developed with dramatic stories and appealing characters (Poppe, personal communication, November 14, 1996).

Monitoring community and clinic projects in the Philippines and Ghana revealed that clients were not reacting positively to newly trained motivators and service providers. Philippine women were not comfortable talking to the male farmer-motivators who had been trained in insurance sales techniques. As a result, the project was quickly revised so that couples rather than men alone talked to other farm couples (JHU/PCS, 1990e). In Ghana, early monitoring of the extensive provider training in the "I Care" program showed that clinic-based health care providers were not treating young people sympathetically. As a result, the training curriculum was quickly modified to emphasize a nonjudgmental approach to young clients who wanted family planning (Huntington, Lettenmaier, & Obeng-Quaidoo, 1990).

Chapter 7

Impact Evaluation

CHOICE OF EVALUATION METHODOLOGY

Lesson 1.   Various research designs are suitable for evaluating the impact of health communication programs.

Lesson 2.   The randomized control group design has limited value for communication program evaluation because it is usually not feasible and because by itself it does not provide information about the underlying processes of change.

Lesson 3.   Because most communication programs now use mass media to try to reach the entire population, the most rigorous design available is the one-group, before-after longitudinal design with multivariate statistical controls.

Lesson 4.   An interrupted time-series analysis of service statistics provides additional evidence of communication impact, especially when one of the objectives of the program is to promote service providers.

Lesson 5.   Evaluations can benefit from asking audience members for their own opinions about the impact of communication.

THEORY-DRIVEN EVALUATION

Lesson 6.   Evaluations that include subobjectives based on theoretical models such as the Steps to Behavior Change provide evidence of impact on behavior and useful feedback to improve future programs.

Lesson 7.   A thorough evaluation of the impact of communication includes an analysis of its indirect effects as well as its direct effects on health behavior.

Lesson 8.   Exposure to communication and the steps to behavior change have cumulative effects on behavior much like cumulative risk and dose response in epidemiologic research.

Lesson 9.   Aggregating survey data by local units of analysis such as villages or sample clusters reveals the impact of communication on local culture in addition to its impact on individuals.

Lesson 10.   Path analysis can depict and test the direction and strength of all the relationships measured in a communication program evaluation.

EVALUATING CLIENT-PROVIDER COMMUNICATION

Lesson 11.   Because of the interactive nature of interpersonal communication and counseling, innovative research methods are needed for effective evaluation.

COLLABORATION AND DISSEMINATION OF FINDINGS

Lesson 12.   Collaborating with other organizations for program evaluation can provide substantial benefits.

Lesson 13.   Evaluation results can be presented at various levels of complexity to suit different audiences.

Evaluation is the systematic application of scientific procedures to assess the conceptualization, design, implementation, impact, and cost-effectiveness of social interventions (Bertrand & Kincaid, 1996). The purpose of evaluation is to measure the process and the impact of a program against the objectives established in the strategic design in order to contribute to decision-making. *Measurement* requires methods for collecting information and assessing the changes specified in the program objectives. *Process* refers to what takes place as the program is implemented. *Impact* refers to program outcomes. *Decision-making* means applying the findings of an evaluation to improve ongoing or future programs.

Evaluation is easy to ignore until a project nears the end but impossible to carry out effectively unless it is planned from the start. Parallel with the P Process itself, evaluation in fact begins along with the preliminary analysis that provides background information and baseline data. It takes further shape in the strategic design phase, where specific, measurable (SMART) objectives and supporting subobjectives are established. Evaluation issues also arise in the pretest, development, and implementation stages, where evaluators determine whether the process described in the design document is actually taking place and whether the outputs are understood by the audience. Eventually, at the close of the program or at some milestone in an ongoing program, evaluation assesses impact on the intended audience or the entire population, measuring and analyzing changes specified by the original objective. This chapter focuses on that impact evaluation. Ultimately, evaluation findings, disseminated both within a program and externally, provide the basis for decision-making to correct deficiencies, build on program successes, and plan for continuity (see Chapter 8). The entire evaluation process is illustrated in the Communication Design and Evaluation System (CODES) diagram (see Figure 7.1).

Figure 7.1
Communication Design and Evaluation System (CODES)

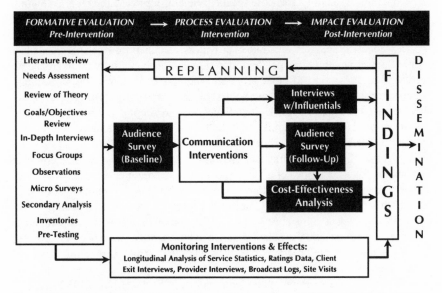

Note: CODES has evolved out of the Media Impact Research System (MIRS) originally developed
    by D. Lawrence Kincaid for JHU/CCP/PCS in 1990.
Source: JHU/CCP/PCS, 1995.

Evaluating any social program is difficult. To make the most convincing case that the program was responsible for the observed outcome, eight criteria are important (Bertrand & Kincaid, 1996; Hill, 1971; Mohr, 1992; Schlesselman, 1982). It is difficult to satisfy all eight criteria in a single study. Fortunately, they are not all required in order to make a valid conclusion about impact. The more that apply, however, the greater the confidence in the conclusion.

- Measurement of a change or difference in the population of interest (variation in outcome).
- Correlation between exposure to the program and the intended outcome (covariation).
- Evidence that exposure to the program occurred *before* the observed change in the outcome (time-order).
- Control of the effects of confounding variables that might also influence the outcome (spuriousness).
- Observation of an abrupt, large impact in the absence of other major influences (magnitude).
- A direct and close causal connection specified by theory between a program and its outcome (proximity).
- Impact that increases in proportion to the level or duration of communication exposure (dose response).
- Consistency with the evidence from previous communication program evaluations (replication with variation.)

Communication programs pose special problems for evaluators. It is a daunting task to demonstrate that communication programs themselves make a difference to health behavior—both apart from other program functions, such as availability of services, adequate supplies, and trained providers, and apart from secular trends that may influence health behavior. First, communication is not only an independent function but also a part of other program functions from counseling to training. Second, most communication has both short-term and long-term effects. Many short-term campaigns in the United States—for example, promoting smoking cessation or use of automobile seat belts—have been evaluated as failures (McGuire, 1986), and yet over the last decade smoking has declined and seat belt use has grown. In fact, both practices are now social norms. People often consider information for a long time before they take action, making impact evaluations over a short time span invalid predictors of the long term. Third, communication may have both intended and unintended effects. Since program communication never takes place in a vacuum but always in a context, and often in competition with other messages, communication evaluation may need to identify unintended effects, not just those anticipated in program objectives, and also to track competing messages or activities in order to assess the net impact of the program.

The experience of Population Communication Services since 1982 suggests that the eight basic criteria can be most easily met and the special problems of communication evaluation resolved when the programs under evaluation are intensive, multimedia programs that take place over relatively short time periods, albeit repeatedly. The reason is that, when communication suddenly increases from a very low to a very high level and then is suddenly eliminated, while very few, if any, changes occur in the other family planning program components, it is easier to attribute the outcome to the communication component. The converse is also true: When a communication program consists of a very diffuse set of activities conducted over a long period of time (more than one year), its impact is difficult to separate from that of other programs or social influences. Therefore long-term multimedia programs are presumably likely to have broad, cumulative impact that will require an extra effort to detect. The impact of intensive short-term campaigns will be easier to detect, but similar campaigns will have to be repeated periodically to have lasting effects.

Population Communication Services tried initially to evaluate specific print materials or selected community meetings and to differentiate between the impacts of one product or channel and another, but these efforts have gradually been abandoned in favor of comprehensive evaluation of major communication programs that will be repeated over several years. Although some pilot projects on interpersonal communication within the family or training in client counseling are still being evaluated separately, major evaluation resources now go to large-scale, continuing programs. Within these larger evaluations, it is often possible to compare the differential impacts of specific activities in a fairly simple and inexpensive way.

A useful rule of thumb is that an evaluation should cost about 10 percent of the total cost of the program being evaluated. There is little to be gained by spending any more than this on evaluation, since the resources would be better spent to expand the program and increase its (measurable) impact. This rule has an implication for small projects: If the project is very small—for example, US$50,000—evaluation is not worthwhile because 10 percent ($5,000) is not enough to pay for an adequate evaluation; at the same time, the program probably is not strong enough to have a measurable impact. Important exceptions to the 10 percent rule are new programs or pilot projects for which very little previous research has been done. In such cases a disproportionately large expenditure on research may be warranted, since the results may have long-term implications. Evaluation of client-provider interaction and counseling is an example of this (see Lesson 11).

Thus the lessons learned from 15 years of PCS program evaluation come primarily from major evaluations of several large country programs. The Bangladesh experience has been especially instructive because it covers a span of almost 10 years and includes innovations in communication linked directly to service delivery. It is less directly linked to mass media than other projects. Evaluations in Kenya, the Philippines, Tanzania, and Uganda show primarily how multimedia campaigns can be evaluated. In each case, the purpose of the evaluation was not only to determine whether the program achieved its preestablished objectives but also to learn what worked and what did not work within the program so that future activities could be improved.

Lessons about evaluation can be grouped under several summary lessons:

- **Choice of evaluation methodology.** No one evaluation design is ideal for all programs. The choice of design depends on the nature of the program, its objectives, and the data that can be collected. The most revealing evaluations combine multiple designs and measurements to address different issues and reinforce one another.
- **Theory-driven design.** Evaluation design that is theory-based and uses the same theory of behavior change that underlies the program itself can produce findings with powerful practical applications for improving future programs.
- **Collaboration and dissemination of findings.** Collaborating with other organizations saves time and money, introduces new ideas, and facilitates sharing information. The results of evaluation must be disseminated to important people at different decision-making levels, but they must be presented in ways appropriate to people's needs and knowledge at each level.

CHOICE OF EVALUATION METHODOLOGY

LESSON 1.

Various research designs are suitable for evaluating the impact of health communication programs.

Several major types of research design have been used by Population Communication Services to evaluate program impacts. They have been applied in evaluating mass media campaigns, community-based projects, counseling, and counseling training. They have been used primarily with individuals as the units for analysis but in a few cases with various geographic units or with groups. While every design has limitations, these designs, when adapted and applied in appropriate situations, can evaluate the impact of communication programs on behavior:

- **Randomized control group design**, sometimes called the "classical" experimental design, randomly assigns individuals, groups, or geographical areas either to an experimental treatment or to a control group. Random assignment helps to ensure that the two groups are equivalent. The differences that appear over time between the treatment group and the control group are then the measure of program impact. This design can be applied most readily in evaluating the training and performance of service providers, where a large number of providers, clinics, or clients can be assigned randomly to a treatment or control group.
- **Nonequivalent control group design** is similar to classic experimental design except that, instead of random assignment, the groups are matched as closely as possible on characteristics thought to affect the outcome.
- **One-group, before-after design with sample surveys** of the population of interest is appropriate to evaluate a communication program implemented for an entire population. A representative sample of that population is surveyed before and after the program. Differences between "before" and "after" findings measure how much change

occurred during the interval and whether people who were exposed to the program changed more than those who were not exposed. The survey data can be used to control statistically for the influence of confounding variables. This is the design most often used by PCS for mass media or large-scale, full-coverage interventions. For example, it was used to evaluate both of the Zimbabwe male motivation campaigns (Piotrow, Kincaid, et al., 1992; Y. M. Kim, Marangwanda & Kols, 1996) and the Bolivian Reproductive Health Campaign (Valente, Saba, et al., 1996), as well as Turkish, Philippine, Kenyan, and Ugandan campaigns and many others.

One-group, before-after designs can use one of at least three different types of surveys: (1) independent surveys, using a different random sample of respondents for each round of data collection, which is the most common approach; (2) longitudinal (panel) surveys, using the same random sample of respondents repeatedly for each round; and (3) another type of longitudinal survey using the same random sample of clusters, but interviewing a different random sample of individuals in each cluster at each round. Longitudinal surveys can show which came first—interest in and use of contraceptives or exposure to the communication program being evaluated. Assessment of the time-order relationship can either strengthen or undermine the inference that exposure to the program caused the intended change. Panel surveys have been used in PCS evaluations in the Philippines, Bangladesh, and Peru. A panel survey was also carried out by Westoff and Bankole to evaluate the impact of mass media family planning efforts in Nigeria (Westoff & Bankole, 1996).

- **Interrupted time-series design** measures behavior at many intervals over an extended period of time, usually with sales or service statistics. This design is useful in evaluating health communication programs, such as the mass media vasectomy campaigns in Brazil (Kincaid, Payne Merritt, et al., 1996), for two reasons: first, communication activities, unlike services, can be started and stopped at distinct intervals that can be compared with the time-series data; second, family planning and most health services already maintain service statistics. When unusually high demand for services coincides with the communication activities, as was the case in Brazil, the evidence for a causal link between the two is strengthened (see Lesson 4, below). Service statistics can, of course, also be used to evaluate other forms of communication such as counseling, interpersonal communication training, and community events, as was done in Nigeria (Piotrow, Rimon, et al., 1990). When providers are trained to ask clients directly what prompted them to come for services, these source-of-referral data can strengthen the conclusions drawn from the analysis of service statistics.

In theory each of these designs is distinct, but in practice evaluations sometimes can combine more than one methodology or measurement. The Bangladesh evaluation, discussed in Lessons 2 and 6 through 10, includes elements of a randomized control group design and one-group, before-after design with longitudinal sample surveys. Kenya evaluations involved one-group, before-after surveys and an interrupted time-series design using service statistics. The more that different designs and measurements can be used, the greater the confidence that the observed outcome can be attributed to the communication program.

LESSON 2.

The randomized control group design has limited value for communication program evaluation because it is usually not feasible and because by itself it does not provide information about the underlying processes of change.

Effective evaluation accomplishes both goals of evaluation—measurement of the *process* and the *impact* of communication—in a manner that provides useful information to improve future programs. The classical experimental design can yield the most definite conclusion about the impact of a program, but unless it is supplemented by other methods, it provides no information about the underlying causal processes that lead to that impact (Campbell & Stanley, 1963; Cook & Campbell, 1979; Rossi & Freeman, 1989; Mohr, 1992; Bertrand & Kincaid, 1996). Theory plays an indispensable role in evaluation because it is used to identify the expected causal processes, to suggest ways to measure those processes, and to incorporate them into program design. This is why program evaluation is now described as either method-driven or theory-driven (Chen & Rossi, 1987; Chen, 1990). To accomplish both goals of evaluation, evaluation research needs to be driven by rigorous methods *and* by valid theories.

To understand this important lesson requires a clear understanding of the strengths and weaknesses of the classical experimental design. It was developed for use in agricultural research stations in the early part of the century, in a situation where theory was weak or nonexistent, and then adopted by psychologists, social scientists, and program evaluators for the same reasons (R. A. Fisher, 1956; Gigerenzer et al., 1989).

The three main weaknesses of the classic randomized control group design when it is applied to field experiments are not usually given enough emphasis in the textbooks.

1. The level of control implied by the logic of the design is rarely achieved in field settings.

In field settings the experimental treatment (in this case the program) may actually change over time and from place to place as it is being implemented. The longer the experiment lasts, the more likely these changes will occur. Ironically, flexibility in public health programs is both necessary and beneficial from the point of view of developing an effective program, but it negates the experimental design's assumption of a "uniform treatment" and interferes with the goal of assessing impact. This natural variation in treatment that occurs in field settings makes it difficult to say *what* the treatment was that led to the observed impact.

2. It is weak in external validity—the generalization of its results to future implementations on a full-scale basis.

A partial-coverage program tested under relatively controlled conditions will usually not be the same as the one that is later implemented full-scale. Nor should it be. The program should be improved first. Many policy-makers are aware of this lesson, and they say, "Don't give us another pilot experimental project. It takes too long, costs too much, and, when you're done, you still don't know how it will work on a full scale." Less well understood is that, if a program is comprised of several diverse components, then, technically speaking, separate experiments or experimental treatment groups would have to be organized to test each one. This level of experimentation takes too much time and money for most social programs, such as those in public health.

3. Unless supplemented with other methods, the experimental design provides no information about the processes of change that are necessary to improve the program.

The classic experimental design provides a macro-level indication of impact without specifying what happens at the micro level inside the experimental group. To illustrate this strength and weakness, a field experiment from Bangladesh is described below. Lessons 6 through 10 describe supplemental methods that can be used to measure and test the underlying, micro-level processes in program evaluation.

Evaluation researchers must select a research design that satisfies as many of the eight criteria for a causal attribution (described above) as possible given the nature of the program. As noted, one of the key issues that the research design addresses is whether or not the outcome would have happened anyway without the program. The *strength* of the classic experimental design is that it readily satisfies this criterion. It includes a control group that does not receive the program. Each unit of interest (individual, village, school, etc.) is randomly assigned to either a control group or a treatment group. The assignment by means of a random process ensures that the two groups will be statistically equivalent before the program is implemented. If the outcome in the group that received the communication program is significantly different from the outcome in the one that did not receive it, then the difference can be attributed to the program, since all other influences should be the same for both groups.

This type of experimental design was used to evaluate the newly developed *jiggasha* approach to family planning/health promotion in Bangladesh (Kincaid, Das Gupta, et al., 1993). *Jiggasha*, a Bangladeshi term meaning "to inquire," was the name given to an innovative interpersonal communication intervention developed to improve the effectiveness of the government family welfare assistants (FWAs), who for over 15 years have been visiting village women in their homes in Bangladesh (see Box 3.2, in Chapter 3).

In the experiment 24 villages in Trishal thana[1] were rank ordered in terms of contraceptive prevalence (any method), and after a random starting point in the list every other village was assigned to the treatment group and the remaining ones were assigned to the control group. The 12 villages in the treatment group received the new *jiggasha* approach to family planning communication. Individual women or households were not assigned to experimental groups because the smallest unit in which the program could be conducted was a village.

Even when whole villages are assigned to groups, there is still a possibility of "contamination" between the experimental and control villages. Field workers or individuals from the experimental treatment villages may inadvertently tell those living in the control villages what they are doing or what they have learned. The other villages may even try to emulate the intervention on their own. In many evaluation situations it is so difficult to find units that are appropriate or numerous enough for random assignment to groups that the comparative experimental design cannot be used.

In the *jiggasha* experiment the villages were far enough apart that contamination did not become a problem. There were no policy or ethical constraints, either. Women in the control villages were not prevented from receiving health information and services. The *jiggasha* approach was designed to *improve* the work of the existing family planning field workers, so the 12 villages assigned to the control group continued to receive their normal services during the experiment. The experimental test, then, was whether or not the new approach would have any *added* advantage over the regular government program. Until this could be demonstrated, there would be no reason to expand the approach to other villages.

Table 7.1 shows the outcome of the program in terms of increasing modern contraceptive use, the primary objective of the project. In the 12 *jiggasha* villages the mean rate of modern method use increased from 1989 to 1992 by 11.4 percentage points, from 13.5 percent to 24.9 percent, while the mean rate of modern contraceptive use in the control villages rose by only 5.3 percentage points, from 24.8 percent to 30.1 percent. The increase in the villages with the *jiggasha* approach was more than twice as great as in the control villages. The intervention succeeded in helping these villages "catch up" to the level of the control villages in terms of modern contraceptive use.

Table 7.1
Mean Percentage of Married Women Using Modern Contraceptives, by Village Intervention Status: Trishal, Bangladesh, 1989 and 1992

Village Intervention Status	1989	1992	Change*
Jiggasha *villages (N=12)*	13.5	24.9	11.4
Control villages (N=12)	24.8	30.1	5.3

Note: A panel of 1,372 married women interviewed before and after the intervention (repeated measures) aggregated into 24 village units for statistical analysis.
*1992 minus 1989. The difference of 6.1 percentage points between the pre-post changes in *jiggasha* and control villages is statistically significant (t = −2.95 with 22 d.f., p < 0.01).
Source: Kincaid, Das Gupta, et al., 1993.

The substantial initial difference in modern contraceptive use between the *jiggasha* and control villages is an example of what is sometimes called "unhappy" randomization in experimental designs (Mohr, 1992). With a relatively small number of units, in this case just 24, there is greater likelihood that a random assignment will not produce equivalent groups. A close examination revealed that the median levels of contraceptive use of the two groups were very close. When the very high and very low prevalence villages were randomly assigned, however, by chance the mean level of the control group was skewed upward, and the mean level of the *jiggasha* group downward. An examination of the initial levels of any method use (modern and nonmodern) illustrates the problem of having only 24 units. There was no statistically significant difference between the groups in terms of *any* method use, but the difference was still substantial (22.2% v. 33.3%; F = 3.59, p = 0.0715). For the *jiggasha* experiment it was not feasible to conduct the program in more than 12 villages with the available time and personnel.

The experimental design confirmed that the communication program was a success in terms of the primary objective, but this knowledge by itself offered nothing that could be used to improve the program in the future. The experimental design—which answers the success/failure question so well—by itself only provides an "outer shell" for evaluation, within which more precise measures of the processes related to the change must be measured and analyzed in greater depth (Cronbach, 1982). This lesson applies whether the project has been found to be a success or a failure. When the results of an evaluation indicate no significant impact, policy-makers want to know why and how to do it better next time. Even if the impact of an experiment can be successfully demonstrated, when it is implemented under changed conditions on a wider scale, the policy-maker still needs to know what conditions and changes would make it work better the next time (Cronbach, 1982).

The next set of lessons describes alternatives to the classic experimental design that are practical for full-coverage communication programs. Then Lessons 6 through 10 describe methods for incorporating theory and measures of causal process into communication program evaluation.

LESSON 3.

Because most communication programs now use mass media to try to reach the entire population, the most rigorous research design available is the one-group, before-after longitudinal design with multivariate statistical controls.

Today the broadcast mass media can reach almost everyone. When the program is designed to reach as many people as possible, no group can be used as a control. Instead, the only possible comparison is between those who were actually exposed to the communication and those who were not. Follow-up sample surveys of the population can determine who was actually exposed and what happened to them as a result. Because exposure to family planning communication usually ranges from 40 percent to 70 percent, a comparison group is still available in one-group research designs.

Unfortunately, two serious threats arise that make it difficult to estimate the impact of communication in a one-group design where only part of the population is exposed: confounding effects and selectivity bias. *Confounding effects* mean that behavior change may not have actually occurred because of exposure to communication but rather because of the influence of other variables that also happen to determine exposure. Exposed persons more often own or have access to radio and television, for example. They usually are of higher socioeconomic status, have more education, live in cities where electricity is available rather than in villages, are younger, and so forth. Because these variables are often related to use of family planning, which is the outcome variable, any statistical finding that shows a relationship between exposure and family planning is confounded by these other differences. In other words, family planning practice and communication exposure may both be due to higher socioeconomic status or education.

Selectivity bias arises because those who are exposed to family planning messages may already practice family planning or may be predisposed to practice, so they are already more motivated to attend to and to recall family planning messages than those who are not exposed to the messages or who paid no attention because they were not interested in family planning. If so, prior family planning attitudes and behavior may influence exposure to communication rather than the other way around. The time-order criterion may be violated.

Both confounding effects and selectivity biases can be taken into account by the type of survey design and analysis that is used. If a randomized control group design is not feasible, then the best way to deal with confounding variables is to control or adjust for them later by means of multivariate statistical analysis, such as multiple linear regression or multiple logistic regression. An evaluation of the Uganda National Interpersonal Communication and Counseling Program illustrates this type of analysis (Kiragu, Galiwango, et al., 1996). A representative follow-up survey of 1,323 men and women ages 20–40 was conducted in the urban and peri-urban areas of four districts that were designated as the intended area for the family planning communication program. Six distinct communication media were used: a radio drama, posters, pamphlets, newspapers, a special yellow flower logo, and a yellow flower advertisement. A dose response (see Lesson 8) was found for exposure to the six communication media: The level of modern contraceptive use among men and women exposed to none or only one medium was 10.9 percent. This increased to 25.9 percent for those exposed to two to four media, and to 37.2 percent for those exposed to five or six media (Kiragu, Galiwango, et al., 1996). This relationship was statistically significant, but there was no control for the influence of confounding variables. What if both use and exposure are simply a result of living in the urban areas as opposed to the peri-urban areas or of being able to afford to own a radio and television?

A multiple logistic regression analysis was conducted to control (or adjust) for the effects of eight potential confounding variables: urban residence, district, education, age, television or car ownership, radio ownership, number of children, and family planning attitude. The results confirmed that a dose response to the six media was still statistically significant *after* controlling for the effects of the other eight variables. Women exposed to two to four media were 2.4 times more likely to use modern contraceptives than women exposed to one or none (the reference group). (See Table 7.2.) Women exposed to five or six media were 4.2 times more likely to use modern contraceptives than those in the reference group.

This type of multivariate regression analysis is the most rigorous kind of statistical analysis that can be done with survey data. It can eliminate the possibility of confounding variables, but only for variables that are measured in the survey and

Table 7.2
Multiple Logistic Regression of Modern Contraceptive Use Among Ugandan Women on Campaign Exposure and Eight Control Variables

Variable	Odds Ratio	95% Confidence Interval
Campaign Exposure		
0–1 materials	1.00	
2–4 materials	2.40	1.24–4.63*
5–6 materials	4.24	1.95–9.22*
Location		
Urban	1.00	
Peri-urban	0.91	0.59–1.39
District		
Kampala	1.00	
Jinja	1.00	0.58–1.72
Mbarara	1.42	0.80–2.51
Masaka	1.52	0.89–2.59
Education Level		
None/primary	1.00	
Secondary	1.74	1.11–2.72*
Beyond secondary	1.65	0.91–3.03
Age		
20–24	1.00	
25–29	1.37	0.85–2.20
30–34	1.56	0.89–2.73
35–40	2.97	1.20–7.41*
Owns TV/Car[a]		
Owns neither	1.00	
Owns one of the two	1.60	1.03–2.47*
Owns both	1.72	0.90–3.30
Owns a Radio		
No	1.00	
Yes	1.11	0.66–1.89
Number of Children		
Less than 3	1.00	
3 or more	1.74	1.09–2.78*
Attitude Toward Family Planning		
Opposed	1.00	
Favorable	1.90	1.22–2.95*

*$p \leq 0.05$. N = 643; unadjusted data.
[a]An indicator of socioeconomic status.
Source: Johns Hopkins University/Center for Communication Programs and
Family Planning Association of Uganda, Uganda Family Planning
Promotion Project (Kiragu, Galiwango, et al., 1996, p. 85).

included in the regression. Other confounding variables not identified may still account for some of the observed relationship between communication exposure and family planning behavior. Knowing that these eight are not confounding variables, however, considerably increases confidence that the campaign did have an impact on modern contraceptive use among Ugandan women.

Regression analysis of follow-up survey data only still suffers from the threat of selectivity bias. Those who already used modern methods may simply have paid more attention to the campaign than those who did not, and therefore they reported higher exposure. The best way to overcome selectivity bias in a full-coverage program is with longitudinal analysis—to collect panel data on the same individuals before and after some have been exposed to the communication program. Then it is possible to control for prior family planning behavior (Moffitt, 1991).

Population Communication Services used a longitudinal survey design to evaluate the 1993 National Communication Campaign in the Philippines. Three waves of data were collected from the same men and women before, during, and after the campaign (Kincaid, Coleman, & Rimon, 1995). This allows for multiple regression analysis to control for the prior status of any outcome variable, including contraceptive use (see Table 7.3). The dependent variable, current contraceptive use, assumed three values—0 for nonuse, 1 for traditional contraceptive use, and 2 for modern contraceptive use—so multinomial logistic regression was used for the statistical analysis. Both traditional and modern contraceptive users were compared with nonusers. The relative risk ratios indicate how much greater the proportion of method use is among those who are high on a predictor variable, such as campaign exposure, compared with those who are low on that variable.

Because the longitudinal design consisted of three waves of panel survey data collected from the same men and women, it was possible to estimate the effect of campaign exposure on contraceptive use at wave 2 and wave 3 while controlling for the influence of contraceptive use at each previous point in time as well as for the effect of other confounding variables.

Before the campaign began (wave 1), the best predictor of traditional method use was a positive attitude toward the rhythm/NFP (natural family planning) method, as indicated by perceptions that the method was healthy, effective, safe, moral, and easy to use. Those with a positive attitude toward rhythm/NFP had a probability of using a traditional method 1.63 times greater than those who had a negative attitude, after the effects of all of the other variables are controlled. The best predictors of modern method use in wave 1 (before the programs) were a positive attitude toward oral pills and a negative attitude toward rhythm/NFP.

Analysis of the survey data at wave 2, after the first phase of the campaign, showed that exposure to communication had a statistically significant impact on both traditional and modern method use. At wave 2, respondents were 1.45 times more likely to use traditional methods and 2.23 times more likely to use modern methods if they had been exposed to the campaign, after all other variables including prior method use are controlled. At wave 3, respondents exposed to the campaign during the second and third phases were 1.57 times more likely to use a traditional method and 1.9 times more likely to use a modern method.

Table 7.3
Multinomial Logistic Regression of Contraceptive Use on Campaign Exposure, Attitudes, and Sociodemographic Characteristics, Philippines, 1994

Variable	Wave 1 (N=1,421) RR Ratio	95% Confidence Interval	Wave 2 (N=1,486) RR Ratio	95% Confidence Interval	Wave 3 (N=1,105) RR Ratio	95% Confidence Interval
		Traditional Method Use				
Campaign exposure	—	—	1.45	1.05–2.01	1.57	1.09–2.25
Pill attitude	NS	—	0.64	0.47–0.86	NS	—
Rhythm attitude	1.63	(1.26–2.11)	2.16	1.61–2.89	1.38	1.00–1.92
Prior modern use	—	—	5.61	3.29–9.58	2.01	1.15–3.51
Prior traditional use	—	—	6.94	5.12–9.41	4.44	3.14–6.29
		Modern Method Use				
Campaign exposure	—	—	2.23	1.44–3.45	1.90	1.22–2.95
Pill attitude	2.15	(1.62–2.86)	1.50	1.03–2.20	2.35	1.30–3.45
Rhythm attitude	0.70	(0.53–0.94)	NS	—	0.62	0.42–0.91
Prior modern use	—	—	86.38	50.1–149.0	25.54	15.25–42.76
Prior traditional use	—	—	2.98	1.86–4.70	2.01	1.28–3.16

RR Ratio = relative risk ratio.
NS = not significant.
Note: All RR ratios are also controlled for age, sex, education, rural-urban residence, and socioeconomic status. All RR ratios shown are statistically significant beyond the .05 level.
Source: Kincaid, Coleman, & Rimon, 1995.

It is clear from this analysis that previous use of either type of method was the best predictor of subsequent method use. In other words, past behavior was the best predictor of future behavior. At wave 3, for example, respondents were 4.44 times more likely to use a traditional method if they already used one at wave 2, but also 2.01 times more likely to use a traditional method if earlier they had used a modern method. This indicated that some Filipinos were switching methods over time. Respondents who used a modern method at wave 1 were 86 times more likely to use one at wave 2, and those who used a modern method at wave 2 were 25.5 times more likely to use a modern method at wave 3. These findings have major implications for program design since they suggest that more attention should be paid to prior users and their reasons for discontinuation.

LESSON 4.

An interrupted time-series analysis of service statistics provides additional evidence of communication impact, especially when one of the objectives of the program is to promote service providers.

Service statistics as an evaluation tool were discredited early in the history of national family planning programs because the data were unreliable. Program statistics on new and continuing family planning clients were often inflated by the pressure of national targets or wishful thinking. Definitions of both new and continuing clients differed. Even more often, records were inconsistently and erratically maintained and not correctly aggregated from different facilities.

Nevertheless, in some cases where model clinics and fee-for-service providers keep service or sales statistics current, an interrupted time-series analysis based on these statistics can be a useful extension of the one-group research design. This design is especially appropriate when one of the objectives of the program is to increase use of family planning services at a defined number of facilities that have reliable statistics. In an interrupted time-series design the same group in effect serves as its own control group at an earlier point in time. Any changes in the direction or rate of change in service use after a communication program— especially abrupt changes—can be attributed to that program if no other known events or influences could have caused a change of the size observed.

Evaluation of the impact of three different communication activities over 12 years in the history of the Pro-Pater vasectomy clinic in São Paulo, Brazil, is an example of how this type of longitudinal analysis can be used to gauge impact (Kincaid, Payne Merrit, et al., 1996) (see Figure 7.2; see also Box 5.1 in Chapter 5). Each of the abrupt and substantial increases in vasectomies performed after the three mass media campaigns was statistically significant.

LESSON 5.

Evaluations can benefit from asking audience members for their own opinions about the impact of communication.

Rigorous design, theory, and analysis are necessary to demonstrate the impact of communication, but the opinions of the audience also are important. Most evaluation researchers discount this type of data because it is based merely on opinion. Opinion can be biased, especially in the case of survey respondents who may know that the purpose of the study is to evaluate the intervention and may want to please the interviewer.

Some of these problems with opinion data can be eliminated or reduced by a careful wording of questions, however. Open-ended questions that do not lead the

Figure 7.2
Effect of Media Events on Number of Vasectomies Performed per Month,
and Poisson Regression, Pro-Pater Clinic, São Paulo, Brazil, 1981–1992

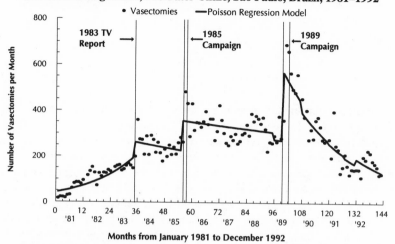

Source: Kincaid, Payne Merritt, et al., 1996.
Reproduced with the permission of The Alan Guttmacher Institute from D. Lawrence Kincaid,
et al. "Impact of a Mass Media Vasectomy Promotion Campaign in Brazil." *International
Family Planning Perspectives.* Volume 22. Number 4. December 1996.

respondent or indicate the desired answer are better than closed or precoded
questions that do. Once exposure to a mass media campaign has been established,
it is better to ask what, if anything, the survey respondent did as a result of hearing
the messages rather than to ask directly, "Did you visit the health clinic as a result
of hearing the message?" Later questions may confirm that the same respondent
visited a clinic during the campaign, but only the respondent is in a position to say
whether she thinks that the campaign was one of the reasons that led her to do so.

The opinion of the participants is worthwhile even if it is somewhat biased. It
is especially valuable as a complement to other types of evidence. On one hand, if
none of the audience members exposed to the program's communication say that
it influenced them to do anything, then the other evidence regarding the effects of
communication is suspect. On the other hand, if a significant portion of those
exposed can confirm that the communication made a difference for them, then the
other findings are reinforced.

The evaluation of the *jiggasha* approach in Trishal, Bangladesh, did ask the
266 participants for their opinions (Kincaid, Kapadia-Kundu, et al., 1994). Over
half of the participants said that as a result of the *jiggasha* group meetings they
discussed family planning and the *jiggasha* experience itself with their husbands
and with other women. About 30 percent said that they adopted a modern
contraceptive method; 22 percent said that they decided to continue using their
current method; 17 percent said that they visited a family planning clinic; and 7
percent said that they switched to another method as a result of participating in
jiggasha meetings. These opinions were consistent with the other conclusions of the

evaluation, thus confirming that the *jiggasha* intervention had an impact. If used in conjunction with other types of evidence, asking the opinion of participants—even if all bias cannot be eliminated—is better than not having their opinions at all.

THEORY-DRIVEN EVALUATION

LESSON 6.

Evaluations that include subobjectives based on theoretical models such as the steps to behavior change provide evidence of impact on behavior and useful feedback to improve future programs.

To measure the process of communication and behavior change, evaluation should be not only *method-driven* but also *theory-driven*—that is, based on theories of change that explain or predict why and how individuals will respond to the program (Chen & Rossi, 1983 & 1987; Chen, 1990; Shadish, Cook, & Leviton, 1991). In family planning and health communication, these theories specify the causal links between exposure to communication and the behavior change intended. For evaluation purposes, these causal links should be the same ones used to develop the communication strategy for the project.

For communication projects, the Steps to Behavior Change model describes a clear set of intervening steps that are expected theoretically to take place in response to communication and that are expected to lead to sustained behavior change. Achieving these intervening steps should be treated as *subobjectives* of the project. Appropriate indicators can then be devised to measure these steps as well as the primary objective of behavior change. If the subobjectives are achieved as predicted by theory, and if these steps can be shown to be related to the desired outcome (behavior change), then the evaluation not only has evidence of success or failure but also has a more precise explanation of *why* that outcome occurred and with whom. This is the kind of information that can be used to improve the strategic design of future communication projects. This basic approach to evaluation, of course, can be used with other theoretical models of change.

In the *jiggasha* experiment described above, longitudinal sample surveys of the same women in all 24 villages were conducted by Mitra and Associates before and after the program. Thus, in addition to identifying differences in outcome between the experimental and control areas, the evaluation also could identify many other differences among individual women. The surveys collected information from each woman that corresponded to several of the subobjectives specified by the Steps to Behavior Change model. Statistical analysis of these variables revealed which steps were most closely related to individual behavior.

As Table 7.4 shows, the women who rated high or positive on each of the five steps measured were more likely to be using a modern contraceptive method than

Table 7.4

Steps to Behavior Change and Their Relationship to Modern Family Planning Use Among Married Women, Trishal Thana, Bangladesh, 1992

Intervening Variable	% High or Yes	% Using Modern Method When Intervening Variable Is:		Crude Odds Ratio*
		Low/No	High/Yes	
Unaided knowledge of 4–6 modern FP methods	68.3	15.4	30.2	2.4
Positive FP attitude	57.5	18.2	30.9	2.0
Discussed FP with other women	43.9	17.0	36.3	2.8
Discussed family size or contraceptives with husband	67.5	12.4	31.9	3.3
Husband approves of FP practice	74.8	5.7	32.1	7.8

FP = family planning.
*N = 1,705 to 1,707; all differences are statistically significant beyond the .001 level of probability.
Source: Kincaid, Das Gupta, et al., 1993.

those who rated low. Of the five steps that were measured, husband's approval was their husbands approved of their practicing family planning, 32.1 percent were using a modern method, compared with only 5.7 percent of women whose husbands disapproved. In other words, women whose husbands approved were 7.8 times more likely to use a modern method. (The odds-ratio calculation is useful because it best indicates the relative strength of each variable compared with the others.)

All five variables—positive attitudes, high levels of knowledge, discussions with other women, discussions with husband, and husband's approval—come from the Steps to Behavior Change model. There is a theoretical basis for predicting that each of these variables would be related to the intended behavior. Indeed, that was the same theoretical basis for designing the *jiggasha* concept of group discussion and networking from the start. Because it helps to explain *why* the difference occurred, the findings that, in practice, the *jiggasha* approach was associated with the results predicted by theory, strengthen the conclusion that the program was in fact responsible for the differences measured in the experimental design. It also helps to dismiss the possibility that some other event may have caused the difference (spuriousness).

In addition, this theory-based evaluation provides useful conclusions for future programs: All of these variables should continue to be emphasized in the future, but, since husband's approval made more difference to contraceptive use than the other four, even more attention should be given to that aspect of the *jiggasha* approach. The men of Bangladesh, often neglected in maternal and child health programs, should become a more important focus for future communication activities.

LESSON 7.

A thorough evaluation of the impact of communication includes an analysis of its indirect effects as well as its direct effects on health behavior.

Evidence that these theoretical linkages are indeed related to the desired behavior outcome contributes substantially to the evaluation of impact, but evaluation must also show that exposure to the communication had an impact on these theoretically linked variables. In Bangladesh, did the *jiggasha* intervention itself make a difference in the attitudes and knowledge of participants? If so, then the communication had an indirect effect on behavior, through its effect on these causal links, as well as a direct effect. In terms of analysis, the five theoretical variables (steps) operate as *intervening variables* between exposure to communication and behavior (see Figure 7.3). The analysis of the *jiggasha* experiment in Lesson 6 showed that selected subobjectives (steps) were strongly related to modern

Figure 7.3
Schematic Diagram of the Direct and Indirect Effects of Communication

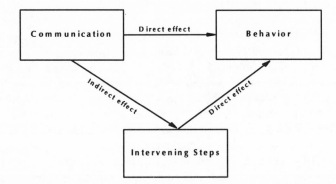

contraceptive use. Further analysis shows whether and to what extent the individual women who actually participated in *jiggasha* sessions differed, with respect to these five selected variables, from women who did not participate.

As Table 7.5 indicates, *jiggasha* participation had a statistically significant relationship with all but one intervening variable. *Jiggasha* participation appears to be most strongly associated with discussion of family planning with other women. Participants were 3.1 times more likely than nonparticipants to discuss family planning with other women. The *jiggasha* participants also were 2.1 times more likely to recall more than four modern methods, 1.7 times more likely to discuss family planning with their husbands, and 1.4 times more likely to have highly positive attitudes. Thus, four of the five subobjectives (steps) found to be related to modern contraceptive use also were significantly related to *jiggasha* participation. Evidence of indirect effects such as this increases confidence that communication had an impact on contraceptive behavior *in ways that were expected theoretically*.

Table 7.5
The Impact of *Jiggasha* Participation on the Intervening Steps to Behavior Change
Among Married Women, Trishal Thana, Bangladesh, 1992

Intervening Variable	% Rated High on Intervening Variable by *Jiggasha* Participation		Crude Odds Ratio[a]
	Did Not Participate	Did Participate	
Positive FP attitude	56.5	63.8	1.4*
Unaided knowledge of 4-6 modern FP methods	66.0	80.3	2.1**
Discussed FP with other women	39.9	67.0	3.1***
Discussed family size or contraceptives with husband	65.7	76.6	1.7**
Husband approves of FP practice	73.7	79.4	1.4

FP = family planning.

Note: The 229 *jiggasha* participants represented 12.2 percent of the 1,877 women surveyed in all 24 villages in the follow-up survey in 1992, and 24.0 percent of the women surveyed in the 12 villages where the *jiggasha* intervention was implemented.

[a]Level of statistical significance: *p < 0.05; **p < 0.01; ***p < 0.001.

Source: Kincaid, Das Gupta, et al., 1993.

This information has immediate implications for improving the *jiggasha* intervention because it provides evidence on *why* and *how* the intervention influenced modern contraceptive use. For example, the data show that the strongest intervening variable for contraceptive use, husband's approval, was *not* significantly related to *jiggasha* participation at the individual level. Perhaps this was because participants and nonparticipants both had fairly high husbands' approval, 79.4 percent versus 73.7 percent. Still, it suggests that the *jiggasha* did not help women win their husbands' approval for family planning. For the 25 percent or so of these Bangladeshi women whose husbands disapproved, this disapproval appears to be an important constraint: 94 percent of these women do not currently use modern contraceptives.

These findings suggest that the *jiggasha* intervention could be improved to address this issue further. What can be done in *jiggasha* meetings for men, as well as for women, to influence the remaining opposing husbands to change their minds? Is it acceptable to talk openly about this during *jiggasha* meetings? To identify wives whose husbands still object, find out why they object, and what can be done to change their minds? Perhaps male opinion leaders in the village would be willing to talk to these men about it. Perhaps just informing the disapproving husbands that a majority of men already approve might be persuasive. Ideas such as these are now being incorporated into the revised field worker training curriculum for the next phase of the program.

LESSON 8.

Exposure to communication and the steps to behavior change have cumulative effects on behavior much like cumulative risk and dose response in epidemiologic research.

In research on communication, the concept of cumulative effects or impact is analogous to the concept of cumulative risk in epidemiological studies of disease and to a dose response in medicine (Schlesselman, 1982). In communication evaluation, cumulative impact means that the greater the number of steps to behavior change that apply to any individual, the greater the probability that the individual will adopt that health behavior. Thus an evaluation that shows this provides powerful evidence of impact. Such evaluation also is useful in determining the marginal utility of seeking to achieve each additional step.

As indicated in Chapter 2, the Steps to Behavior Change model depicts a process. But all individuals do not necessarily pass through the steps in the same order, nor do all individuals necessarily pass through all of the steps before they change their behavior. For example, a woman may talk to her husband and friends about family planning before she knows much about contraceptive methods or without necessarily having a positive attitude about practicing family planning. She may even try the first method she hears about, discontinue it, and then try others until eventually she finds one that is suitable. Meanwhile, her knowledge increases and her attitudes toward contraceptive use become more positive as she learns the benefits first hand or through talking with other women. Such complex adaptive behavior is not fully captured by staged models of communication and behavior. What matters, however, is that the important steps are identified and that in combination they make a difference to behavior.

Several Johns Hopkins evaluations in different cultures have demonstrated that each of the steps to behavior change *by itself* usually has a statistically significant association with contraceptive use (as already shown for Bangladesh in Table 7.1). It has now been demonstrated, in addition, that these steps, regardless of their order, have a cumulative impact on behavior (Kincaid, 1995a; Kincaid, 1996). The measures of the steps to behavior change are usually so closely correlated with one another that they meet the statistical criterion to be combined into a single, underlying factor. If the number of steps (variables) that apply to an individual are simply summed, the resulting measure of *how many* intervening steps apply represents the strength of that factor. Analysis of the cumulative measure of the steps to behavior change can show how much impact each additional intervening variable has on behavior. Evaluation of family planning communication is the first area of communication research where this phenomenon has been demonstrated (Kincaid, 1995a; Kincaid, 1996).

In Bangladesh, when the *jiggasha* project was replicated in three new thanas, and a one-group, before-after longitudinal panel survey was used for evaluation (Kincaid, 1996), there were 1,479 women in the 1994 baseline survey and 1,058 of these women in the 1996 follow-up plus a supplemental sample. The same five

Figure 7.4
Modern Contraceptive Use Among Eligible Married Women by the Cumulative Number of Steps to Behavior Change, Bangladesh, 1994

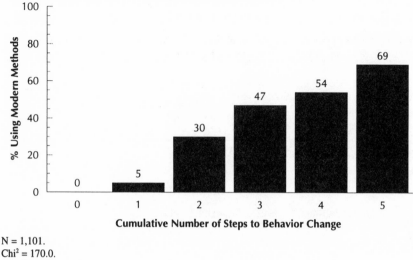

N = 1,101.
Chi^2 = 170.0.
p < .0001.
Source: Kincaid, 1996.

intervening steps or variables were used as described in Lessons 6 and 7—women's knowledge, approval, discussion with other women, discussion with husband, and husband's approval.

As the bar graph in Figure 7.4 above illustrates, the percentage of eligible married women using modern methods increased cumulatively and significantly with each additional step to behavior change that applied. Most strikingly, the level of use of modern contraceptives among women who rated low on all five steps is *zero*—no users whatsoever. Among women who have taken just one step, the prevalence rate is 5 percent. With two steps, prevalence jumps to 30 percent, and then up to 54 percent with four steps. Women to whom all five steps apply have a modern contraceptive use rate of 69 percent, which is about the level of contraceptive use in many developed countries.

A comprehensive evaluation can identify a cumulative impact of communication similar to a dose response. As Table 7.6 shows, women who were exposed to a strong communication intervention—*jiggasha* discussion groups led by a family welfare assistant—were most likely to use modern contraceptive methods: almost 75 percent did so. These are the cumulative direct effects of communication activities on the behavior outcome. Some 56 percent of those who were visited by a family welfare assistant at home but did not attend *jiggashas* were modern method users, but only 17 percent of women exposed to neither *jiggasha* nor home visits.

A similar dose response effect is evident in the indirect impact of exposure on the intervening steps to behavior change. Of the women who participated in *jiggasha* discussion groups, 88 percent ranked high (with four or five steps) on the steps to behavior change. In comparison, only 35 percent of women exposed to neither intervention and about 68 percent of those visited by a field worker at home only ranked high on the five steps.

Table 7.6
Modern Contraceptive Use and Level of Steps to Behavior Change Among Eligible Married Women in Bangladesh by Level of Family Planning Communication[1]

Variable	None (%)	Home Visit by FWA (%)	*Jiggasha* with FWA (%)	Total (N)
		Level of Family Planning Communication		
Direct Effect: Modern Contraceptive Use[2]				
No	83.0	44.0	25.5	556
Yes	17.0	56.0	74.5	545
Indirect Effect: Number of Steps to Behavior Change[3]				
Low (0–3)	64.8	32.3	11.7	408
High (4–5)	35.2	67.7	88.3	693
Number of Cases	253	703	145	1,101

FWA = family welfare assistant.
[1]Sample consists of married women ages 12–49 who are eligible for family planning: not pregnant, breastfeeding, or infertile.
[2]$Chi^2 = 155.2; p < .0001$.
[3]$Chi^2 = 130.4; p < .0001$.
Source: Kincaid, 1996.

The same type of analysis can be used to evaluate predominantly mass media communication programs. In Kenya the *Haki Yako* family planning campaign was evaluated through a 1994 national sample survey of 4,459 men and women. Communication activities were divided into four principal channels: a radio serial drama, radio in general, print materials, and visits by community-based workers. The evaluation showed a similar dose response to levels of communication exposure and a similar cumulative impact—both direct and indirect—of the steps to behavior change (Kincaid, 1995a). The results are presented in the form of three related bar graphs in Figure 7.5.

The first bar graph shows the direct cumulative effect of exposure to family planning messages through the four communication channels. There is a clear dose response: The greater the number of channels of exposure to family planning messages, the higher the rate of modern contraceptive use. The prevalence rate is only 10 percent for men and women with exposure to none of the four channels. The rate increases steadily with each channel added, reaching a high of 43 percent using modern methods among those exposed to all four channels.

The second bar graph shows the direct effect of six selected steps to behavior change on modern contraceptive use. Men and women for whom none of the six

Figure 7.5
Direct and Indirect Effects of Family Planning Communication Among Men and Women in Kenya, 1994 *

Direct Effect of Communication Exposure on Behavior

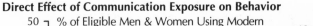
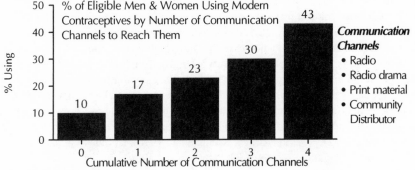

% of Eligible Men & Women Using Modern Contraceptives by Number of Communication Channels to Reach Them

Communication Channels
• Radio
• Radio drama
• Print material
• Community Distributor

Direct Effect of the Number of Steps to Behavior Change

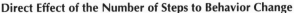
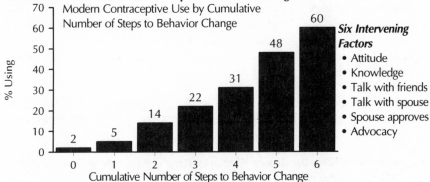

Modern Contraceptive Use by Cumulative Number of Steps to Behavior Change

Six Intervening Factors
• Attitude
• Knowledge
• Talk with friends
• Talk with spouse
• Spouse approves
• Advocacy

Indirect Effect of Communication Through the Intervening Steps

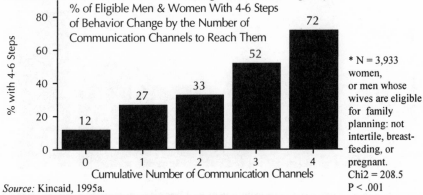

% of Eligible Men & Women With 4-6 Steps of Behavior Change by the Number of Communication Channels to Reach Them

* N = 3,933 women, or men whose wives are eligible for family planning: not intertile, breast-feeding, or pregnant.
Chi2 = 208.5
P < .001

Source: Kincaid, 1995a.

intervening steps applies have a modern contraceptive use rate of just 2 percent. The rate increases dramatically with the addition of each new step. The use rate reaches 31 percent for those to whom four steps apply, which exceeds the national modern contraceptive prevalence rate of 20.4 percent. The men and women to whom all six factors apply have a modern prevalence rate of 60 percent.

The third bar graph shows the strong dose response of the number of channels on the six intervening steps related to contraceptive adoption. Only 12 percent of respondents with no communication exposure have high levels (4 to 6) on the steps to change. The percentage of respondents who are at high levels increases very rapidly with the addition of each channel of family planning communication: 72 percent of those exposed to all four channels of communication have high levels on the steps. Similar dose responses to communication exposure have been found in evaluations of family planning communication programs in Zimbabwe (Piotrow, Kincaid, et al., 1992), Nigeria (Kiragu, Krenn, et al., 1996), Bolivia (Valente, Saba, et al., 1996), and Uganda (Kiragu, Galiwango, et al., 1996).

Even where separate surveys are not fielded to evaluate communication impacts, other surveys, such as Demographic and Health Surveys, can be analyzed to identify a dose response or cumulative impact of communication. In Tanzania, for example, a 1994 national sample survey of 4,225 women ages 15 to 49 (Weinstein et al., 1994), conducted by the Tanzanian Bureau of Statistics and Planning Commission, showed that during the preceding two years the modern contraceptive prevalence rate had nearly doubled, rising from 5.9 percent to 11.2 percent. A statistical analysis of the cumulative effect of seven family planning channels used during those two years (the *Zinduka* radio serial drama, other radio programs, the family planning logo, newspapers, posters, brochures, and

Figure 7.6
Modern Contraceptive Use Among Women by Level of Exposure to Communication Channels, Tanzania, 1994

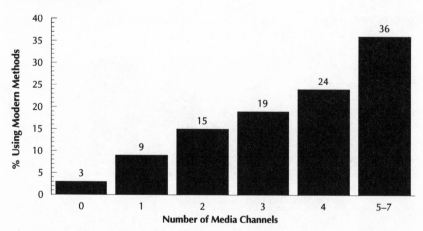

N = 4,225 women ages 15–49.
Source: Adapted from Jato, Simbakalia, et al., 1996.

television) showed the expected stairstep pattern with modern contraceptive use (Jato, Simbakalia, et al., 1996). (See Figure 7.6.) The contraceptive prevalence rate among women not exposed to any channel was only 3 percent; this increased to 24 percent for those exposed to four channels and peaked at 36 percent for those exposed to five or more channels. Thus the modern contraceptive use rate for women exposed to family planning messages through more than five channels was three times higher than the national rate of 11.2 percent.

LESSON 9.

Aggregating survey data by local units of analysis such as villages or sample clusters reveals the impact of communication on local culture in addition to its impact on individuals.

Most Population Communication Services evaluations involve surveys to measure individual behavior change. These, like most other surveys, are carried out with samples designed to select a certain number of independent individuals with a known probability. For economic and practical reasons, large surveys are conducted by multistage cluster sampling procedures. That is, through systematic or simple randomized sampling methods, certain geographical units within a country are selected first, followed by a second randomized sample of smaller units within the larger area, such as villages and urban neighborhoods or blocks. Within these units, maps are usually drawn of all of the households, and then a randomized sample of households is selected. Households are then selected so that they are geographically dispersed in order to reduce the interdependence that occurs due to communication and other shared cultural influences among individuals who live in close proximity. A final randomized selection procedure ensures that every eligible individual within each household has an equal probability of being selected. As a result, the sample is representative of the population from which it is drawn. The smallest geographical unit—the village or neighborhood—is usually referred to as a "cluster."

The effects of local culture within these clusters on the individuals who are ultimately sampled cannot be entirely eliminated. Some villages and neighborhoods are wealthier than others, for example, or include more individuals with higher levels of education or who own radios, so that the average levels of income, education, or radio ownership for that cluster are higher than for other clusters. Also, some clusters are closer than others to roads, schools, and health/family planning service facilities, and hence are visited more often by outreach workers.

For randomized sampling and for analyzing individual behavior, these local cultural effects are a nuisance, and efforts are usually made to adjust the statistical analysis for such effects. For understanding social and cultural change, however, cluster effects are quite informative. Although it may seem obvious that the individual is the unit who adopts a new behavior, the evidence and many theories suggest that change also occurs at a higher level, the level of cultural units. Why should this be so? Unless a woman believes that those in her community—friends and neighbors as well as local leaders—publicly endorse a new technology or behavior, it is difficult for her to adopt it. Stated another way, once the new behavior seems socially acceptable, it is easier for individuals to adopt it (Fishbein & Ajzen, 1975). This phenomenon is one of the rationales for conducting community mobilization programs in public health and for including discussion and advocacy of family planning in the Steps to Behavior Change model.

PCS evaluations have identified a strong village cluster effect on use of family planning in Bangladesh. In the 1989 baseline survey within the socioeconomically homogeneous thana of Trishal, the contraceptive prevalence rates of the 24 villages varied from 7 percent to 58 percent (Kincaid, Das Gupta, et al., 1993). At that time, the national rate and the overall trishal rate were about 32 percent (Kincaid, 1995b). When the *jiggasha* project was replicated in 1994, surveys in 30 villages of three thanas revealed the same wide range of contraceptive prevalence among villages, from 9 percent to 58 percent (averaging 40 percent) (Kincaid, 1996).

Analysis of the 1996 follow-up survey for the *jiggasha* replication found that there was also a village-level relationship between modern contraceptive prevalence and the steps to behavior change. When the individual-level data were aggregated at the cluster level, there was a high correlation ($r = 0.85$) between the modern contraceptive prevalence rate and the women's mean number of steps to change. At the individual level, the comparable correlation was $r = 0.39$, moderately high but much lower than the village-level correlation. In technical terms, this means that 72 percent of the variance in modern contraceptive use was explained by these cumulative steps to behavior change at the cluster or village level of analysis. This relationship, illustrated in Figure 7.7, is linear: the higher the cluster's average level on the intervening steps to behavior change, the higher the rate of modern method use.

Figure 7.7 supports the conclusion that contraceptive adoption varies among local cultural units according to ideational factors, as measured by the five steps to behavior change. This finding implies that family planning adoption occurs at the level of villages as well as individuals. It corresponds to findings on the fertility transitions in Europe described in Chapter 1—namely, that fertility decline spreads first through similar cultural and linguistic areas within countries, regardless of the levels of socioeconomic development (Coale & Watkins, 1986). This finding helped to give rise to the ideational theory of fertility transition, which states that fertility decline spreads primarily through the communication of new ideas (Cleland & Wilson, 1987).

The same cultural effect can be shown in national-level sample surveys of countries where mass media programs play a larger role. Following similar procedures, a 1994 Kenyan national sample survey of 4,459 men and women was aggregated at the cluster level for further analysis. This yielded a total of 268 clusters with an average size of 16.6 individuals per cluster. Figure 7.8a shows the scatterplot and regression line of the modern contraceptive prevalence rate on the average number of the five steps to behavior change among men and women in the 268 Kenyan clusters. Each solid square represents the level of a cluster on the two variables. The correlation at the aggregate level is 0.54. This represents a fairly

Figure 7.7

Regression of Modern Contraceptive Prevalence on Five Intervening Steps to Behavior Change in 30 Bangladesh Villages, 1996

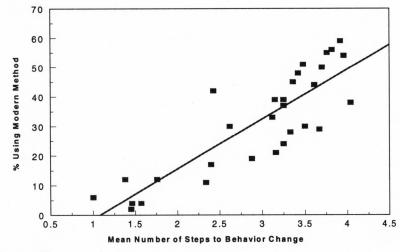

Note: r = .85.

strong linear relationship between local culture (ideation) and family planning practice in Kenya, but not as strong as the relationship reported for Bangladesh. This probably reflects the fact that Bangladesh is a more homogeneous society with less communication among villages.

In Kenya, exposure to family planning messages, via media or in person, also varies by local community, and the community level of media exposure is positively related to local ideational factors (as indicated by the intervening steps to behavior change). The scatterplot in Figure 7.8b shows the relationship between the average number of steps to behavior change and the average cumulative exposure to family planning media in Kenya by cluster. The correlation is 0.55.

The ideational theory and the results from this type of evaluation and analysis in developing countries have important implications for communication programs: Health and family planning communication programs should be strategically designed for communities as well as for individuals. This, too, was one of the primary motives behind the *jiggasha* project in Bangladesh. Changing the field workers' pattern of work from individual home visits to local group meetings was expected to strengthen the community norm supporting family planning and thus stimulate individual practice. For evaluation, the lesson is that, when large national sample surveys are used for individual-level analysis, the results also should be aggregated at the cluster level to examine the impact of programs on social units. Then programs can be developed with the people and leaders of those units to address their concerns.

Figure 7.8a
**Regression of Modern Contraceptive Prevalence on Six Cumulative Steps to
Behavior Change in 268 Clusters in Kenya, 1994**

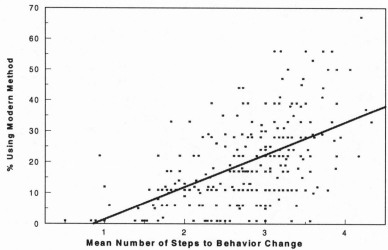

Note: r = .54.

Figure 7.8b
**Regression of Mean Number of Steps to Behavior Change on Media Exposure
in 268 Clusters in Kenya, 1994**

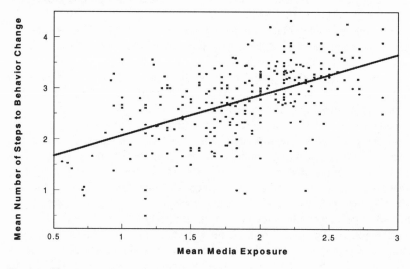

Note: r = .55.
Source: Kincaid, 1995a.

LESSON 10.

Path analysis can depict and test the direction and strength of all the relationships measured in a communication program evaluation.

One of the most advanced methodologies that can be used to represent and test the complex relationships described above is *path analysis*, also referred to as structural equation modeling (Hayduk, 1987; Glymour et al., 1987; Joreskog & Sorbom, 1979). When used with longitudinal survey data and when the theoretical relationships underlying the causal process are understood, path analysis offers a practical compromise. This compromise achieves the internal validity obtained from the randomized control group design and the external validity (generalizability) obtained from the sample surveys used in the one-group, before-after designs. The main disadvantage of using path analysis for evaluation research is that its use and interpretation require a sophisticated statistical background (Chen, 1990). If the path models are kept as simple as possible and can be clearly diagrammed, however, then the method offers many advantages for program evaluation.

In the case of the evaluation of the *jiggasha* approach in Bangladesh, for example, just three program variables and eight control variables were used:

- the outcome behavior (family planning practice),
- communication (*jiggashas* with family welfare assistants—FWAs), and
- the ideation factor (five steps to behavior change).

Communication and the ideation factor each were treated as having direct effects on family planning, and communication was also treated as having an indirect effect on family planning through its effect on the ideation factor. These same relationships were diagrammed as a set of paths in Figure 7.9. To test these relationships rigorously with data, however, it was necessary to control for any confounding variables that may be influencing each of the three variables and to assess time-order and the threat of selectivity (see Lesson 3). To do so required that a multiple regression analysis be conducted for each of the three variables and that the three resulting regression equations be evaluated as a whole set or system. Two computer programs have been developed to make this easier to do: LISREL (Joreskog & Sorbom, 1979) and EQS (Bentler, 1995). Also, a conventional method for diagramming the results has made them easier to interpret.

The longitudinal survey data from the evaluation of the *jiggasha* replication in Bangladesh were submitted to the EQS program to test a path model for family planning use and intention. Five degrees of intention to use (ranging from "definitely will not practice" to "definitely will practice in the future") were combined with traditional and modern contraceptive use to create a seven-point, continuous scale required for the analysis. Ideation comprised the five cumulative steps to behavior change described above, while the measure of communication consisted of no contact, FWA visits at home, and participation in *jiggashas* led by FWAs.

The resulting path analysis is diagrammed in Figure 7.9. Each line in the graph represents a causal influence. The direction of influence is indicated by the arrowhead. The longitudinal (panel) design of the survey makes it possible to assess the efforts of the control variables and program variables measured in 1994 on the three program variables measured in 1996.[2] The paths of influence leading to each variable represent the results of the three multiple regression analyses. Only statistically significant relationships are shown. The three main relationships of interest for evaluation are represented by thicker lines: the direct and indirect effects of the *jiggashas* with FWAs and the direct effect of the ideation factor (five steps to behavior change [SBC]) on family planning use and intention. The numbers next to each arrowhead indicate the *relative size* of the causal influence. Technically, they are the standardized regression coefficients from the regression analysis for each variable. A negative sign next to a number indicates an inverse relationship. Thus, for example, younger women are more likely to participate in *jiggasha* meetings and to practice or intend to practice family planning (−.11 and −.19, respectively), controlling for the effects of number of children and other variables.

The diagram shows that only five variables have significant influences on family planning use and intention after controlling for all other variables. The strongest influence is the ideation/SBC factor (.34), followed by prior family planning use and intention (.22). The *jiggasha*/FWA intervention has the third strongest influence (.18), followed by the two control variables age (−.19) and number of children (.12). Education and socioeconomic status have no direct effect on family planning use and intention. They have influence only through their effects on the ideation factor. Also, socioeconomic status has a negative relationship with ideation. That is, lower-status women are higher on the five steps to behavior change. The strongest influence on ideation comes from *jiggasha*/FWA communication (.33), followed by a woman's prior (1994) ideation level (.21). *Jiggasha* and field worker visits in 1996 are determined mainly by prior FWA visits and prior family planning use and intention.

The path analysis illuminates the causal paths expected by the communication and steps to behavior change theories used to design the *jiggasha* program and to evaluate it. Path analysis controls statistically for the confounding influences of other variables. And because a longitudinal (panel) survey was used, the time-order of the relationships and the problem of selectivity are taken into account. Thus the analysis makes possible this conclusion: Prior family plannning use and intention, as measured in 1994, did influence who participated in *jiggasha* meetings and who was visited by family welfare assistants in 1996, but *jiggasha*/FWA communication in 1996 still had a significant influence on family planning use and intention, even after controlling for this source of selectivity. Using path analysis with longitudinal data accomplishes the two goals of program evaluation discussed throughout this chapter: (1) measuring the impact of communication and (2) specifying the causal process that accounts for that impact.[3]

Figure 7.9
A Path Model of the Direct and Indirect Impact of *Jiggasha* Participation on Family Planning in Bangladesh, 1994–1996

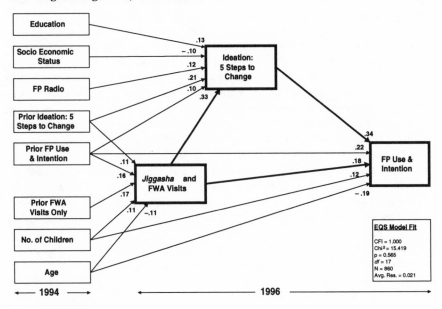

FP = family planning.
FWA = family welfare assistant.
Source: Kincaid, 1996.

EVALUATING CLIENT-PROVIDER COMMUNICATION

LESSON 11.

Because of the interactive nature of interpersonal communication and counseling, innovative research methods are needed for effective evaluation.

Interpersonal communication and counseling (IPC/C) are often crucial components in the process of behavior change. Most people start to use family planning only after counseling sessions with service providers. They also talk with their spouse or partner, friends, and others to seek information, confirmation, or emotional support—usually even before seeing service providers.

It is universally assumed that the quality of client-provider interaction in counseling sessions can influence whether clients use contraceptive methods correctly, and for how long. Therefore much attention is now being given to efforts to improve the quality of counseling. These efforts have included setting standards and guidelines for counseling, upgrading supervision of counseling, providing counseling aids, empowering clients to expect and ask for appropriate information, and, most frequently, training providers in interpersonal communication and counseling skills.

In the past, evaluation of training was often limited to output measures alone: counting the number of providers trained, comparing pre- and post-training test scores, and collecting trainees' reports on their satisfaction with training. More in-depth evaluation of the content and quality of interpersonal communication and counseling has been difficult until recent years because of the lack of standards, the variability in desired outcomes, and the lack of measurement tools. Therefore, the difficult task of evaluating how providers apply the knowledge and skills learned during training when they return to their jobs is rarely undertaken.

To assess limited aspects of client-provider interaction, such as waiting times, use of counseling aids, respect for privacy, and the number of contraceptive methods mentioned, either observation during the session or "exit" interviews with clients afterward are needed. More important, follow-up evaluation of the impact of training or other client-provider communication on the clients' subsequent family planning behavior has been seriously neglected.

To improve the quality and impact of counseling first requires improving understanding of the counseling process. Several innovative methods of studying family planning counseling have been developed over the last 10 years and applied by Population Communication Services. These include:

- refined indicators of counseling skills;
- assessment of clients' perspectives on counseling quality;
- studying the interaction between client and provider during counseling sessions; and
- follow-up of clients' contraceptive behavior after counseling sessions.

Refined indicators of counseling skills. New indicators and corresponding data collection instruments have been developed to assess counseling skills based on the widely used GATHER approach to counseling (greet, ask, tell, help choose, explain, and return/refer) (see Box 4.1, in Chapter 4). Several instruments for observation, client interviews, provider interviews, and study site observation have been used in Nigeria (Y. M. Kim, Rimon, et al., 1992), Ghana (Y. M. Kim, Amissah, et al., 1994), Kenya (Y. M. Kim, Lettenmaier, et al., 1996), Zimbabwe (Y. M. Kim, Marangwanda, & Kols, 1996), and Nepal (Heckert et al., 1996). A generic set of these instruments is available in a manual from Johns Hopkins Center for Communication Programs (Y. M. Kim & Lettenmaier, 1995). The indicators and instruments were also adapted for use by the Population Council in the Situation Analysis studies (A. Fisher et al., 1996).

Client-provider interaction and client behavior. Most efforts to improve and then evaluate counseling quality have focused on what the provider does. The GATHER process, for example, focuses mainly on the actions of the provider. But evaluation of counseling quality should also address the role of the client during the counseling session and examine the dynamics of the interaction between the client and the provider.

Population Communication Services, in collaboration with the Quality Assurance Project, AVSC International, and the Population Council, has developed and continues to refine a technique for "interaction analysis" to better measure and understand the complexity of these interactions. The technique uses transcript analysis. It involves recording audio or videotapes and then coding and analyzing these dialogues using both qualitative and quantitative techniques (Roter & Hall, 1992). The interactions are then studied to determine how clients participate in counseling, how providers respond to clients, and how decisions are made. This technique has been applied in Kenya, Zimbabwe, and Indonesia (Y. M. Kim, Odallo, et al., 1997; Y. M. Kim, Marangwanda, & Kols, 1996; Y. M. Kim, 1997).

Interaction analysis offers several advantages over direct observations or client exit interviews. First, transcripts provide an accurate record and do not rely on human recall of what happened. Second, complex communication can be disaggregated to assess separately the behavior of both clients and providers in the same context. Third, evaluators can use and study the transcripts repeatedly to get a variety of points of view from clients, providers, counseling specialists, program managers, and trainers.

An example from Kenya based on audio transcripts of 178 counseling sessions with women provides the following insights into client-provider interaction and suggests guidelines for improving counseling in the future:

- Providers tend to dominate the sessions and do not allow clients to express or implement their own agendas.
- Providers do not elaborate on the risks or benefits of specific methods.
- Providers do not obtain adequate medical histories to be able to assess the appropriateness of method choices.
- Clients select contraceptive methods according to the conventional definition of "informed choice," but providers do not try to assess whether the decision is based on an accurate understanding of the information provided (Y. M. Kim, Odallo, et al., 1997; Y. M. Kim & Kols, 1996).
- Clients can be taught to take a more active role in the interaction and consequently increase the quality of information they receive and their own satisfaction.

Client perspectives. The client perspective on quality of counseling is important if the client is expected to change her behavior as a result. Exit interviews and focus-group discussions with clients have permitted Population Communication Services to incorporate client values into efforts to upgrade client-provider interaction and counseling. According to client interviews in Nigeria, nurses trained in counseling skills were more likely than untrained nurses to listen attentively to their clients, to make them feel comfortable, and to treat them politely (Y. M. Kim, Rimon, et al., 1992). In the Central Asian Republics, focus-group discussions with men and women revealed that service providers were perceived as unreliable sources of information and as lacking concern for the clients' welfare (Storey, Ilkhamov, & Saksvig, 1997). In Ghana, a study of service quality involved a follow-up of contraceptive acceptors who did not return to the clinic, asking them directly why they did not return (Tweedie, 1995).

Impact evaluation. The most important question is: Does improved counseling have an impact on clients' behavior, and specifically on behavior that reduces unwanted fertility? Indicators now being tested in Kenya include decision to use a method, selection of an appropriate method for the client's reported characteristics, method continuation, compliance with effective use procedures, timely return visit for resupply, and method switching that avoids the risk of pregnancy. The study uses clinic records to follow clients over a 42-month period (Y. M. Kim & Kols, 1996). Because of the nature of the data, specialized statistical routines of longitudinal regression analysis will be used, including general equation estimation (Diggle, Liang, & Zeger, 1994). In Nigeria, the indicator of impact, collected from client records, was the timely return of new clients for the first follow-up appointment. The clients who had been attended by nurses trained in counseling were more likely to return to clinics than those attended by untrained nurses (Y. M. Kim, Rimon, et al., 1992). This was one of the first evaluations to link provider training with subsequent client behavior.

Figure 7.10a
Nature of Clients' Active Participation in Counseling, Kenya

Figure 7.10b
Providers' Responses to Clients' Active Participation, Kenya

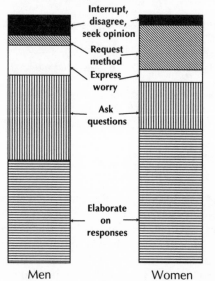
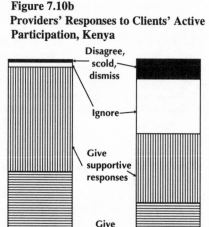

N = 65 men and 173 women.
Note: Based on transcript analysis.
Source: Y. M. Kim, Odallo, et al., 1997.

Methods for assessing the quality of client-provider interaction have been developed primarily with women, but they can be modified and applied to men, couples, or adolescents of either sex. In Kenya, for example, both observation and transcript analysis indicated the following:

- Male clients participate more actively than women in counseling sessions when they come alone for counseling.
- When both partners are present in counseling sessions, women become more passive than when they are alone.
- Providers give more supportive responses to men than to women.
- Providers ignore and disagree more with women than with men (Y. M. Kim & Awasum, 1996; Mwarogo, Kim, & Kols, 1996). As Figures 7.10a and 7.10b illustrate, when clients take an active role in the counseling session, men are more likely than women to ask questions but less likely to request a family planning method and less likely to elaborate on their responses to a provider's questions. For their part, the providers' responses to their clients' active participation also varied by the sex of the client. Providers were more likely to ignore women's statements and more likely to give men supportive responses and technical information.

In Zimbabwe, youth counseling sessions were evaluated using expert observation and exit interviews. They found the following:

- Young people, ages 12 to 24, were very uncomfortable in dealing with sexuality and reproductive health issues. Younger clients were more anxious, embarrassed, or shy, and giggled nervously instead of answering questions during the session. Providers had to be more patient in dealing with young clients.
- Young people were more passive than adults in counseling sessions. Providers had to make considerable efforts to obtain essential information or to determine the client's agenda for the session.
- Despite being passive or even nonresponsive during the sessions, many young people wanted the sessions to last longer and to provide more information, according to their exit interviews.
- Young people were concerned about a number of issues that were not related to reproductive health, such as school, dating, friendships, and alcohol (Y. M. Kim & Marangwanda, 1996).

Innovative research such as this makes it possible to understand better the impact of provider interaction interventions on client behavior; to provide specific guidelines to improve the provider training curriculum, materials, and audiovisual aids; to develop client education at service facilities and campaigns that can increase clients' participation during counseling; to improve the methodologies for studying client-provider interaction; and, above all, to improve the services provided.

COLLABORATION AND DISSEMINATION OF FINDINGS

LESSON 12.

Collaborating with other organizations for program evaluation can provide substantial benefits.

Just as effective health programs require a broad base of collaboration, evaluation also benefits from collaboration in the following ways:

- reducing costs by avoiding duplication in design and data collection;
- reducing the time required for design and data collection;
- creating opportunities for multiple points of view and different analyses;
- increasing utilization of results by involving implementing organizations in the evaluation process; and
- increasing credibility, public scrutiny, and application of evaluation results to future programs.

Collaboration can vary considerably. Collaborating institutions can include a wide variety of agencies, from government statistical offices to market research firms to university faculty. Different mechanisms can be used to plan this collaboration, including workshops and seminars, technical advisory groups, periodic updates for collaborators, and circulation of materials for review and comment. While extra effort is usually involved in ensuring appropriate timing, comparable samples, or satisfactory questions, generally the advantages of collaboration outweigh the disadvantages. In practice, collaboration can take place at four stages of evaluation implementation: research design, data collection, analysis, and utilization of data.

Research design. Communication program evaluations should incorporate a broad base of institutional and expert participation in the research design and in the development of research instruments. This collaboration can help to ensure a common conceptualization of the problems, the theoretical model, the objectives, and the subobjectives and to win full support for the evaluation. In Zambia, for example, an Information, Education, and Communication Subcommittee of the Government's Intertechnical Committee on Population helped to review research designs and two sets of survey protocols. The committee provided high-level policy review of the evaluation. Later, based on the evaluation results, the committee helped to develop a set of program recommendations that became guidelines for future program implementation.

Data collection. Since data collection is often the most expensive, time-consuming, labor-intensive, and quality-sensitive component of evaluation, collaboration at this stage is especially useful. It can include sharing technical staff, field operations resources (vehicles, field workers, and area managers), organizational resources (sample frames, questionnaires, computers and software, accounting and financial systems), and, of course, costs. In Zimbabwe, the primary survey for a new youth communication initiative was funded by the German Agency for Technical Development (GTZ). The design and analysis were guided by Population Communication Services. The Zimbabwe National Family Planning Council carried out the program.

A powerful and cost-effective way to collaborate in data collection is by participation in country-specific Demographic and Health Surveys (DHS). At the request of Population Communication Services, several countries have incorporated additional communication questions into their surveys to establish baselines for communication programs. In Tanzania, for example, the 1995 Demographic and Health Survey included questions on recognition and comprehension of the national family planning logo and a radio social drama with family planning messages (see Lesson 8). The 1997 Demographic and Health Survey in Jordan includes a survey of men, at the request of the government, to facilitate evaluation of a planned communication campaign to promote men's participation in family planning. Collaboration between Population Communication Services and the Demographic and Health Surveys was formalized when PCS developed a detailed communication module for optional inclusion in future surveys. PCS also collaborates with the Demographic and Health Surveys to improve the analysis of communication issues using survey data.

Communication researchers also can include questions on recurring consumer surveys, generally called omnibus surveys. Market research firms put together questions from a number of clients who then pay for the answers to their specific questions. Firms will perform simple bivariate analysis of clients' questions in relation to common background variables. Because such surveys usually are carried out quarterly, they can provide data periodically. While the audiences might not be precisely those intended and the survey quality might vary, omnibus survey questions are relatively inexpensive. They can be used to augment and help interpret data from other sources. In Kenya, Nigeria, and Zimbabwe, omnibus surveys have been used to measure national exposure to communication interventions, such as radio programs or logos.

Analysis. Collaborating with other agencies in data analysis can provide valuable opportunities for developing-country researchers as well as ensuring that evaluation results will become known to host-country counterparts. The Zimbabwe National Family Planning Council, one of the few family planning associations with a trained Research and Evaluation unit, often collaborates with Population Communication Services in analyzing Zimbabwe data.

Conversely, Population Communication Services also has collaborated in analyzing data collected by other organizations. For example, in Ghana the Population Council carried out a Situation Analysis, observing family planning services at different facilities. The data were then analyzed by the Population Council, the Ministry of Health, and Population Communication Services to assess clinic education and counseling activities, to improve training, and to support advocacy for an expanded role for communication in the Health Education Unit of the Ministry of Health.

Utilization. One of the most cost-effective forms of collaboration is to allow other researchers to use data for additional secondary analysis. This opens the way for new perspectives, peer review of work, and application in broader and perhaps unanticipated program areas. To facilitate additional secondary analysis and utilization, Population Communication Services has established an archive of quantitative and qualitative data sets from its program evaluations. The archive maintains copies of data collection protocols, reports, and analysis as well as the computer files of the actual data, searchable by region, country, study population, date of study, and the variables covered by the study. Approximately three dozen data sets are currently available for independent analysis by other researchers, students, donors, and program planners. Some of these have been used for doctoral dissertations at Johns Hopkins University and elsewhere.

LESSON 13.

Evaluation results can be presented at various levels of complexity to suit different audiences.

Like any other message, evaluation results are useless unless they are communicated, understood, appreciated, and applied by the intended audiences. The audiences for evaluation are usually policy-makers, donors, program managers, and eventually other communication and social science researchers and evaluators.

At the policy level, the challenge in presenting evaluation results is to make a convincing case that the communication program changed behavior without overwhelming officials with complex statistics. Policy-makers are usually very busy, interested mainly in "the big picture" and the implications for future programs, and expert in areas other than statistics. Moreover, they always want to see evaluation results as soon as possible.

Researchers and academic experts, in contrast, want to be sure that evaluation methodology, theory, and analysis are sound. They will apply various tests for causal inference. They will make comparisons with evaluations they have undertaken themselves. And, in the always lively spirit of intellectual debate, they will look for points to criticize.

To meet the demands of such diverse audiences, evaluation results need to be presented in at least three different ways.

Key findings need to report major program results in a timely way. These reports need to summarize briefly the program objectives and subobjectives, the basic program strategies, the messages and materials produced and distributed, and the nature of the evaluation, as well as its findings. Statistics should be simple and clear. Graphics might consist of a single line graph, a bar graph, or a pie chart to illustrate a main conclusion. The format should lend itself to presentations at official meetings or workshops, to press releases, and to notices on the Internet. The PCS Key Findings Series began in 1997.

Field reports need to describe background and program issues as well as reporting in more detail on findings and results. Ranging from about 20 to 60 pages, field reports on major projects can be illustrated and printed. A field report should serve as a guide to program managers, highlighting what happened, as well as what was effective and what was not, and recommending improvements for the future. When time and space allow, a field report should provide a comprehensive record for future reference including relevant data tables. To date, PCS has issued 10 formal field reports and several dozen informal ones. These are listed in POPLINE, the computerized database, and single copies are usually available on request.

Journal articles, presentations at professional meetings, or *book chapters* usually require the presentation of complex statistical analysis. Several articles may focus on different issues within a single comprehensive program evaluation. In fact, journal articles and presentations rarely can present a comprehensive picture of a major program and its impacts. Instead, they often present in-depth analysis of a particularly interesting aspect of a program.

During the process leading from key findings to journal articles, the type and complexity of statistical analysis presented usually increases. Within this chapter alone, for example, the type of statistical analysis has progressed from comparisons of mean village contraceptive rates in percentages, to simple bar graphs, crude odds ratios, and scatterplots with linear regression, to multiple logistical regression, conditional multinomial regression with panel data, Poisson regression with longitudinal service statistics, and path analysis. The simpler methods—linear regression, percentages, and crude odds ratios—are easier to present and to understand; the more complex methods are necessary to compensate for alternative sources of influence and selectivity that are inherent with one-group research designs and to elaborate the causal pathways.

A close look shows, however, that even complex analyses can be presented in simple ways—that is, through odds ratios and bar graphs. Figure 7.5 (see page 155) on Kenya, for example, illustrates the complex relationship among three different sets of variables—modern contraceptive use, exposure to communication, and intervening steps to behavior change—in three fairly simple bar graphs. Meeting the increasing demand for rigorous and relevant evaluation of communication programs requires presenting even the most complex statistical analysis in a form that is accessible to everyone.

NOTES

1. In Bangladesh, a *thana* is an administrative subdivision equivalent to a U.S. county.

2. The terms, "control variables" and "program variables" are used to remain consistent with the terminology used in the rest of this chapter. In structured equation modeling terminology the variables on the left-hand side measured in 1994 are referred to as "exogenous" variables, and the variables on the right-hand side measured in 1996 are referred to as "endogenous" variables.

3. The EQS analysis provides several indicators of the fit of the path model to the data (lower right-hand box). The comparative fit index (CFI) is 1.000, indicating an almost perfect fit of the model to the data, and the Chi^2 goodness of fit test indicates that there is no statistically significant difference between the model and the data. The average correlation

among the residuals of each variable is 0.021, indicating that there are no variables left out of the model that might still be determining any of the relationships shown in the model. The covariances among the exogenous variables measured in 1994 are omitted for ease of presentation, as are the residual terms, E, for the three endogenous variables. The amount of variance in family planning use and intention that is explained by the path model is 36 percent, so residual coefficient was .80. Thirty-one percent of the variance in ideation (5 SBC) is explained by the model, so the residual coefficient was .83, and 14 percent of the variance in *jiggasha*/FWA communication is explained by the model, so its residual coefficient is .93.

Chapter 8

Planning for Continuity

SCALING UP

Lesson 1.   Planning for continuity begins with a review of changing environments and an analysis of how ongoing programs can adapt to these changes.

Lesson 2.   Follow-on programs should be designed to scale up successful activities and programs.

Lesson 3.   Follow-on programs should apply and benefit from the lessons learned in pilot projects.

Lesson 4.   The mistakes of the past provide guidance for the future.

SUSTAINABILITY

Lesson 5.   Financing for follow-on programs must be identified early in the review and planning process.

Lesson 6.   Planning a follow-on project must consider cost-effectiveness and sustainability.

Lesson 7.   Building broader coalitions and promoting a wider range of services can enhance sustainability.

Communication is an ongoing process, not a onetime effort. Just as individuals talk to one another continually and businesses advertise their products over and over again, so also health communication needs to be continuous.

Continuity is important for many reasons. First, repetition per se is a fundamental part of learning, since few people remember a onetime message. Second, there are many different audiences to be reached, from adolescents to in-laws, health care providers to policy-makers. Different audiences are best reached through a series of different materials, messages, and campaigns, phased in over time. Third, different people move through the steps to behavior change at different speeds, and therefore a single, onetime message will not influence an entire audience, even if everyone is exposed to it. Fourth, people's circumstances and needs change over the years—and thus their receptivity to family planning messages changes; the messages should be there when people grow ready for them. Fifth, over the years new people enter their reproductive years, while others leave. Sixth, continuity allows programs to expand, scaling up from pilot projects to regional or national efforts. Seventh, continuity creates opportunities for sustainability, by permitting program managers to seek additional support for programs and events that have proved popular. Finally, with continuity, program managers can apply the lessons learned from the past to improve and expand future efforts.

Without communication, the impact of health communication is much diminished. As the evaluation of the Pro-Pater mass media promotion illustrated (see Figure 7.2, in Chapter 7), interest in vasectomy peaked during each campaign. Although interest remained higher after each campaign than before, it dropped when promotion ended.

Planning for continuity is therefore important to link past experience with present and future needs. This planning can help communication programs scale up to meet the growing needs of ever-larger populations. In the process, planning for continuity can enhance the overall quality and impact of health communication.

SCALING UP

LESSON 1.

Planning for continuity begins with a review of changing environments and an analysis of how ongoing programs can adapt to these changes.

Plans for follow-on communication programs should begin, like the initial program, with a review or analysis of current policies, programs, audiences, and options to see how they may have changed over the life of the initial program. Overall, major changes have occurred in the last decade. For example, on the policy level, the 1994 International Conference on Population and Development in Cairo emphasized the broad field of reproductive health, including HIV/AIDS, STDs, safe motherhood, and the empowerment of women (Alcalá, 1995). On the program level, contraceptives such as injectables and Norplant subdermal implants are becoming more readily available. Moreover, many programs have improved their ability to deliver good-quality services. Intended audiences are both expanding—for example, to include younger people at risk and men—and at the same time becoming more segmented, to focus on specific subgroups such as women who have an identified unmet need for family planning or those who intend to adopt family planning in the future. Finally, the spread of communication technologies, especially radio and television, has created new opportunities to influence community norms and stimulate informed individual choices.

In addition to these global changes, the policy environment in many countries has changed, usually in a manner favorable to voluntary family planning programs. For example, a new president elected in Bolivia in 1993 made it possible to transform a low-key, mainly private-sector reproductive health communication initiative into a national program with much more government leadership and support, first from the Minister of Health and then from the vice-president. In the Philippines, a popular president elected in 1992 and a strong Minister of Health were willing to promote reproductive health and family planning issues more vigorously than their predecessors, despite continuing resistance from the Catholic Church. Thus, while Juan Flavier was Minister of Health, a major new outreach campaign was developed.

Audiences, too, evolve, and new ones emerge. In part because of past and current health communication campaigns, people are progressing continuously through the steps to behavior change from awareness to action. In countries as diverse as Egypt and Ghana, communication campaigns have shifted emphasis from awareness of family planning, which is now close to 100 percent among married women of reproductive age (El-Zanaty et al., 1996; Ghana Statistical Service [GSS] & Macro International, Inc. [MI], 1994), to promotion of specific facilities where family planning services or specific methods are available. Behavior change is now an openly acknowledged objective. The use of logos to identify facilities where people can take action as a result of their new knowledge and attitudes is now a key program element in countries as different as Bolivia, Burkina Faso, Egypt, Ghana, Indonesia, Mexico, Nigeria, Peru, Tanzania, and Uganda (see Chapter 4, Lesson 15).

Finally, the nature of health programs, and especially family planning and reproductive health programs, is changing worldwide. Both donor agencies and national governments are developing comprehensive country strategies that seek to integrate training, supplies, management, service delivery, and communication in coherent packages or frameworks. These involve, for example, new links between public- and private-sector programs, pre-service and in-service training, and suppliers of contraceptives and other commodities. Communication strategies will need to find their own specific niche within these overall strategies, a niche broad enough to include both the aggressive marketing tactics of social marketers and pharmaceutical companies and the concern for informed choice, quality, and access among service providers. Communication programs for behavior change, as contrasted with communication projects designed to produce pamphlets, brochures, or mass media advertising, can play an important part in national health strategies—but only if both communication experts and health leaders recognize the full potential of strategic health communication.

A comprehensive example of how public health officials can review changing environments and redesign communication projects to respond to new opportunities can be found in Burkina Faso. The Ministry of Health and Social Action and Population Communication Services cooperated for 10 years on an effort to promote use of modern family planning. In the early 1990s they sought to reinvigorate and refocus efforts on the basis of experience, the results of recent household surveys, and the changing policy environment. The adjustments made were tantamount to a total overhaul of the project, with major changes in six areas:

- With awareness of family planning now widespread, program managers decided that messages meant to increase knowledge of family planning were no longer needed. Instead, they concentrated on creating messages to encourage Burkinabes to take action—for example, to talk with their spouses about family planning or to visit a clinic.
- Because Burkinabes had proved to be especially receptive to family planning messages aired on radio and television, program managers placed new emphasis on broadcast media. For example, a theater troupe that successfully conveyed family planning messages in live performances during earlier campaigns now had their performances taped for broadcast.
- Three groups with limited awareness of family planning—youth, the less educated, and Muslims—were identified as new audiences. The shift to broadcast media would help reach these groups. For example, less-educated women and men would benefit more from radio programs than from print materials.
- Most Burkinabes were still familiar with only one family planning method: the Pill. To inform people about a wider range of family planning methods that were becoming available, project managers decided to reprint more leaflets about multiple methods.
- While a large proportion of Burkinabes now approved of family planning, most continued to believe that their partners disapproved. So the program encouraged spouses and other sexual partners to talk with one another, an important step in the process of behavior change. It particularly encouraged the involvement of men by distributing posters that showed couples discussing family planning and by airing broadcasts designed to interest men.
- Data showed that most adults had seen the project logo, but few understood its link to family planning. Managers therefore decided to place new emphasis on the logo, printing it on bags, key chains, and other objects. The project also sponsored theatrical performances promoting the logo as the national family planning symbol.

LESSON 2.

Follow-on programs should be designed to scale up successful activities and programs.

Unless review and analysis suggest a need for radical changes, follow-on programs should reinforce and expand ongoing programs. This reinforcement or expansion can take different forms—increasing the volume of current activities, expanding from urban and peri-urban to rural areas, moving into other geographic regions, or adding new program elements. Identifying and meeting unmet communication needs should have high priority. Basically, continuity should involve scaling up—that is, transforming initial projects into larger programs that can have greater impact, usually at a lower cost per person reached and over a longer period.

Some of the most effective follow-on communication programs have simply extended earlier accomplishments, recognizing that providing more of the same often makes sense. Since dissemination is often short-changed, especially when funds are limited, reprinting and distributing existing materials in larger volume can be both useful and cost-effective in follow-on projects. In Cameroon, for example, a logo and a campaign slogan, *Le signe de bonheur* (The sign of happiness), were developed in 1992 during the second phase of the Cameroon Child-Spacing project. During the third phase, the project was expanded. Planners wanted to encourage potential clients to seek services. A major effort was made to disseminate the logo and slogan more widely, first doubling and then tripling the number of clinic signs, billboards, posters, and television and radio spots featuring them (JHU/PCS, 1994g). While the materials were essentially the same, plans for the follow-on project were detailed and specific about using additional mass media to reach urban audiences and involving existing women's community groups (tontines) to reach semi-urban and low-income women. In Tanzania a radio soap opera heard by 22 percent of the population during its first year was extended for another year. Also, the Green Star Tanzania family planning logo, designed for the first phase of the project, was reprinted for display on additional billboards and clinic facilities in the second phase. In each case, personnel who played a major role in designing and implementing the initial projects provided continuity by playing a key role in the expansion.

Expanding geographically can be an important goal of follow-on efforts. Many other examples can be cited. In Ghana, for example, health communication campaigns that began in just three regions were expanded to cover six additional regions (Ghana MOH/HEU & JHU/PCS, 1993a). In India, the training and promotion of members of the Indian Medical Association initiated in Gujarat State are now being replicated in the larger state of Uttar Pradesh. In Nigeria, where traditional dramas performed by local artists and followed by question-and-answer sessions proved popular in Benue State, a follow-on project replicated this approach in other state programs. In both Benue and Ogun States, attendance at local clinics increased after these performances (Babalola et al., 1993; Kiragu, Zhang, et al., 1994). In Latin America, second-phase programs moved from urban areas to rural areas in Bolivia, Mexico, and Peru.

In some programs, contraceptive use will increase for a time and then level off, or plateau. What can health communication do to rejuvenate family planning programs when they reach plateaus? There are several possible solutions, not mutually exclusive. One is to improve the performance of existing activities, by upgrading the quality of communication as well as services and by removing policy and program barriers to improve access. Another approach is to add new elements:

a new method of contraception, a new type of provider, or a new form of promotion. Promoting new contraceptive methods is a major feature of new communication projects in Nepal, for example. In the past the major method in Nepal was voluntary sterilization. This served the needs of women who wanted no more children but did not serve women who wished to space births. Therefore promotion of temporary methods, such as pills, injectables, and even IUDs, became the focus of a follow-on communication project while providers continued to provide long-term methods as appropriate. In Ghana, a new form of provider was developed. Literacy facilitators were trained to become community-based distributors of various contraceptives. Already part of the community, they easily assumed this new task and welcomed the radio and press publicity that accompanied it (Institute for Adult Education, University of Ghana & JHU/CCP, 1995).

LESSON 3.

Follow-on programs should apply and benefit from the lessons learned in pilot projects.

Planning for continuity means planning for continuous improvement, based on lessons learned from smaller pilot projects. Many communication programs start on a fairly small scale. At that level, research-based efforts that pay attention to audience reactions can determine what works best and what adjustments may be needed when scaling up to a larger program.

The Minya Initiative, the governorate-level community mobilization project in upper Egypt, taught several major lessons that are being applied in follow-on activities (Kemprecos et al., 1994). These lessons emphasize the importance of:

- geographic concentration,
- time concentration,
- clear focus on audience needs and concerns, and
- coordination among agencies.

Geographic concentration. The success of the Minya Initiative attests to the wisdom of concentrating efforts in one geographic region at a time. Contraceptive prevalence rates in Minya in 1992 were low (21.9 percent) relative to the overall rate in Egypt (47 percent) but increased significantly, to 30.2 percent, during the 11 months of the project (Kemprecos et al., 1994). This lesson is being used in the Select Village Initiative, which concentrates on rural Egyptian villages with low use rates rather than on rural Egypt as a whole. While the original plan was to add 50 villages to the project every six months, it soon became clear that such a pace would allow neither adequate resources for the newly involved villages nor an effective level of follow-on activities in existing Select Villages to sustain increased use rates. Therefore the decision was made to reduce the pace of expansion to new villages and instead to concentrate follow-on community mobilization activities in the existing Select Villages.

Time concentration. "Health Weeks," five-day community mobilization campaigns implemented in the Minya governorate, demonstrated that concentrating activities in a short time period can attract the most attention and foster a high demand for family planning services. Therefore the Select Village Initiative adopted this approach. A similar approach is being used in Morocco, with two well-publicized family planning weeks each year.

Focus on audience needs. To reach the most underserved audiences—that is, those living farthest from the capital city—specific follow-on strategies in Minya included training and supervision of female outreach workers and creation of more mobile teams to work in remote areas. Emphasis was placed on the type of community meetings that had proved most effective: for women, clinic meetings, because family planning services were offered afterward; for men, Enter-Educate events and village meetings. Specific messages were used to counter the most prevalent rumors and misinformation. For example, messages emphasized that a woman can become pregnant while breastfeeding and that modern contraceptives do not cause sterility.

Coordination among agencies. In the Minya Initiative the Ministry of Health and Population and the State Information Service worked in tandem to create teams that included female physicians and communication specialists. These teams conducted joint meetings in village clinics, with family planning services available immediately afterwards. Joint meetings are now common practice in the Select Village Initiative.

Coordination among agencies has become even closer in Egypt's new Quality Improvement Project (QIP). The project is carried out jointly by the Ministry of Health and Population, through the training of providers and strict adherence to quality indicators at the clinic level, and by the State Information Service, promoting the Gold Star logo through mass media and community mobilization (see Chapter 4, Lesson 5). These communication activities are intended to direct potential clients to services offered by the newly improved, high-quality clinics.

LESSON 4.

The mistakes of the past provide guidance for the future.

Admitting failure is difficult when evaluating projects, but it is invaluable to planning future activities. In many cases the best prospect for achieving greater impact in the future comes from looking specifically for the causes behind disappointments in the first round. Among communication programs, one example of a problem that was specifically taken into account for future programs comes from the Ghana family planning promotion campaign. While the first project in Ghana expanded use of contraception, use of oral contraceptives fell sharply midway through the campaign. As noted (Chapter 4, Lesson 8), evaluation revealed that contraceptive supplies in Ministry of Health clinics were not adequate to meet the demand generated by the campaign. Thus, the stock of oral contraceptives plummeted at a time when campaign activities were still at a high level. The follow-on Ghana program made specific plans to avoid stock-outs during future campaigns through closer coordination between the logistics and communication efforts.

Another project that had limited impact was a radio soap opera on AIDS in Zambia. Designed to encourage condom use and discourage sexual relations with multiple partners, the project was hampered by problems with logistics and coordination with other AIDS-prevention activities throughout Zambia. As a result, the radio drama—a single effort rather than part of an integrated campaign—influenced knowledge and attitudes, but it did not significantly influence men's condom use, although it did encourage women to reduce their number of partners (Yoder, Hornick, & Chirwa, 1996). The impact was greatest among those who listened most often to the drama (Valente, 1996b). The lesson was clear: a single, freestanding show not supported by grassroots community mobilization activities or other forms of social mobilization has a relatively small impact. In the follow-on Zambian project, a coordinated multimedia effort is planned. Reinforcing radio soap operas and other mass media entertainment with additional promotion and community activities is now standard procedure for Population Communication Services.

SUSTAINABILITY

LESSON 5.

Financing for follow-on programs must be identified early in the review and planning process.

Like all other fields of development, health communication has a history of pilot projects that were to some degree successful but, for lack of funding, were never continued or expanded. There are many reasons for this lack of funding. Personnel changes can alter program direction. Some family planning communication programs operate for periods too short to allow the projects to become self-sustaining before the original momentum is lost. All donors prefer to support innovative, new projects rather than recurring costs, even in projects that have proved successful. Private donors and foundations often expect governments to take over support of innovative or research-oriented projects that their private money has initiated. Government donors sometimes face policy changes, such as the USAID decision in 1993 to close more than 20 overseas missions, that may curtail even the most successful projects. Government donors also face funding cuts resulting from internal economic or political problems. Finding follow-on funding for programs started by other donors requires considerable ingenuity and persuasion. Many developing-country project directors cannot easily undertake this task on their own.

Thus identifying resources to sustain future operations is a key step in planning follow-on programs. In countries where USAID support is relatively long-term, such as Bangladesh, Bolivia, Egypt, Indonesia, and the Philippines, communication programs have received continued support with which they could be expanded, revised, and improved with the benefit of experience. These programs continue to show appreciable impact. Similarly, projects carried out by family planning associations such as PROFAMILIA in Colombia, the Family Planning Association of Kenya, and the Planned Parenthood Federation of Nigeria, which receive continuing support from the International Planned Parenthood Federation, can compensate for shifts in funding by government donors. In contrast, mass media communication projects initiated by Population Communication Services were not continued in either Pakistan or Turkey as a result of changing policies by the major donor, despite their demonstrated impact on family planning knowledge, attitudes, and behavior. (One of the Turkey projects, the television series featuring a rural midwife, was taken up later independently by UNICEF, although without strong family planning messages) (Government of Turkey & UNICEF, 1991).

Many donors are more willing to support direct service delivery or commodities essential for program survival than to support communication, and especially mass media communication, which is still regarded in some quarters as an extravagance. Thus, when an original donor is not willing to support a communication effort over the long term, special effort, personal interventions, persistence, and a collaborative spirit are required to find other donors who will pick up ongoing costs. For example, in Cameroon, when USAID funding was cut off, the personal intervention of a key communication professional made it possible for the United Nations Population Fund (UNFPA) to continue much of the work begun with USAID funding. Where long-term support from a single donor seems unlikely, program officials need to pay special attention from the start to building links that can ultimately lead to support from other sources.

LESSON 6.

Planning a follow-on project must consider cost-effectiveness and sustainability.

While innovative health communication projects often cannot focus at the start on sustainability or revenue generation, follow-on projects must give additional attention to sustainability—that is, to the ability of the project to pay at least a part of recurring costs over the long term. Today, both governments and donors are putting increased emphasis on sustainability. In the field of health communication, emphasis on sustainability requires attention to five elements:

- free air time and news coverage,
- production of collateral material,
- commercial sponsorship,
- co-production, and
- cost-effectiveness.

Free air time and news coverage. Free air time and news coverage can contribute significantly to sustainability, especially when it is prime-time or front-page coverage. In the Enter-Educate projects in Mexico, Nigeria, and the Philippines, the value of free air time and press coverage alone amounted to between three and four times the production cost of the popular songs promoted. In Nigeria, for example, during the first six months after the two songs "Choices" and "Wait For Me" were launched, the value of the free air time amounted to US$325,000 compared with production costs of about US$43,118 (JHU/PCS, 1993f). Press coverage focusing on the relationship between singers King Sunny Adé and Onyeka Onwenu (a common rumor with celebrity performers) included front-page stories in papers and magazines. These stories generated sales and drew public attention to the songs. In Turkey both the television serial on a family migrating to the city, *Sparrows Don't Migrate*, and the minidrama on the rural midwife, *Hope Is Always There*, generated considerable news coverage. These dramas, plus video spots starring Turkey's top comedian, attracted prime-time news coverage not only because of the quality of the productions but also because of the celebrity status of the performers involved.

Collateral materials. When commercial or other sources provide collateral materials, communication projects can become more sustainable. For example, in the Philippine Multimedia Campaign for Young People, commercial firms such as Nike footwear, Pepsi-Cola, and Close-Up toothpaste produced posters, T-shirts, cue cards, and other materials in support of Lea Salonga's popular songs advocating responsible sexual behavior. The Philippine long-distance telephone company sponsored the Dial-A-Friend hotline to advise young people on boy-girl relationships and sexual issues at no cost to the project after the initial funding had expired (Rimon, Treiman, et al., 1994). This sponsorship, which began in August 1990, is still continuing after seven years (P. L. Coleman, personal communication, November 5, 1996).

Commercial sponsorship and co-production. In the long run, the most effective form of sustainability is for commercial firms to take over production, distribution, and sponsorship of the products or services launched initially by health promotion campaigns. A first step may be commercial sponsorship of a drama or serial. The underwriting of television soap operas such as *Simplemente Maria* in Peru, sponsored by the Singer Sewing Machine Company, and *Hum Log* in India, sponsored by Maggii Instant Noodles, is an example of the important role that commercial sponsorship can play in making Enter-Educate materials not just self-sustaining but even profitable for their sponsors (Noel-Nariman, 1993). Among recent Population Communication Services–assisted follow-on projects, local businesses have assumed some of the costs of health communication in Kenya, where Johnson & Johnson is contributing to continuation of the popular *Youth Variety Show*; Indonesia, where Indonesian Television and Radio in 1993 assumed half the production costs of the *Equatorial Trilogy* on environment and population, and a television station in 1995 assumed the full production costs of *Alang, Alang*, a full-length film about the importance of girls' education; and in Uganda, where a local newspaper paid the Family Planning Association to prepare a monthly supplement for youth called *Straight Talk*.

Co-production can be an effective way to share costs. In Bolivia a television series (Open Dialogue) was produced in partnership with the International Planned Parenthood Federation, the Center for Research, Education, and Services (CIES)—a local nongovernmental agency—and the National Secretariat of Gender. The series focused on gender and youth issues and was broadcast through the national television station. A commercial sales strategy built into the project design helped to defray broadcasting costs and generate revenue that offset some production costs (Saba, personal communication, November 12, 1996). Programs that include messages for young people are especially attractive to sponsors because young people are the most likely to become long-term consumers. Current Enter-Educate programs in many countries are seeking commercial sponsors, as well as other donors, to sustain their work.

In the long run, to the extent that manufacturers or service providers, such as pharmaceutical companies, private fee-for-service providers, and even various media channels, see a boost in sales of their products from popular health promotion programs, they will help to support these programs. Indeed, with effective initial promotion and marketing to potential sponsors, some health communication projects can become entirely self-sustaining.

Cost-effectiveness. Demonstrating cost-effectiveness is vital for follow-on projects. Many donors who are willing to support service delivery or grassroots organizations remain skeptical about the value of strategic communication. Thus it is important from the start to measure the overall cost of specific communication campaigns and activities and to calculate, from pre- and post-survey data or service statistics, the number of people reached and influenced by communication interventions. When it is possible to show that a large population can be reached with persuasive family planning messages at a small cost per person—as, for example, in the Zimbabwe male motivation campaign—a strong argument can be made for expanded use of the mass media (Piotrow, Kincaid, et al., 1992; Y. M. Kim, Marangwanda, & Kols, 1996) (see Table 4.1, in Chapter 4).

It is not easy to document the impact of a single health communication project on specific knowledge, attitudes, and behavior, but such findings, when based on objective and reliable data, become a powerful argument for continuation of communication activities. Such calculations are, of course, very common in the commercial sector, where marketers pay close attention to the sales return for every dollar expended on promotion. But they are much less common in the health field or among medical personnel. Even within the health field, much less attention is paid to returns from investment in communication than to returns from training, equipment, or other technical inputs.

LESSON 7.

Building broader coalitions and promoting a wider range of services can enhance sustainability.

Initial or pilot communication projects usually involve only a few organizations and address only one or two health issues. While limited objectives and a clear focus are helpful at the start, over time health communication projects need to scale up if they are to survive as full-fledged, continuing programs. In addition to expanded volume, greater geographic reach, and new program inputs, follow-on communication activities can also

* build larger coalitions to implement larger projects;
* integrate specific family planning promotion with promotion of other, related reproductive health activities; and
* cooperate with environmental and other concerned organizations.

Coalition-building. As pilot projects move to become larger programs, working with a coalition, rather than seeking to carry forward a project as a single institution, is almost always necessary. Even when, as in Bolivia, the government comes to assume a leadership role, the participation of other institutions and private-sector stakeholders is important. In Bolivia the original Technical Committee of 10 organizations more than doubled in size even as the Ministry of Health assumed a larger role. In Ghana the initial health and family planning information project began by forging partnerships with several other organizations, including the Ghana Registered Midwives Association, the National Audiovisual and Film Technical Institute (NAFTI), and the Planned Parenthood Federation of Ghana. These coalitions were further reinforced and expanded as the program extended nationwide.

The *jiggasha* project in Bangladesh was carried out initially by the Ministry of Health with Population Communication Services assistance. As recognition of its impact spread, other organizations, including Pathfinder International, expressed interest in replicating the project in other thanas. To carry out the project in these other areas, a broader coalition is being formed that involves not only support from other nongovernmental organizations but also support from other donors such as the World Bank and the United Nations Population Fund. Extensive training materials, including a six-part training video, were developed to help collaborating organizations train field workers. The training helps field workers communicate with women's groups and community networks as well as individual clients. Coalition-building, with the gradual inclusion of a growing number of different organizations, becomes more and more necessary as second- and third-generation communication projects expand their outreach to a wider area.

Integration of family planning and reproductive health promotion. Besides expanding the number of collaborating organizations, continuity can be enhanced by integrating other health messages with the original family planning messages.

Promoting safe motherhood, child survival, and HIV/AIDS prevention as well as family planning builds wider community, religious, and political support. Moreover, adding messages about other aspects of reproductive and sexual health to family planning messages not only attracts a wider clientele but also appeals to clients already using health facilities for other services. In Bangladesh, for example, the Green Umbrella logo publicizes the wide range of reproductive health services "under a single umbrella" in stationary facilities—prenatal and postnatal care, immunization, and other elements of maternal and child health as well as family planning.

For larger health facilities, the "Inreach" approach has been developed by AVSC International. It is designed to extend the reach of family planning promotion beyond clients who come expressly for family planning services to those who may come for child immunization, treatment of sexually transmitted diseases (STDs), or any other problems (Lynam, Dwyer, & Bradley, 1994). In this approach, family planning posters, brochures, and other client materials will be available from other services, where providers will refer clients to family planning units for counseling and supplies. While single-purpose health promotion projects and simple messages may be necessary to start a new program, as programs mature (in health communication as in service delivery), it makes good sense to add other components to attract a wider clientele at a lower cost per client. Which components to include, how to phase them in, and, for health communicators, how to promote them without overwhelming the audience with an information overload will be a continuing challenge.

Cooperation with environmental organizations. Moving beyond the issues of health service delivery, family planning programs have natural allies among agencies and individuals concerned with protecting the environment, preserving natural habitats, and ensuring sustainable agriculture and industry. In Guatemala, Population Communication Services helped the family planning association, APROFAM, to develop a regional video production center. The center then produced 10 five-minute videos on environment, population, and development issues. The videos were presented to the presidents of the Central American countries in 1989, who in turn showed their support by passing a resolution to create a Central American Commission for Environment and Development (JHU/PCS, 1989a). More of this type of collaboration can take place worldwide.

Another effective and appropriate way to cooperate with environmental organizations and to promote integrated reproductive health services is through Enter-Educate projects. Productions that begin with a focus on family planning issues can easily be extended to cover other health issues ranging from childhood accidents to STDs and environmental issues. The *Equatorial Trilogy* film series in Indonesia was co-sponsored by the Ministry of the Environment and emphasized increasing environmental degradation and population pressures as they affected poor families. In serial dramas, the need for continuing and complex plots creates a constant demand for new issues and for new dangers to be surmounted by the characters (role models) in the drama (de Fossard, 1997).

Thus planning for continuity must focus, much more than initial project development, on the potential for reaching larger audiences through closer relationships with other types of health services and related programs. Such an approach is, of course, not only cost-effective but also entirely consistent with the mandates of the 1994 International Conference on Population and Development to address a wide range of reproductive and environmental health issues.

Planning a new, expanded program essentially repeats all the steps of the initial program. While building on the initial analysis, follow-on projects still require a review of changing conditions, based on a sound evaluation of the impact of the original project. They require audience identification and segmentation, strategic design, specific guidance for implementation, vigilant monitoring, objective evaluation, and, more than ever, attention to sustainability.

Planning for programs to continue to scale up, to reflect changing policy priorities, to become more cost-effective over time, and to play a strategic role in comprehensive national reproductive health strategies is the last stage in the P Process of communication program development.

Chapter 9

Challenges and Opportunities for the 21st Century

Family planning programs have made great progress since the government of India announced the first national program in 1952 (Mauldin & Sinding, 1993; Rogers, 1973; Ross & Mauldin, 1996). By September 1994, the time of the International Conference on Population and Development in Cairo, 168 governments had national population policies and some form of family planning program (UNFPA, 1995). Moreover, total fertility rates in the developing world have declined from an average of 6 children per woman in the 1970s to 3.4 in 1997, in large part thanks to those national family planning programs (Population Reference Bureau, 1997; UNFPA, 1995).

Family planning communication also has made great progress (see Chapter 1). A practice that was once too private to discuss—except perhaps with one's personal physician or a nurse (and occasionally within the family)—is now regularly publicized in mass media news, feature stories, and entertainment, and openly discussed among friends. Family planning communication, once mainly simple brochures and flipcharts to supplement lectures and counseling, now encompasses national communication strategies for multimedia promotion of reproductive health—strategies that combine the reach of the mass media, the immediacy of interpersonal communication, and the social influence of community action. Once limited to the objective of increasing awareness of contraceptive methods, communication now aims to spread new community norms and encourage new individual behavior. Once concentrated on meeting targets for numbers of new acceptors, family planning communication now focuses on enabling informed individual choice. Once an ad hoc "let's-print-a-poster" approach, family planning communication programs now follow a tested, step-by-step process that is goal-oriented, audience-focused, systematic, and responsive to feedback. Once an appendage of service delivery, family planning and reproductive health communication has matured as a discipline of its own, with scientific theory influencing program design and with program experience, in turn, stimulating the evolution of theory. Overall, communication has become a more prominent, more scientific, and a more strategic component in family planning and reproductive health programs. Indeed, health communication has progressed so much that now it can be a steering wheel for family planning programs rather than a spare wheel (see Chapter 4, Strategic Design).

With adequate funding and priority, progress will continue. The next decades will see continuing rapid demographic, political, and technological change. As they have over the last several decades, family planning and reproductive health communication programs will adapt to:

- changing audiences,
- changing channels of communication,
- changing behavioral science theory and research,
- changing values and mandates,
- changing organizational structures, and
- changing political environments and resources.

Many of these changes are interrelated, creating a new context for future family planning and other public health programs.

CHANGING AUDIENCES

Audiences for reproductive health communication will be changing demographically in at least three important respects: size, age structure, and location. In some countries there may be other changes as well—in religious and ethnic composition, in literacy, in employment, in economic status. Many of these changes will be substantial.

Size. Population size will increase massively, from about 5.84 billion in 1997 to over 8.036 billion in the year 2025—unless there is a dramatic shift in current trends. About 98 percent of this expected increase will take place in the developing countries of Asia, Africa, Latin America, and the Near East (PRB, 1996 & 1997).

This expected increase is the result of demographic momentum, of course—the large number of births that occurred 15 to 30 years ago, before family planning programs achieved their present strength, offspring of the large number of parents who were themselves born before programs had even started. As a result, up to 40 percent of the population in developing countries is still under age 15 and, although not yet having children of their own, soon will be. By the year 2025 there will probably be about 3.6 billion men and women of reproductive age (15 to 44) in the developing world compared with 2.4 billion in 1995 (UN, 1994; Center for International Research/Bureau of the Census, 1994).

To reach and serve such a large population will require massive new communication programs—hundreds of millions of additional sessions for counseling and other forms of interpersonal communication, millions of copies of print materials, and a whole array of new mass media programming, community activities, and training programs. As the audience grows in numbers, only efficient, large-scale approaches and popular, easily replicable community activities are likely to have impact sufficient to meet the need.

Age structure. The most notable change in the age structure worldwide is the increasing proportion of young people in the population. As of 1995, one person in every five was between the ages of 15 and 24 (UN, 1995a). These young people are now somewhere on the way from virginity to parenthood. Two patterns are clear:

• In much of the world, both developing and developed, more young people are postponing marriage and engaging in sex before marriage.
• When they have sex, many are not protecting themselves from pregnancy or sexually transmitted diseases (McCauley & Salter, 1995).

For example, the Young Adult Reproductive Health Surveys, conducted in Costa Rica, Haiti, Jamaica, and 10 cities in five other Latin American countries since 1985, found that 30 to 75 percent of boys ages 15 to 19 had engaged in sex before marriage, as had 12 to 59 percent of girls in the same age range. Among these youths, as many as 30 percent of boys and 40 percent of girls had used no contraceptive the first time they had sex (Morris, 1992). Similarly, in Kenya, surveys of 13- to 16-year-olds found that nearly half of these adolescent boys and more than one-fifth of the girls were sexually active. Fewer than half of the young women having intercourse had ever used contraceptives, and fewer than one-third had used contraceptives in their most recent sexual encounters (Kiragu, 1991). The consequences? More than 10,000 young Kenyan girls are expelled from school each year because they are pregnant (Ferguson, Gitonga, & Kibira, 1988). These patterns are repeated, to differing degrees, in much of the world.

What does this mean for family planning communication? Clearly, no audience gets more conflicting and confusing messages about sex—from peers, parents, and the mass media—or at so crucial a time, when the behavior patterns of a lifetime are taking form (McCauley & Salter, 1995). Thus a major challenge is competing successfully with so many and such conflicting messages. Successes with young audiences on three continents suggest that Enter-Educate approaches will offer some of the best opportunities.

A further challenge is how to segment the potential audiences effectively. Those audiences include the adults who serve as gatekeepers, the young people who are already sexually active and need practical advice, and the young people—usually even younger—who are not yet sexually active and need to know how to avoid sex until they are ready. In other words, programs will need to create messages that adults find acceptable and young people in different situations find relevant (McCauley & Salter, 1995).

Location. People will be in different places in the 21st century—sometimes easier to reach, sometimes harder. As the 21st century begins, more people will be living in urban and peri-urban areas. By the year 2025, 61 percent of the global population is expected to live in urban and peri-urban areas, compared with just under 45 percent in 1994. The move to the cities is fastest in developing countries. In these countries city dwellers accounted for 37 percent of the population in 1994. They are expected to account for 57 percent in 2025 (UN, 1995a & 1995b).

Also, people are becoming more mobile. Not only does increasing urbanization involve more rural to urban movement, but it involves more return visits to rural home areas. More people are traveling long distances for work, too, living apart from their spouses for months at a time. International migration is increasing, stimulated by the need for labor on the part of the developed countries and the desire for better jobs on the part of ambitious developing-country populations. At the same time, ethnic and religious conflicts, often aggravated by rapid population growth, are creating millions of refugees around the world, in camps, on the move, or settling temporarily in new places.

These changes in the distribution of populations—and especially among young people, who are often the first to migrate—will pose new challenges for all forms of health communication. Mobile populations are hard to reach and hard to provide with continuing services. Political backlash, especially against international migrants, may limit the family planning, health education, and other preventive services that they most need in the long run. Migrants may not know about services in new areas or may not qualify for them immediately. In urban areas some forms of communication will reach even more people—large meetings, television, telephones, and other electronic media—but more communication may be with strangers or other new and therefore less credible sources. Providing credible information and recognizing the unique needs of refugees, migrants, and recent arrivals will create both challenges and opportunities.

CHANGING CHANNELS OF COMMUNICATION

Among the most conspicuous challenges to health communication will be the changes in the channels of communication themselves. The world is undergoing a communication revolution. Publications, radio, and television are now reaching billions of people around the world in what is increasingly a global communication network and market. U.S. magazines are read around the world. Latin American soap operas attract fans in Asia and eastern Europe. Music blending styles from all regions of the world now sells throughout the Western Hemisphere as World Beat music. Millions of households across the globe, in countries as different as India and Cameroon, suddenly have direct, unrestricted access to radio and television broadcasts as local entrepreneurs build satellite dishes and set up neighborhood cable transmission (Aldhous, 1995). Databases, accessible via the Internet or on

CD-ROM, may replace libraries or go where no libraries eve
linked an estimated 8.5 million people at the end of 1995. '
doubled in 1996, reaching 19 million, and the rate of inc
(E-Land, 1996). The world has moved from print space to
within a few decades. Especially for pacesetters and infl
telecommunications technology and computers may bypass ь
communication just as airplanes have bypassed railroads.

By the year 2000, television receivers, virtually nonexistent in the developing world in 1965, will number 2 billion. In fact, in the five-year period between 1995 to 2000, the number of radio and television receivers in these countries is projected to double (see Figure 1.1, in Chapter 1). Low incomes may not stand in the way, as families give priority to consumer goods and entertainment and consumer credit systems expand to meet and fuel consumer demand.

All this new access to information revolutionizes the way many people communicate, forging direct links among groups and individuals on a scale never before conceived. For example, doctors in China, mystified by a dying woman's illness, posted her symptoms on the Internet and put out a general call for advice to hospitals around the world. Within the same day a U.S. doctor sent the correct diagnosis, and it was confirmed by 80 other doctors from different parts of the world (Gunby, 1995).

As more channels of communication become available, audiences will have more choices for information gathering and information sharing. Thus health communicators will have to work harder to attract audiences' attention. At the same time, the growing number of channels means that messages can be more easily addressed to specific audience segments. In radio and television programming, this practice is now referred to as "narrowcasting," in contrast to "broadcasting." For health communicators, this increasing self-segmentation creates a need for more diverse materials or productions. There will also be more misinformation circulating, as the ability to broadcast messages, as well as to receive them, comes to more and more people. Thus health communication will have to correct and explain more than ever, and more effectively, to anticipate and preempt rumor through aggressive public information campaigns.

Of course, access to electronic information is not equal. Some governments or commercial firms will try to restrict access; others will try to monopolize access. Furthermore, the gap in access to information between rich and poor will widen, at least until cheap new user hardware becomes available. Since those with the greatest need for public health services will have the least access, health professionals and policy-makers will have to serve as their advocates on issues of communication policy, technology, and infrastructure development.

Already, greater access to information and new ideas is inspiring clients to ask for health services and information that they never knew existed before and to expect more from health care providers. Family planning communicators are beginning to encourage this budding consumerism as a path to informed choice and a way to inspire the performance of service providers. At the same time, they are ning service providers to respond to this demand with more service-oriented attitudes and better quality of care.

For training, new communication technologies will reach further and yet be more personal. Distance-learning technologies, from live teleconferencing to self-paced tutorials on CD-ROM or the Internet, will make the best instructors and the best instructional methods available across the globe. At the same time, they will offer the student more interaction than is possible even in the conventional classroom. Interactive computer software such as Johns Hopkins' SCOPE combines "high tech" with "high touch" to enable trainees to participate directly with their colleagues and mentors in developing communication strategies and messages (see Box 6.2, in Chapter 6).

As new technologies and new approaches to communication create new expectations, both mass media and client-provider communication will need to become more participatory, more engaging, and less didactic. The audiences of the future will want—and expect—communication to be a dialogue, not a lecture.

CHANGING BEHAVIORAL SCIENCE THEORY AND RESEARCH

Even as health communication recognizes the importance of theory (see Chapter 2), some of the theoretical models of communication and behavior change are being modified. Major theoretical issues facing designers, managers, and evaluators of health communication programs include the following:

- How can intended audiences best be segmented?
- How can entertainment—whether in the media or live—be used more effectively for educational purposes?
- What are the most appropriate units of analysis—individuals, couples, client-provider pairs, or communities?
- How can time and change be taken into account?
- Can a community's research empower the community?

Audience segmentation. Although audience segmentation is an established principle in marketing and advertising (see Chapter 3), the bases for segmentation keep evolving. As discussed in Chapters 2 and 4, beyond simple demographic variables such as age and sex, or geographic variables, the most common bases for audience segmentation are stages of behavior change—knowledge, approval, intention, practice, and advocacy. Recently, however, some theorists have suggested that addressing individual traits of character and personality, such as self-esteem, willingness to take risks, and perceived self-efficacy, may be more important—a more powerful way to segment audiences and develop messages (Novelli, 1988). One result is psychographic profiles. These profiles often address propensity to change, contrasting innovators with traditionalists, for example. The power of these two approaches to segmentation suggests that the next step is combining the two to understand the differing dynamics of change in different personality types.

Entertainment for health education. Why is entertainment such a good way to communicate social messages? A variety of viewpoints contribute to our understanding, from Bandura's social learning theory (Bandura, 1977, 1986, & 1995) through the historical—and, no doubt, prehistorical—reliance of all cultures on storytelling and performance arts to transmit social values (Bruner, 1990; Burke, 1945; W. R. Fisher, 1987; Goffman, 1974; V. Turner, 1982) to experimental evidence that release of adrenaline and noradrenaline, triggered by emotional events in a story, enhances memory of those events (Cahill et al., 1994). Better synthesis of these varying viewpoints would improve the ability to communicate messages that will help people adopt healthier behavior.

Units of analysis. Western society usually considers the individual to be the primary unit of decision-making and thus of analysis. But in other cultures—and perhaps in the West more than is recognized—the decision-making unit often is not an individual but a couple, extended family, or social group, especially for family and reproductive decisions (Kincaid, 1987). Already communication programs are putting more emphasis on stimulating male involvement and improving communication between sexual partners. Researchers will want to focus on the dynamics of decision-making at the level of the couple, the extended family, and even the community.

In both Western societies and developing countries, new research suggests that perceived community norms—that is, what people think other people expect them to do—may influence their behavior more than knowledge of reproductive physiology and contraception (Fishbein & Ajzen, 1975; Rogers & Kincaid, 1981; Saba et al., 1994). As research in Bangladesh suggests, community norms about family planning may be so strong that an entire village could be described as practicing—or not practicing—family planning (see Chapter 7, Lesson 9). In other words, what one researcher might describe as individual behavior, another might describe as community or group behavior. Network analysis, drawing upon early research on diffusion of innovations, offers new ways to determine who, within any community, informs and influences whom about what kinds of behavior (Valente, 1995).

Accounting for time and change. Nesselroad and Hershberger (1993) describe research as defined in three dimensions: persons, content, and occasions (i.e., time). If one is emphasized, the others usually must be curtailed. Thus sociologists and demographers, interested in "persons"—that is, the characteristics of large populations—conduct surveys of thousands of people. Usually limited to at most a one-hour interview with each respondent, they sacrifice depth for breadth. In contrast, anthropologists and psychologists are concerned more with "content," seeking a depth of knowledge about persons and their culture. Spending more time with each person, they observe or measure more variables, but they sacrifice sample size and sometimes generalizability to larger populations. None of these disciplines, however, has paid much attention to change over time, although new methods for research and analysis have emerged during the last 10 years (Diggle, Liang, & Zeger, 1994; Eerola, 1994; Finkel, 1995; Hagenaars, 1990).

Taking account of time is especially important to the study of fertility and family planning. Family planning behavior is a "complex adaptive process"—that is, most people go through a process of trying a method, discontinuing, and switching, interspersed with intended and often unintended pregnancies, as their lives change. Large cross-sectional surveys and short-term in-depth research do not reveal enough about this process or what influences its path.

Furthermore, recording the sequence of events is valuable for proving causality. Cause must precede effect. But this obvious truth hangs like a dark cloud over cross-sectional analysis: When a survey finds that discussion of family planning between spouses is associated with their use of family planning, are they discussing because they are using, or using because they are discussing? Knowing which came first would help. Until research methodologies can sort out the direction(s) of causality in large populations, skeptics will continue to question the role of organized communication and to cast doubt on the impact of specific programs.

Ultimately, research approaches that give us valid information on persons, context, *and* occasions will be needed to advance the understanding of communication and the measurement of its impact on behavior. For example, surveys can incorporate more "content" questions. Also, despite their difficulty, longitudinal studies are needed to follow people over years or to look in on them periodically.

Community research for community mobilization and local advocacy. Research in group dynamics finds that a group takes action when its members become dissatisfied with the gap between their current state and some moderate, feasible goal (Zander, 1971). As community members volunteer for and assign tasks to accomplish an agreed-upon goal in an agreed-upon time period, the community mobilizes to close the gap. But the community's first step toward change is to assess where they are and where they want to be.

Similarly, manufacturing plants in Japan have improved productivity by teaching assembly line workers elementary statistics and probability theory so they can monitor the quality and quantity of their own work (Walton, 1986). The workers then have responsibility for taking action if these indicators fall below standard—action that can range from making recommendations to shutting down the assembly line—and they receive a share of profits that reflect their work.

Together these two models suggest a locally controlled, self-motivated community approach to family planning and health improvement, in which community members conduct their own research on their own needs, set goals, take collective action, monitor changes over time, and assess the outcomes. For example, if hand-washing with soap in a greater and greater percentage of households can be shown to reduce the incidence of diarrhea, then the community will redouble its efforts to encourage hand-washing. No doubt all communities already conduct some monitoring of critical resources such as water supply, crop yield, or rainfall. If professional researchers are willing to give up control over the conduct of research, they can teach communities how to monitor more aspects of their own situation more effectively and more usefully. If many communities adopted this approach, outsiders would need only to collect data for each unit and aggregate it to report to government and international agencies. This decentralization of research offers a promising approach to community mobilization in family planning and other public health programs.

CHANGING VALUES AND MANDATES

In the 1980s family planning programs and related communication campaigns were charged with reducing high-risk fertility, stimulating informed choice of family size, and increasing the use of effective contraceptives. By the early 1990s concern over HIV/AIDS created a new demand for communication to encourage sexual responsibility, limiting the number of sexual partners, and using condoms regularly. To these mandates the 1994 International Conference on Population and Development in Cairo and the 1995 United Nations Fourth World Conference on Women in Beijing added more emphasis on quality of care, a broader definition of reproductive health (to include safe motherhood and protection from sexually transmitted disease), and more concern for the rights and well-being of women, including protection against domestic and political violence (UNFPA, 1995).

What might be the new mandates of the future? There are many different points of view. On one hand, some programs and health promotion strategies already implicitly or explicitly focus on meeting unmet need—addressing first the needs of those who are already motivated to space or limit pregnancies but for various reasons are not using family planning. On the other hand, some donors and other institutions are emphasizing long-term structural changes intended to increase motivation for smaller families, especially more education, employment, and other opportunities for women.

On one hand, many from a health and human services background emphasize the need to maximize access to services, to improve the quality of services, and to integrate family planning more closely with other maternal and child health services. On the other hand, some donors and economists are beginning to emphasize the need for sustainable programs, that is, programs that can begin paying for themselves as soon as possible—a major challenge for any preventive health service.

On one hand, many health workers see family planning as a way to improve maternal and child health and to reduce the incidence of abortion, while, on the other hand, some political and religious spokesmen see family planning organizations as the main advocates for abortion. They would cut back family planning programs, not recognizing that the result would be more unsafe abortions, with all their adverse health consequences.

Still, to paraphrase the American saying that "all politics is local politics," it is also true that "all health is personal health." This is especially so of reproductive health. Whatever the national goals or mandates, people usually act on the basis of their own personal needs and not on the basis of public health mandates. The challenge for public health communication will be to translate those broader mandates into specific benefits that appeal to individuals and families and that they in turn as advocates, will seek from their communities and governments.

CHANGING ORGANIZATIONAL STRUCTURES

Worldwide, a wave of decentralization and privatization is under way. Whereas governments once emphasized national programs either to foster nation-building or to create a social safety net within a welfare state, today many governments are turning away from highly centralized approaches. Whether driven by financial limitations or by declining confidence in large central institutions, more and more countries are encouraging local government units, community-based nongovernmental organizations, and commercial firms to take over services that were once seen as central government responsibilities. This process is under way in places as different as Bolivia, Mexico, the Philippines, Uganda, Zimbabwe, much of the former Soviet Union, and the United States.

How will decentralization affect family planning programs and family planning communication? The first requirement will be to build effective local advocacy for family planning programs. Emphasis must shift away from advocacy for national policies, directed at national officials, and toward advocacy within communities and by local citizens, organized by grassroots leadership and directed at local officials; away from advocacy on behalf of others and toward advocacy for family planning for the benefit of one's community, family, and self; away from public advocacy exclusively for policy change and toward personal advocacy as the final step in behavior change. In other words, to change others, people may need to change themselves. In more decentralized systems, the people themselves will have to give family planning and reproductive health high priority and apply their own time, effort, and resources to ensure that the community provides services, or take action for themselves. To do this, people must appreciate the direct and personal benefits of family planning or any other health practice. The challenge for health promotion is clear: Messages must be even more immediate, attention-getting, personal, and convincing, and they must help people in the community to express their consensus that healthy practices are both accepted and expected.

A second requirement for effectively decentralizing communication programs will be more training for community, grassroots, and private-sector workers. Local government personnel, community activists, field workers, and private-sector employees will need to learn how to design and manage communication activities. Just as communities can collect, analyze, and take action based on their own research, communities can analyze local information needs, develop strategies, and carry out communication efforts.

Decentralization may also mean more privatization of communication functions. In the future, as mass media communication about health becomes increasingly welcome, and if incomes rise, many more people will buy their own health products. Commercial firms will also make more effort to advertise to them. Indeed, worldwide spending for advertising is increasing rapidly. Expressed in 1989 dollars, world expenditure on advertising grew from about $100 million in 1970 to $256 million in 1990, an increase of more than 150 percent in 25 years (L. Brown, Kane, & Ayres, 1993). Advertising related to family planning and other reproductive health will be part of this trend. Advertising can position family planning products (social marketing) or health care providers (the PRO Approach) to fill various market niches. Advertising can use a global image, such as the Coca-Cola logo, to promote even the smallest retail store. And advertising can make the personal benefits of a product more appealing to consumers, thus increasing their willingness to buy.

Paradoxically, decentralization may bring not only more commercial activity but also more volunteer activism. In general, people, especially professionals, expect to be paid when they work at the national level, but they are much more likely to volunteer to help family, friends, and neighbors. To be effective at the local level, health communication programs will have to recruit more volunteers and mobilize them for campaigns and promotion—as has been done in Egypt, Ghana, Indonesia, Zimbabwe, and elsewhere.

Finally, to be most effective, communicators in decentralized programs will need to link local needs and events with the rest of the world, which now impinges so deeply on people's daily lives through the mass media. Health communication programs can take a local event, such as a school health drama contest, and broadcast it nationally or even internationally. Conversely, good managers can take an international event, such as the World Cup Soccer Tournament, and transform the national "Dream Team" into role models of responsible behavior for local athletes and young people. Although the world is becoming a global village, people will still follow the "village leaders" they know and trust personally.

CHANGING POLITICAL ENVIRONMENTS AND RESOURCES

As the 21st century nears, family planning programs may be approaching a financial crisis. More countries are implementing programs; more people want a wider variety of services; the number of potential clients is increasing; program objectives are expanding; technology is improving; and knowledge of how to design effective programs is growing. All this costs money. The Program of Action developed at the Cairo International Conference on Population and Development in 1994 called for US$17 billion in constant 1993 dollars by the year 2000 for population-related programs. About $10 billion would be needed for family planning alone. One-third—$5.7 billion—would come from donor countries, the rest from local governments and users (Conly, 1996). Yet, just as the magnitude of the need is being recognized, financial support for these programs may be diminishing. As a result, the high goals set in Cairo may be out of reach.

Why should funding for family planning and related programs fail to keep pace with the need when all evidence points to both the importance and the success of these efforts? A major threat is that donor nations may become more concerned with their own domestic deficits and social security. As these governments cut domestic social welfare programs, they may make comparable or even greater cuts in international development assistance, which already stands at a much lower level. This danger is real. The U.S. Congress cut more than one-third from U.S.

international population programs in 1996 and almost one-quarter from development assistance overall; Japan also has reduced its population assistance (Conly & Rosen, 1996; "Japan's ODA Growth," 1996).

At the same time, some of the developing countries with the highest population growth rates may be overwhelmed by their own immediate and interrelated domestic problems—social, economic, religious, and political—and unwilling to invest in long-term population programs. Many will not compensate for declines in donor funding. Some of the economically more advanced developing countries in East Asia, the Near East, and Latin America could provide more assistance through South-to-South programs. But will they?

There are at least four different ways in which better communication can maximize the impact of current resources and generate new ones over the next few decades:

• increasing the volume of clients using currently underutilized services,
• encouraging clients to pay for services,
• cost-sharing and generating revenue through Enter-Educate strategies, and
• expanding advocacy for family planning.

Increasing volume. Family planning and reproductive health services in many countries are underutilized. Strategic communication programs could encourage more use of these services, thus lowering unit cost, in numerous ways: Better promotion—including more open discussion of family planning benefits in the mass media and the community—could attract more clients; clients who come for one service could be referred to other services in the same facility; and satisfied clients can be mobilized to recruit new clients.

Moreover, many services could be demedicalized—that is, unnecessary medical barriers could be removed (Shelton, Angle, & Jacobstein, 1992). There is much to be learned from the business world about how to win more customers. Convenience is a major concern to most consumers, but medical services or health programs rarely consider patient convenience. Lessons and techniques learned from business can increase the flow of clients and improve efficiency. In particular, every business knows that it is more cost-effective to retain a current client, subscriber, or user than to recruit a new one. Family planning programs are beginning to recognize the importance of continuation rates and satisfied users, as the Philippine data show (see Chapter 7, Lesson 3 and Table 7.3). The next step will be to develop plans to improve continuation by meeting users' ongoing and changing needs and to assess the cost-effectiveness of alternative ways to do so.

Operations research in countries as different as Belize, Guyana, Ecuador, Zaire, and Indonesia suggests that better promotion, both in the community and within multipurpose health facilities themselves, can substantially increase the number of clients for family planning services (Ahmed, 1996; Bertrand, 1988; Buana et al., 1990; Gass & Barber-Madden, 1990; Mosley, personal communication, July 11, 1996). Likewise, promoting providers through the Blue Circle campaign in Indonesia, the Gold Star campaign in Egypt, and elsewhere shows that, where programs reach a plateau or the number of dropouts begins to equal the number of new users, strategically designed communication can make a difference.

Encouraging clients to pay for services. Faced with more demand and smaller subsidies, many family planning programs have instituted charges for their services and products. Indeed, social marketing experts have argued for years that, even aside from generating revenue, charging a small fee is a good idea: people appreciate a service or product more when they pay for it (Harvey, 1993, 1994, & 1996).

Experience shows that imposing a small charge for previously free services or raising the price slightly on health products does diminish use temporarily, but good promotion and sound positioning can minimize or in time overcome that drop. In the second Zimbabwe male motivation campaign, for example, energetic promotion helped to arrest the decline in contraceptive use that occurred in 1992 after government facilities imposed fees (Y. M. Kim, Marangwanda, & Kols, 1996). In the Bangladesh social marketing program, sharp increases in the price of condoms and pills reduced retail sales in 1990 but, with systematic promotion and some price rollbacks, the Population Services International program succeeded eventually in boosting both sales and revenue (Ciszewski & Harvey, 1991; Lande & Geller, 1991).

It is axiomatic that people who are sick will pay whatever they can for curative care, but healthy people will not pay for preventive care such as family planning—not unless they appreciate its immediate and important personal benefits. All too often in public health programs, however, the promotion and public education that can create that awareness are the first components to be cut when money is short, even though they might produce the higher volume of clients that would increase revenue and reduce unit costs. To communicate these benefits so that more people are willing to pay for them will be a major challenge for health communication and health financing in the coming years.

Sharing cost and generating revenue. If public funds for family planning and family planning promotion do not increase, new strategies to share costs and to generate revenue from other sources will be essential. One of the best ways to enlist new sources of support is the Enter-Educate approach (see Chapter 4, Lesson 12).

The strategy of incorporating health information into entertainment and products that consumers or sponsors will pay for is a win-win proposition. While making social messages popular, songs developed with help from Population Communication Services in Latin America, Nigeria, and the Philippines have generated free air time and press coverage worth several times the direct cost, while commercial firms contributed collateral material such as posters, cards, T-shirts, and hats. In fact, demonstrated success can inspire a commercial firm to take over supporting outreach efforts, as when the Philippine Long Distance Telephone Company provided support for the Dial-A-Friend telephone hotline long after support from Population Communication Services had ended (Rimon, Treiman, et al., 1994). Similarly, soap operas in Egypt, India, Indonesia, Kenya, Mexico, Nepal, the Philippines, Tanzania, the United States, Zambia, and Zimbabwe—in fact, almost everywhere—have conveyed important messages about family planning,

AIDS, immunization, women's empowerment, and other reproductive health issues. Whether created especially to tell a family planning or AIDS story or incorporating these themes into ongoing series, some of these soap operas have found commercial sponsorship (Kaiser Family Foundation, 1996). In fact, one of the first such soap operas, the Indian drama *Hum Log*, was also one of the first television programs in India with a commercial sponsor (Singhal & Rogers, 1989). In a time of limited resources, the potential is obvious: The ability of the Enter-Educate approach to draw large and young audiences at low cost per person reached can attract sponsors seeking name recognition and an opportunity to contribute to public welfare.

Expanding advocacy. The importance of reducing population growth and protecting health calls for more and better advocacy on behalf of family planning and reproductive health. To maintain or increase resources, advocacy, like other family planning and reproductive health communication, needs to be systematic and strategic; the lessons and processes outlined in this book will have to be applied to advocacy.

When it comes to arguing for resources, family planning and reproductive health programs should not have to stand alone. They are too important to overall health, to environmental protection, to women's progress, and to economic and social development. Partnerships and coalitions can be built with all those organizations and interests that stand to lose by continued rapid population growth and ill health. That number is massive. It includes all maternal and child health programs; educators trying to teach in overflowing classrooms; manufacturers who cannot sell products to customers too poor to buy; government officials trying to maintain services for ever-growing constituencies; scientists and conservationists working to prevent environmental degradation and conserve resources; job-seekers looking for a living wage—and many more. In fact, it can be argued that everyone stands to lose, that everyone will suffer unless population growth is checked and unwanted pregnancies avoided. Or, to put it positively, family planning helps everyone, and everyone should mobilize to support it.

Partnerships can take many forms, involving both nonprofit and commercial interests. Partnerships can include coalitions with shared interests such as women's groups, environmental organizations, and community activists. They can also include employer-funded health education and service programs, insurance plans that cover family planning, and schools that cover reproductive health as part of the curriculum. To cohere, such coalitions require reciprocity; family planning advocates owe their support in return to the causes of their coalition partners.

CONCLUSION

When national family planning programs began about 35 years ago, no one knew whether they could have any impact. When family planning communication programs began to assume a more distinct role some 20 years ago, no one knew what strategies would be effective or even acceptable. Even a decade and a half ago, when the Population Communication Services project began, no one knew what a national communication strategy was or how to combine mass media, community mobilization, and interpersonal communication synergistically to help people adopt healthier behavior.

Much has been learned about family planning and health communication in recent years, as this book has described. Many lessons from family planning communication apply to other fields of public health as well. HIV/AIDS prevention and control efforts also deal with reproductive health and with private, sexually motivated behavior (see Box 9.1). Child survival programs depend upon changing community norms—in diet, in home-based care, and in preventive measures such as immunization, for example—that in turn will prompt behavior change in every home. And safe motherhood programs, like family planning services, require a network of responsive, well informed, technically trained service providers with adequate supplies to meet immediate needs. Many public health programs depend on accurate information, communicated to the public as well as to providers in a sufficiently practical and memorable way that the knowledge will be used when

Box 9.1
Hits for Hope in Uganda

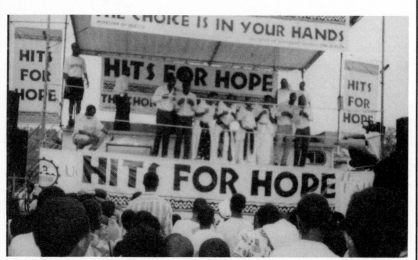

On a mobile stage in Uganda, amateur performers compete in Hits for Hope, a nationwide contest to choose a theme song for a national AIDS-prevention campaign. Organized by the IEC Division of the Delivery of Improved Services for Health (DISH) project, supported by USAID, Hits for Hope featured local contest finalists in each of seven districts in shows run by Group Africa, a firm that stages musical performances, sells time to sponsors, and stages its shows throughout the country. Thus the 1995 program combined entertainment, community participation, and commercial enterprise to take the AIDS-prevention message to the public.

needed. Thus the lessons learned from communication programs that are effective in changing reproductive health practices can well be applied to address the broad range of other behavioral or life-style health issues that the world will face in the 21st century.

But family planning and reproductive health are unique in the degree of commitment they require from individuals and couples in the face of powerful sexual urges and social customs. For millennia these urges and customs were advantageous to survival, but now they can be detrimental. To be effective in changing old practices, family planning communication about reproductive health must engage audiences at all times, must offer clear and compelling information, and, above all, must listen and respond to the personal needs of individuals and couples.

For the next few decades family planning communication will face many challenges. But with each challenge comes opportunity. With determination, professional skills, and, above all, a willingness to learn from experience, family planning and health communication programs will achieve their goal—to make family planning a household word, a community norm, and an informed individual choice for everyone.

Appendix: Organizations Collaborating with the Johns Hopkins Center for Communication Programs, 1982–1996

INTERNATIONAL AND US-BASED AGENCIES

Academy for Educational Development (AED)
Advocates for Youth
AIDS Public Health Communication Project (AIDSCOM)
Alan Guttmacher Institute
Annenberg School for Communication, University of Southern California
Asia Foundation
Australian International Development Associates Bureau
AVSC International
Basic Support for Institutionalizing Child Survival (BASICS)
CARE
Carolina Population Center, University of North Carolina
Center for Development and Population Activities (CEDPA)
Center for Health and Population Research (formerly ICDDR,Bangladesh)
Charles A. Dana Foundation
Columbia University, Center for Population and Family Health
Compton Foundation
Cowell Foundation
Demographic and Health Surveys (DHS) Project, Macro International
Development Associates, Inc.
Development through Self-Reliance, Inc. (DSR)

Dillon Fund
East-West Center
Educational Foundation of America
Ernie Petrich & Associates, Inc.
The EVALUATION Project/Carolina Population Center at the University of
    North Carolina, Chapel Hill
Family Health International (FHI)
Florida A & M University (FAMU)
Ford Foundation
The Futures Group International
Georgetown University, Institute for International Studies in Natural Family
    Planning
Helen Keller International
Hewlett Foundation
International Center for Diarrhoeal Disease Research (ICDDR)
International Development Research Center (IDRC)
International Planned Parenthood Federation (IPPF)/Western Hemisphere
    Region (WHR)
International Red Cross and Red Crescent Societies
International Science and Technology Institute (ISTI)
International Youth Foundation
INTRAH (Program for International Training in Health, University of North
    Carolina at Chapel Hill)
Japanese International Cooperation Agency (JICA)
Japanese Organization for International Cooperation in Family Planning
    (JOICFP)
JHPIEGO, Inc.
John Snow, Inc. Research and Training Institute
Kempner Fund
Levinson Foundation
Macro International/Demographic and Health Surveys
Management Sciences for Health (MSH)
Manoff International, Inc.
Margaret Sanger Center
Marie Stopes International
National Council on International Health (NCIH)
Near East Foundation
Omani-American Joint Commission
Options Project for Population Policy
Packard Foundation
Pan American Health Organization (PAHO)
Pathfinder International
Peace Corps
Peat, Marwick, Main and Company
Planned Parenthood Federation of America*

Population Communications International
Population Council
Population Initiatives for Peace
Population Reference Bureau (PRB)
Porter/Novelli Incorporated
Princeton University, Population Studies Center
The PROFIT Project, Deloitte Touche
Program for Appropriate Technology in Health (PATH)
Prospect International
Public Welfare Foundation
Research Triangle Institute
Rockefeller Foundation
Save the Children
Service Expansion and Technical Support (SEATS)/John Snow, Inc.
Social Marketing for Change (SOMARC)
United Nations Food and Agriculture Organization (FAO)
United Nations Children's Fund (UNICEF)
United Nations Education, Scientific, and Cultural Organization (UNESCO)
United Nations Population Fund (UNFPA)
United Nations World Health Organization (WHO)
United States Agency for International Development (USAID)
United States Bureau of the Census
United States Centers for Disease Control and Prevention (CDC)
University of Chicago, Community & Family Study Center
University of Michigan, International Population Fellows Program
University of New Mexico, Department of Communications and Journalism
University Research Corporation (URC)
Winslow Foundation
World Bank
World Learning
Worldview International Foundation

AFRICA

Africa—Regional

African Center for Professional Journalists and Communicators (Tunisia)
    (Centre Africain de Perfectionnement des Journalistes et Communicateurs
    —CAPJC)
Center for African Family Studies (CAFS), Nairobi, Kenya and Lomé, Togo
Center for Applied Research on Population and Development (Centre d'Etudes
    et de Recherche sur la Population et le Développement—CERPOD)
Economic Commission for Africa
Research International East Africa, Ltd. (RIEA) (Kenya)

Union of National Radio and Television Organizations of Africa (URTNA)
    (Kenya and Senegal)
USAID REDSO/ESA, Kenya
USAID REDSO/WCA, Côte d'Ivoire

Benin

Benin National Committee for Promotion of the Family

Burkina Faso

Burkinabè Midwives' Association (Association Burkinabè des Sages Femmes
    —ABSF)
Burkinabè Family Welfare Association (Association Burkinabè pour le Bien-
    Etre Familiar—ABBEF)
Burkina Faso Theater Workshop (Atelier-Théâtre Burkinabè—ATB)
Department for the Promotion of the Family, Ministry of Health and Social
Action (Direction de la Promotion de la Famille—DPF)
Department of Family Health, Ministry of Health and Social Action (Direction
    de la Santé Familiale)
Farmers' Self-Help Research and Support Group (Groupe de Recherche et
    d'Appai pour l'Auto-promotion Paysanne—GRAAP)
Horizon FM
Ministry of Social Action and the Status of Women (Ministère de l'Action
    Sociale et de la Condition Féminine, formerly part of the Ministry of Health)
National Health/IEC Center
National School of Social Work (Ecole Nationale des Services Sociaux—ENSS)
Radio Nationale Burkinabè
Télévision Nationale Burkinabè
Women and Health, Regional Station/West Africa (Projet Femmes et Santé,
    Antenne Régionale/Afrique de l'Ouest)
Women—Health—Development in Sub-Saharan Africa Associaiton
    (Association Femmes—Santé—Développement en Afrique Sub-saharienne
    —FESADE)
Zama Publicité

Cameroon

ABC Bikanda
Cameroon National Association of Family Welfare (CAMNAFAW)
Cameroon Radio and Television (CRTV)
Directorate of Family and Mental Health
Fondation Roger Milla et Felen
International Breastfeeding Association (IBFAN)
Luma Graphics

Soyoko Recording Studio
Women's Organization for Security and Development of Cameroon
(Organisation des Femmes pour la Sécurité et le Développement du
Cameroun)

Central African Republic

Ministry of Public Health and Social Affairs (Ministère de la Santé Publique et
des Affaires Sociales)

Chad

Maternal and Child Health/Family Well-Being Unit, Ministry of Public Health
(Ministère de la Santé Publique Cellule Santé Materno-Infantile/ Bien-Etre
Familial)
National Radio
Radio Sarh

Côte d'Ivoire

Center for Teaching and Research in Communication (Centre d'Enseignement et
de Recherche en Communication—CERCOM)
Côte d'Ivoire Radio and Television
Dialogue Productions
Ivorian Assoication for Family Welfare (Association Ivoirienne pour le Bien-
Etre Familial—AIBEF)
PANAFCOM

Ethiopia

Family Guidance Association of Ethiopia
National Office of Population/Ministry of Economic Development and
Cooperation

The Gambia

The Gambia Family Planning Association (GFPA)
Radio Gambia
Studio A Multi-Media Resources

Ghana

Apple Pie Publicity
DAPEG Advertising Agency
Ghana Broadcasting Corporation (GBC)

Ghana Home Sciences Association
Ghana Institute of Journalism (GIJ)
Ghana Institute of Management and Public Administration (GIMPA)
Ghana Ministry of Health/Health Education Unit (formerly Health Education
    Division)
Ghana Registered Midwives Association (GRMA)
Ghana Social Marketing Foundation (GSMF)
Lintas: Ghana Ltd.
Management Development and Productivity Institute
Media and Social Research Institute, Ltd. (MSRI)
National Film and Television Institute (NAFTI)
National Population Council (NPC)
Planned Parenthood Association of Ghana (PPAG)
Population Impact Project (PIP)
Research International
31st December Women's Movement
University of Ghana, Institute of Adult Education (IAE)

Kenya

ACE Communications, Ltd. (formerly Broadcast Productions, Ltd.)
African Medical and Research Foundation (AMREF)
Center for the Study of Adolescence (CSA)
Crawford Ellis Associates, Ltd.
Family Care International
Family Planning Association of Kenya (FPAK)
Family Support Institute (FASI; formerly Wamama African Research &
    Documentation Institute—WARDI)
Foundations Papers, Ltd.
Fox Theaters (EA), Ltd.
Innovative Communication Systems (ICS)
Kenya Association for the Promotion of Adolescent Health (KAPAH)
Kenya Broadcasting Corporation (KBC)
Kenya Institute of Mass Communication (KIMC)
Kenya Medical Association (KMA)
Kenya Medical Women's Association
Progress for Women (Mandeleo Ya Wanawake Organization—MYWO)
Ministry of Health/Division of Health Education
Nation, Ltd. (newspaper)
National Council for Population and Development (NCPD)
Omni Company
Programme Exchange Center, URTNA
Reprographics Press Ltd.
Research Evaluation and Training Consultancy, Ltd. (RETCO)
Standard (newspaper)

Steadman & Associates
Thunder & Associates
TOPCOM Productions, Ltd.
Topi Communications, Ltd.

Liberia

Family Planning Association of Liberia

Madagascar

Family Planning Association of Madagascar (Fianakaviana Sambatra—FISA)
Horizons Communication
Malagasy National Radio and Television
Ministry of Population
National Youth and Popular Education School (Ecole Nationale de la Jeunesse
     et de l'Education Populaire—ENTEP)

Mali

Center for Audiovisual Production Services
Mali Association for the Protection and Promotion of the Family (Association
     Malienne pour le Protection et la Promotion de la Famille—AMPPF)
Mali National Radio and Television
National Union of Malian Women (Union Nationale des Femmes Malienne)

Niger

Department of Family Planning/Ministry of Health and Social Affairs (Direction
     de la Planification Familiale/Ministère de la Santé et des Affaires Sociales)
National Center for Family Health (Centre National de la Santé Familiale)
Niger State Council for Arts and Culture

Nigeria

Anambra Broadcasting Service
Association for Reproductive and Family Health (ARFH)
Family Health Services (FHS)
Federal Ministry of Health, Department of Population Activties (FMOHDPA)
Federal Ministry of Health, Health Education Branch (FMOHHEB)
Federal Radio Corporation of Nigeria
Fertility Research Association of Nigeria
Fertility Research Unit of the University of Ibadan, Oyo State
Imo Broadcasting Company
Insight Communication, Ltd.

Kano Broadcasting Corporation
National Council for Population and Environment Activities (NCPEA)
Nigerian Television Authority
Obafemi Awolowo University, Family Planning Operations Research Unit, Ile
    Ife
Pharmaceutical Society of Nigeria
Planned Parenthood Federation of Nigeria (PPFN)
Research and Marketing Services (RMS)
Rivers State Broadcasting Corporation
St. Clairs Agency
School of Health Technology, Minna, Niger State
Sunrise Marketing Communication, Ltd.
University of Nigeria Teaching Hospital, Nsukka
Women in Nigeria (WIN)

Senegal

Family Health and Population Project (Projet de Santé Familiale et de la
    Population—PSFP)
Senegal Radio and Television Bureau

Sierra Leone

Planned Parenthood Association of Sierra Leone
Sierra Leone Broadcasting Services

Somalia

Somali Family Health Care Association

Sudan

Sudan Fertility Control Association

Swaziland

Family Life Association of Swaziland

Tanzania

Advert International
Family Planning Association of Tanzania (UMATI)
Family Planning Unit/Ministry of Health
Great Muungano Cultural Troupe
Health Education Division/Ministry of Health

Organization of Tanzanian Trade Unions (OTTU)
Population and Family Life Education Project (POFLEP)
Radio Tanzania Dar (RTD)
SCANAD Tanzania, Ltd.

Togo

Togolese Family Welfare Association (Association Togolaise pour le Bien-Etre
   Familial—ATBEF)

Uganda

The AIDS Information Centre (AIC)
The AIDS Support Organization (TASO)
African Medical Research Foundation (AMREF)
Allied Industries Ltd. (printers)
AVSC Uganda
Bugosa Diocese Family Life Education Program (FLEP)
Capital Radio
CARE Uganda
Central Broadcasting Services (CBS)
East African (newspaper)
East Ankole Diocese Family Life Education Program
Ernie Petrich & Associates
Family Planning Association of Uganda (FPAU)
Federation of Uganda Employers
Imageset Ltd.
Intermedia Advertising, Publicity and Public Relations
INTRAH
JHPIEGO Uganda
Makerere University Institute of Social Research (MISR)
Marie Stopes International
Media Consultants, Ltd.
Media Forum, Ltd.
Ministry of Health AIDS Control Programme
Ministry of Health, Health Education Division
Ministry of Health, Maternal Child Health /Family Planning Division
Ministry of Health, Sexually Transmitted Diseases (STD) Unit
Ministry of Information Family Life Education Project
The Monitor (newspaper)
New Vision Ltd. (Newspaper)
Pathfinder International
PEARL Project
Polytechnic of Information Technology Limited
The Population Secretariat

Poyen Printers
Radio Sanyu
Radio Uganda
Reprographics Ltd.
Safe Motherhood
Sanyu TV
School for Media Development and Graphic Arts
SOMARC Uganda
Steadman & Associates
Straight Talk
Uganda AIDS Commission
Uganda Private Midwives Association (UPMA)
Uganda TV
UNFPA Uganda
UNICEF
Voice of Toro (VOT)

Zaire

Family Planning Services Project (Projet des Services des Naissances Désirables
    —PSND)
Rural Health Project of Zaire (Santé Rurale—SANRU)

Zambia

Copperbelt Health Education Project (CHEP)
Environment and Population Center
Ministry of Health
Planned Parenthood Association of Zambia (PPAZ)
Zambia Information Service (ZIS)

Zimbabwe

Amkhosi
Lintas Zimbabwe
Media for Development Trust
Roots Media
Zimbabwe Association of Community Theater
Zimbabwe Broadcasting Company
Zimbabwe National Family Planning Council (ZNFPC)

ASIA

Asia Regional

Asia Foundation
Asian Development Bank
Asian Institute for Management
Depth News
Economic and Social Commission for Asia and the Pacific (ESCAP)

Bangladesh

Action Aid
ADCOMM, Ltd.
A D F I L M
ADSHOP
Associates for Communication Options (ACO)
Associates for Community and Population Research (ACPR)
Association of Development Agencies in Bangladesh (ADAB)
AVCom Productions
Bangladesh Association for Voluntary Sterilization (BAVS)
Bangladesh Betar
Bangladesh Institute of Development Studies (BIDS)
Bangladesh Institute of Research for the Promotion of Essential and
    Reproductive Health and Technologies (BIRPERHT)
Bangladesh Integrated Nutrition Project (BINP)
Bangladesh Population Health Consortium (BPHC)
Bangladesh Rural Advancement Committee (BRAC)
Bangladesh Television
Bangladesh Unnayan Parishad Center for Research and Action on Environment
    and Development (BUP)
Bangladesh Women's Health Coalition (BWHC)
Baree Pear & Khan
BASICS
Bureau of Health Education, Directorate of Health Services, Ministry of Health
    and Family Welfare
CARE, Bangladesh
Center for Sustainable Development (CSD)
Children of the World
Concerned Women for Family Planning
Department of Mass Communication, Ministry of Information
Dhaka University
Directorate of Family Planning
Directorate General of Health Services

Expanded Program on Immunization Project (EPI)
Family Planning Association of Bangladesh (FPAB)
Family Planning Management and Development
Family Planning Services and Training Center (FPSTC)
Film Development Corporation
Grameen Bank
Information, Education, and Motivation Unit, Directorate of Family Planning
Lipi Printers and Packages
Local Initiatives Program/MSH
Management Development Unit—Third Population & Family Health Project of
     the World Bank/Bangladesh
Media, Inc., Bangladesh
Ministry of Health and Family Welfare
Mitra and Associates Bangladesh
Mohammedpur Fertility Services and Training Center
National Health Education, Information, and Communication Center (NHEICC)
National Institute of Population Research and Training (NIPORT)
National Institute of Preventive and Social Medicine
National Nutritional Council (NNC)
NGO Affairs Bureau
Pathfinder International, Bangladesh
Population Council, Bangladesh
Press Institute of Bangladesh
Program Communication and Information Section/UNICEF/Bangladesh
Program for Appropriate Technology in Health (PATH)/Bangladesh
Social and Marketing Research Services (SOMRA) Ltd.
Social Marketing Company/Population Services International (SMC/PSI,
     Bangladesh)
Stride Plus
University Research Corporation/Bangladesh (URC/B)
Voluntary Health Services Society (VHHS)

India

All India Women's Development Social Organization (AIWDSO)
AudioVisual Consultants
Center for Media Studies
Indian Institute of Health Management Research
Indian Institute of Mass Communications
Indian Medical Association (IMA)
Jain Satellite Television Studios
Literacy House
Medical Communications Network, India
Ministry of Health and Family Welfare (MOHFW), Government of India

Ministry of Health and Family Welfare (MOHFW), Government of Uttar
    Pradesh
National Institute for Health and Family Welfare
Operations Research Group (ORG)
Parivar Seva Sanstha India
Project Smita Society
Scientific Illustration and Education Technology
Social and Rural Research Institute
State Innovations in Family Planning Services Agency (SIFPSA)
Thompson Social
Uttar Pradesh Academy of Administration
Voluntary Health Association of India

Indonesia

Delima Mekar-Production House, Inc.
ERPRO
Frank Small & Associates
Indonesia Association for Secure Contraception (PKMI)
Indonesia Doctors Association (IDI)
Inter-Ksatrya Film
Ministry of State for Environment
Ministry of State for Population
National Family Planning Coordinating Board/Bureau of Information,
    Education, and Motivation
National Family Planning Coordinating Board/International Training Program
    (BKKBN/ITP)
National Family Planning Coordinating Board/Training Bureau
Paranti House
Radio Republik Indonesia (RRI)
Survey Research Indonesia (SRI)
Surya Citra Televisi (SCTV)
Televisi Pendidikan Indonesia (TPI)
Televisi Republik Indonesia (TVRI)

Nepal

Cine Sound
Communication Management Advertising Training, Inc.
Development Alternatives
Development Oriented Research Center (DORC)
Dristi Productions
Educational AV
Family Planning Association of Nepal (FPAN)
Gorkhapatra Corporation

Management Support Services/Nepal
MCH Products
Ministry of Health
Ministry of Population and Environment
Narayan Oriental Research Center
Nepal Contraceptive Retail Sales Company
Nepal Fertility Care Center
Nepal Medical Association
Nepal Red Cross
Nepal Studies Center
Nepal Television
New Era
Public Health Concern Trust (PHECT)
Radio Nepal
Reel Images
Resource Center for Primary Health Care (RECPHEC)
Saanga Video Film Productions
Sarbanam Street Theatre Group
Valley Research Group (VaRG)

Pakistan

Aftab Associates
Agha Khan Medical University
Aurat Publication and Information Service Foundation
Center for Health Communication
Domestic Research Bureau
Family Planning Association of Pakistan (FPAP)
Filmmakers, Ltd.
Films d'Art
International Institute of Population Studies
Menarid Christian Hospital
Ministry of Population Welfare
Pakistan Television Corporation
Population Welfare Division
Raasta Development Consultants
Voluntary Social Welfare Agency

The Philippines

ABS-CBN Foundation
Ago Medical and Educational Center
Agrarian Reform Beneficiaries Association
Amis Print
Ayala Foundation

Benetton Philippines
Bureau of Agrarian Reform
Campaigns, Inc.
Child Hope International
Christian Medical, Dental and Paramedical Association
Commission on Population (POPCOM)
Communicorp Inc.
Consolidated Broadcasting System
Consumer Pulse
Creative Point
Department of Health
Development Academy of the Philippines (DAP)
Development Training and Communication Planning/United Nations
     Development Programme—UNDP
DKT Philippines Inc.
Eagle Broadcasting Corporation
Economic Development Foundation
Enter-Educate Foundation (EEF)
Jose Fabella Memorial Hospital
Family Planning Organization of the Philippines (FPOP)
Federation of Jeepney Operators and Drivers Association
Office of Senator Juan M. Flavier
Foundation for Adolescent Development (FAD)
Fund for Assistance to Private Education
GMA-7
Golden Grove Communications Inc.
G.R. Creative Management Services, Inc.
GUESS! Philippines
Health Action Information Network
Institute for Social Studies and Action
Institute of Maternal and Child Health
Integrated Maternal and Child Health
International Institute for Rural Reconstruction (IIRR)
J. Romero and Associates
Kabalikat
Kapwa Ko Mahal Ko Foundation
Leadcom Asia
Management Sciences for Health (MSH)/Health Financing and Development
     Project (HFPD)
Manila Bulletin
Manila Times
Office of Senator Orlando Mercado
Mowelfund, Inc.
National Economic Development Authority
National Population Commission

Neo Films Philippines
Philippine Center for Population and Development—PCPD (formerly
    Population Center Foundation—PCF)
Philippine Daily Inquirer
Philippine Federation of Natural Family Planning
Philippine General Hospital
Philippine Health Insurance Co.
Philippine Legislators' Committee on Population and Development Foundation,
    Inc. (PLCPD)
Philippine Long Distance Telephone Company
Philippine Non-Governmental Organization Council
Philippine Rural Reconstruction Movemement
Population Service Pilipina, Inc.
Raya Media Services, Inc.
Reach Out
RPN-TV
TODAY
TRENDS-MBL, Inc.
University of the Philippines Los Baños (UPLB)
University of the Philippines Population Institute (UPPI)
Viva Productions, Inc.
Women's Health Care Foundation
Women's Media Circle Foundation, Inc.

Thailand

Population and Community Development Association
Thai Association for Voluntary Sterilization

LATIN AMERICA

Bolivia

Center for Family Orientation (Centro de Orientacion Familiar—COF)
Center for Research, Education and Services (CIES)
Center for Video and Movies (Centro Cine Video)
Educational System on Anti-drugs and Social Mobilization (Sistema Educativo
    Antidrogas y de Movilización Social—SEAMOS)
Foundation for Social Medical Assistance (Fundación de Asistencia Médico
    Social—FAMES)
Grey Bolivia, S.A.
Hospital San Gabriel (HSG)
Ministry of Human Development, Sub-Secretariat for Gender and Ethnic Affairs
    (Ministerio de Desarrollo Humano, Sub-Secretaria de Género y Asuntos
    Generacionales y Etnicos)

Ministry of Public Health and Social Security (Ministerio de Salud Pública y Previsión Social)

National Health Secretariat (Secretaria Nacional de Salud—SNS)

National Population Council (CONAPO)

National Social Security (Caja Nacional de Salud—CNS)

Population Council/Operations Research in Family Planning and Maternal-Child Health in Latin America and the Caribbean (Investicacion Operacional en Planificación Familiar y Atencion Materno-Infantil para America Latina y el Caribe—INOPAL)

Program on Child Survival Coordination (Programa de Coordinación en Supervivencia Infantil—PROCOSI)

Program on Interactive Radio Education (Programa de Aprendizaje por Radio Interativa—PARI)

Program on Radio Education (PER)

Protection of Health (ProSalud)

Radio Counseling Advisory (Consultorio Radial de Orientación—CROF-Bolivia)

Secretariat of Gender Affairs

Surveys and Studies (Encuestas y Estudios—E&E)

Unit of Population Policies (Unidad de Políticas de Población—UPP)

Brazil

Alberto Sabin Children's Hospital

Association of Brazilian Family Planning Agencies (Associacao Brasileira de Entidades de Planejamento Familiar—ABEPF)

Brazilian Family Welfare Association (Sociedade Civil Bem Estar Familiar no Brasil—BEMFAM)

Ceara Council for Women's Rights

Ceara School of Public Health (Escola de Saude Publica do Ceara—ESP)

Center for Research and Counseling (Centro de Pesquisas e Assessoria—ESPLAR)

Center for Research Assistance to Human Reproduction (CPARH)

Center for Sexual Education (Centro de Educacao Sexual—CEDUS)

Cervantes Group (Street Theater)

Clovis Salgado Center for Research and Studies (Centro de Estudios e Pesquisas Clovis Salgado—CEPECS)

Denison Advertising Sao Paulo Ltd. (Denison Propaganda Sao Paulo Ltda.)

Emilio Odebrecht Foundation (Fundacao Emilio Odebrecht)

Federal University of Minas Gerais (Universidad Federal de Minais Gerais—UFMG)

Health Secretariat for Bahia State (SESAB)

Health Secretariat for Ceara State (SESA)

Import and Commerce of Pharmaceutical Products (Importacao e Comercio de Insumos Farmaceuticos Ltda.—CEPEO/PROFIT)

Ministry of Education
Promotion of Responsible Parenthood (PRO-PATER)
Roquete Pinto Foundation
Schering of Brazil, Chemical and Pharmaceutical Ltd. (Schering do Brasil,
      Quimica e Farmaceutica Ltda.)
School of Arts and Crafts (Bahia Liceu de Artes e Oficios)
Society for Maternal Aid at the Assis Chateaubriand School (SAMEAC)
TV Globo

Caribbean

Concept Advertising Ltd.
The Family Planning Association of Trinidad and Tobago—FPATT
Jamaica Family Planning Association—JFPA
USAID, Regional Office

Colombia

Association for Colombian Family Welfare (PROFAMILIA)
AVSC International/Colombia
Toro Advertising (Publicidad Toro)

Costa Rica

Costa Rican Demographic Association (ADC)
Costa Rican Social Security Institute (CCSS)

Ecuador

Andean University of Communication
Center for Family Obstetrics (Centro Obstétrico Familiar—COF)
Center for Population and Responsible Parenthood Studies (CEPAR)
Ecuadorian Social Security Institute (IESS)
ECUAVISA
The Family Welfare Association of Ecuador (Asociación Pro-Bienestar de la
      Familia Ecuatoriana—APROFE)
Future Foundation
International Center of Advanced Communication Studies for Latin America
      (Centro Internacional de Estudios Superiores de Comunicación para
      América Latina—CIESPAL)
Medical Center for Counseling and Family Planning (Centro Medico de
      Orientación y Planificación Familiar—CEMOPLAF)
Paez and Associates—Consultant (Paez y Asociados—Consultor)
Pro-Day (Pro-Dia)
Women's Network

El Salvador

Child Survival and Maternal Health Project (Proyecto de Salud Materna y
Supervivencia Infantil—PROSAMI)
Ministry of Agriculture and Livestock (Ministerio de Agricultura y
Ganaderia—MAG)
Ministry of Public Health and Social Security (Ministerio de Salud Pública y
Asistencia Social)
National Agricultural Training Center (Centro Nacional de Capacitación
Agropecuaria—CENCAP)
Salvadoran Demographic Association (Asociasión Demographica
Salvadoreña—ADS)

Guatemala

Guatemalan Association for Sexual Education (Asociación Guatemalteca de
Educación Sexual—AGES)
Guatemalan Family Welfare Association (APROFAM)
Importer of Pharmaceutical Products (Importadora de Productos
Farmacéuticos—IPROFASA)
Interamerican Development Advisory Services (IDEAS)/DataPro, S.A.
IPAHO (Instituto de Nutricion de Centro America y Panama—INCAP)
The Population Council (INOPAL Project)
Regional Video Production Center in Guatemala (Centro Regional de
Audiovisuales—CREA)
UNFPA (Fondo de sas Naciones Unidas en Pablacion)
USAID, Regional Office

Haiti

Association for the Promotion of the Family (Association pour la Promotion de
la Famille—PROFAMIL)
Centers for Development and Health (Centres pour le Développement et la
Santé—CDS)
Child Health Institute (Institut Haitien de l'Enfance—IHE)
Community Health Institute for Haitian (Institut Haïtien de Santé
Communautaire—INHSAC)
Foundation for Reproductive Health and Family Education (Fondation de Santé
Reproductive et d'Education Familiale—FOSREF)
Haitian Organization for Family Action
Private Sector Assistance Organization (Association des Oeuvres Privées de
Santé—AOPS)
Professional Management Services
PubliGestion

Honduras

Honduran Family Planning Association (Asociación Hondurena de Planificación
    de Familia—ASHONPLAFA)
Honduran Social Security Institute (IHSS)
Ministry of Health (Ministerio de Salud)
USAID, Regional Office

Mexico

Advisory and Research Gamma S.A. of C.V. (Asesoría e Investigaciones
    Gamma S.A. de C.V.—GAMMA)
Center for the Investigation and Study of Sexuality (Centro de Investigacion y
    Estuios sobre la Sexualidad A.C.—CIESEX)
EMI Capitol de Mexico, S.A. de C.V.
Ford Foundation
GIRE
Institute for Communication Research (IIC)
Intercontinental Resources and Development (Fuentes y Fomento
    Intercontinentales—FFI)
Mexican Academy for Research on Medical Demography (AMIDEM)
Mexican Family Planning Foundation (MEXFAM)
Mexican Federation of Private Family Planning Associations (FEMAP)
Mexican Social Security Institute (IMSS)
National Population Council (Consejo Nacional de Población—CONAPO)
NESA (Novedades Editores, S.A. de C.V.)
Orientation Council for Adolescents (Consejo de Orientación a los
    Adolescentes—CORA)
Pathfinder International
The Population Council—INOPAL
Secretariat of Health (Secretaría de Salud—SSA)
Social Security and Services Institute for Government Employees (ISSSTE)
Televisa S.A. de C.V.
UNFPA (Fondo de Poblacion de Naciones Unidas en Mexico, Cuba y República
    Dominicana)
USAID, Regional Office

Nicaragua

Hilo Productions and Publications
Mejida Godoy Foundation
Ministry of Health
PROFAMILIA of Nicaragua
United Nations Population Fund—UNFPA, Nicaragua

Peru

Advocacy for Population Programs (Apoyo a Programas de Poplación—
    APROPO)
Center Flora Tristan (Centro Flora Tristán)
Iguana Productions
Intercom S.A. of Advertising (Intercom S.A. de Publicidad)
Manuela Ramos Movement (Movimiento Manuela Ramos)
Ministry of Health (MINSA)
Multidisciplinary Association for Research and Teaching on Population
    (Asociación Multidisciplinaria de Investigación y Docencia en
    Población—AMIDEP)
National Population Council (Consejo Nacional de Población—CONAPO)
Peruvian Institute for Responsible Parenthood (INPPARES)
Peruvian Institute of Social Security (IPSS)
Peruvian University Cayetano Heredia (Universidad Peruana Cayetano Heredia)
Programs on Information, Health, Medicine, and Agriculture (PRISMA)
Project Peru 2000
REPROSALUD
Research on Sociology and Marketing (IMASEN)

Trinidad & Tobago

Family Planning Association of Trinidad and Tobago (FPATT)

NEAR EAST

Near East Regional

AGFUND
American University Beirut—AUB
Center of Arab Women for Training and Research (CAWTAR)
International Development research Center (IDRC)
International Planned Parenthood Federation (IPPF)
UNFPA Country Support Team (CST)
UNICEF Middle East and North Africa Regional Office
Yemen Family Care Association

Egypt

Ain Shams University Regional Center for Training in Family Planning, Faculty
    of Medicine
Al-Ahram Media-Buy Research Center

Al-Azhar University, International Islamic Center for Population Studies and
    Research
Americana Advertising Agency
Arab African Promoters for International Conferences
Arab Council for Childhood and Development
Arab Office of Youth and Environment
Bishopric of Public and Social Services/Population and Family Welfare Project
Cairo Demographic Center
Cairo Health Organization
Center for Development Communication
Center for Development Services
Central Agency for Public Mobilization and Statistics, Population Research
    Center
Clinical Services Improvement Project
Coptic-Evangelical Organization for Social Services
Coptic Orthodox Church
Egyptian Advertising Association
Egyptian Family Planning Association
Egyptian Fertility Care Society
Egyptian Junior Medical Doctors' Association
Federation of Islamic Associations
Health Insurance Organization
Institute for Training and Research in Family Planning
Intermarkets Advertising
International Development Resource Council
Look Advertising Co.
MEDTECH
Ministry of Culture
Ministry of Education/Population Education Department
Ministry of Health and Population
Ministry of Health/Quality Improvement Projects/Systems Development Project
Ministry of Information SIS/IEC Center (State Information Service/Information,
    Education and Communication Center)
Ministry of Religious Affairs
Ministry of Youth and Sports
Minya Governorate Office
National Population Council
Palm Press
Pyramid Video Services
RadaResearch and Public Relations
Ro'oya Advertising
Smart Advertising Agency
Social Planning, Analysis & Administration Consultants
Team Misr
Two Stars and Eagle

Wafai and Associates
Women's Committee, Minya

Jordan

Arab Women's Organization
Center for Strategic Studies at the University of Jordan
Development Communication Unit at Jordan Radio and Television
International Center for Studies and Research
Jordan News Agency
Jordan TV
Jordanian Association for Family Planning & Protection
Jordanian Department of Statistics
Jordanian National Population Commission
Jordanian National Women's Commission
Market Research Organization
Middle East Marketing and Research Bureau
Ministry of Awqaf and Islamic Affairs
Ministry of Education
Ministry of Health
Ministry of Youth
Noor Al Hussein Foundation
Queen Alia Fund for Social Work/Princess Basma Center

Morocco

ACT! Communication
ALCO Alternative Consultants
Casablanca Film Productions
Coordination de Projets Internationaux
Leader Management Services and Council
Medias Council
Ministry of Public Health

Oman

Al-Seeb Cultural Center
Al-Seeb Educational Authority
Al-Seeb Sports Club
Arab House for Advertising, PROMOTARGET
Department of Family and Community Health
Department of Health Education
Directorate General of Health Affairs
Middle East Market and Research Bureau
Ministry of Health

Ministry of Information
Ministry of Social Affairs
Muscat Advertising
Muscat Health Directorate
Muscat Municipality
Ministry of Education
National Publishing and Advertising
National Women and Child Care Committee
Omani Scouts Association
Omani Women's Association
Royal Armed Forces
Royal Omani Police
Shoura Council
Sultan Qabus University
Wali Al-Seeb Office

Tunisia

Center of Arab Women for Training and Research—CAWTAR
National Office of the Family and Population

Turkey

Data Processing and Market Research, Inc.
Economic and Social Documentation Research, Inc.
Environmental Problems Foundation of Turkey
Filmeks
Foundation for the Advancement and Recognition of Turkish Women
Haceteppe Institute for Population Studies
Human Resource Development Foundation
Ministry of Health
Turkish Family Health and Planning Foundation
Zet Market Research, Ltd.

Yemen

Ministry of Information
Yemen Family Care Association

NEW INDEPENDENT STATES

Kazakhstan

BRIF: Social Marketing Research Agency

Human Reproductive Center of Almaty
Ministry of Health (MOH)
Totem Television-Radio Broadcasting

Kyrgyzstan

Ministry of Health (MOH)
Pyramid Television-Radio Company
Republic Center for Public Opinion (RCPO)
Republic Health Center (RHC)

Russia

Alter Ego Public Relations Company
Center for Sociological Studies, Moscow State University
Pygmalion Film Company
Russian Family Planning Association
TV Company OBLIK
VideoCosmos Company

Turkmenistan

Ministry of Health (MOH)

Ukraine

National Family Planning Center, Kiev Research Institute of Pediatrics and
    Obstetrics/Gynecology
Ukrainian Social Surveys and Market Research

Uzbekistan

Expert Sociological Research Center
Flamingo Video (FLM)
Fund for a Healthy Generation
Ministry of Health (MOH)

JHU/PCS COLLABORATING ORGANIZATIONS AND KEY PEOPLE, 1982–1996

AFRICA

Africa Regional

Mr. Atsen Ahua, former Director, Program Exchange Center, Union of National Radio and Television Organizations of Africa (URTNA)

Mr. Kassaye Demena, former Secretary General, URTNA

Mr. Pape Syr Diagne, Director, Center for African Family Studies (CAFS)

Mr. Alpha Diallo, Deputy Director, CAFS

Prof. Yaya Drabo, former Director, Francophone Regional Office, CAFS

Mr. François Itoua, former Secretary General, URTNA

Mr. Macharia Kiruhi, Senior Program Officer, IEC, CAFS

Mr. Solomon Luvai, former Director, Program Exchange Center, URTNA

Mr. Efoe Adodo Mensah, Secretary General, URTNA

Mr. Dieudonné Ouédraogo, former Director, Center for Applied Research on Population and Development (CERPOD)

Mr. Baba Traoré, Director, CERPOD

Mr. Edward Ulzen, former IEC Specialist, Program Exchange Center, URTNA

Burkina Faso

Dr. Didier Bakouan, former Director, Directorate of Family Health, Ministry of Health and Social Action (MOHSA)

Dr. Azara Bamba, former Director, Directorate of Family Health, MOHSA

Mrs. Fatoumata Batta, former Director, Directorate of Family Health, MOHSA

Dr. Zeinab Dermé, former Director, Directorate of Family Health, MOHSA

Mr. Prosper Kompaoré, Director, Burkina Faso Theater Workshop

Mrs. Awa Ouédraogo, Director, Department for the Promotion of the Family

Ms. Pascaline Sebgo, Program Officer, Project Femmes et Santé, Antenne Régionale/Afrique de l'Ouest

Cameroon

Dr. David Awasum, former Director, Directorate of Family and Mental Health, Ministry of Public Health

Côte d'Ivoire

Mr. Paul Agodio, Executive Director, Ivoirian Association for Family Welfare

Dr. Hugues Koné, former Director, Center for Teaching and Research in
Communication (CERCOM)
Dr. Régina Traoré Série, Director, CERCOM

Ethiopia

Mr. Asres Kebede, Head, IEC Task Force, National Office of
Population/Ministry of Economic Development and Cooperation
Mr. Opia Mensah Kumah, UNFPA Regional IEC Advisor
Mr. Tewodros Melesse, Pathfinder Country Representative
Dr. Negussie Teffera, Head, National Office of Population/Ministry of
Economic Development and Cooperation

The Gambia

Mr. Yankuba Dibba, Program Manager, The Gambia Family Planning
Association

Ghana

Mr. Alex Banful, Director, Ghana Social Marketing Foundation
Mr. John Barnor, Director, Institute of Adult Education
Prof. Miranda Greenstreet, former Director, Institute of Adult Education
Mrs. Mary Arday Kotei, Head, Ghana Ministry of Health/Health Education Unit
Dr. Richard Turkson, Executive Director, National Population Council

Kenya

Ambassador S.B.A. Bullut, Director, National Council on Population and
Development
Mr. Godwin Z. Mzenge, Executive Director, Family Planning Association of
Kenya
Mr. John Nyoike, Project Coordinator, Innovative Communication Systems
Dr. Emily Obwaka, Chairperson, Kenya Medical Women's Association
Prof. Okoth-Ogendo, Chairman, National Council on Population and
Development
Dr. Khoma Rogo, Director, Center for the Study of Adolescence

Madagascar

Mrs. Monique Andrèas, Director General, Ministry of Population
Mr. Manitra Andriamasinoro, Executive Director, FISA
Dr. Nivoherizo Rakotobe, former Executive Director, Family Planning
Association of Madagascar (FISA)

Dr. Tombo Ramandimbisoa, Director of Population and Social Development,
Ministry of Population

Mali

Mr. Lansina Sidibe, Executive Secretary, Mali Association for the Protection
and Promotion of the Family (AMPPF)
Mr. Eli Simpara, IEC Coordinator, AMPPF

Niger

Dr. Halima Maidouka, Director, National Center for Family Health

Nigeria

Mr. Femi Jarret, Managing Director, St. Clairs Agency
Mr. E. E. Kuteyi, Director, Department of Population Activities, Ministry of
Health
Mr. May Nzerabe, Managing Director, Sunrise Marketing Communication, Ltd.
Mr. Bayo Ola, Head, Health Education Branch, Federal Ministry of Health
Mr. Abiodun Sobanjo, Managing Director, Insight Communications, Ltd.
Dr. A. B. Sulaiman, Executive Director, Planned Parenthood Federation of
Nigeria
Mr. K. A. Tejumola, Managing Director, Research and Marketing Services

Tanzania

Dr. Naomi Katunzi, Executive Secretary, Family Planning Association of
Tanzania
Dr. Godwin Mwaipopo, Head and Co-Director of Green Star Project, Health
Education Division/Ministry of Health
Dr. Edith Ngirwamungu, Coordinator, Green Star Project, Health Education
Division/Ministry of Health
Mrs. Christine Nsekela, former Executive Secretary, Family Planning
Association of Tanzania
Dr. Calista Simbakalia, Director, Family Planning Unit/Ministry of Health

Uganda

Mr. Michael Daugherty, Managing Director, Media Consultants, Ltd.
Dr. Florence O. Ebanyat, Assistant Director for Medical Services, Ministry of
Health (MCH/FP)
Mr. J. K. Gaifube, Assistant Commissioner for Medical Services (PHC/HE),
Ministry of Health

Mr. Michael Galiwango, Managing Director, Polytechnic of Information Technology Limited

Mr. Paul Kaggwa, Deputy Assistant Commissioner for Medical Services (PHC/HE), Ministry of Health

Dr. Elizabeth Madra, Program Manager, STD/AIDS Control Programme, Ministry of Health

Ms. Joy Mukaire, Project Coordinator, Busoga Diocese, Family Life Education Project

Dr. Zikusooko, Executive Director, Family Planning Association of Uganda

Zaire

Mrs. Chirwisa Chiramolekwa, former Director, Family Planning Services Project

Zambia

Mr. Patrick Jabani, Director, Zambia Information Service

Mrs. Margaret Mutamba, Executive Director, Planned Parenthood Association of Zambia

Dr. Mary Shilalukey Ngoma, Head, MCH/FP Unit

Mr. David Olson, Country Representative, PSI/Zambia Social Marketing Project

Zimbabwe

Mrs. Florence Chikara, former Chief, IEC Unit, ZNFPC

Mrs. Caroline Marangwanda, Head, Evaluation and Research Unit (ERU), Zimbabwe National Family Planning Council (ZNFPC)

Kyle Peterson, Director, PSI/Zimbabwe

Mr. John Riber, Director, Media for Development Trust

Mr. Godfrey Tinarwo, Mass Media Manager, IEC Unit, Zimbabwe National Family Planning council (ZNFPC)

Dr. David Wilson, Contractor, Evaluation and Research Unit (ERU), Zimbabwe National Family Planning Council (ZNFPC)

Dr. Alex Zinanga, Executive Director, Zimbabwe National Family Planning Council—ZNFPC

ASIA

Bangladesh

Mr. Md. Nurul Abedin, Additional Secretary, Ministry of Health and Family Welfare, Bangladesh Secretariat, Dhaka

Suhel Ahmed, Director General, NGO Affairs Bureau

Mr. Ali Akbar, Chief, Bureau of Health Education

Dr. M. Alauddin, Country Representative, Pathfinder International

Mr. Muhammed Ali, Secretary, Ministry of Health and Family Welfare Bangladesh Secretariat, Dhaka

Prof. A. K. Nurul Anwar, Director General, Directorate of Health

Dr. Abul Barkat, Sr. Scientist URC, Bangladesh

Ms. G. S. Chowdhury, Chairman and Managing Director, ADCOMM, Ltd.

Dr. Sadia Chowdhury, Director, HPD, Bangladesh Rural Advancement Committee (BRAC)

Dr. Barkat E-Khuda, Project Director, FP-MCH Extension Project, ICDDR, Bangladesh

Dr. A. J. Faisel, Country Representative, Association for Voluntary Surgical Contraception (AVSC)

Mr. Sofiul Haque, Director, Population Cell, Bangladesh Television

Dr. Shamsul Hoque, Director, EPI Project

Md. Shirajul Islam, Director General, Directorate of Family Planning

Mr. Faisal Kader, Managing Director, Social and Marketing Research Services

Dr. Qazi Khaliquzzaman, Chairman, Bangladesh Unnayan Parishad Center for Research and Action on Environment and Development (BUP)

Mr. Tarique Anam Khan, Chief Executive, ADSHOP

Mrs. Mufaweza Khan, Executive Director, Concerned Women for Family Planning

Dr. Rokeya Khanam, EPI Communication Advisor, Basic Support for Institutionalizing Child Survival (BASICS)

Ms. Kirsten Lundeen, Population Program Manager, Asia Foundation

Mr. S. N. Mitra, Executive Director, Mitra & Associates

Mr. Absar Ali Mollah, Director, IEM (In-Charge) Directorate of Family Planning

Mr. M. Muzakkyer, Director, Population Cell, Bangladesh Betar

Mr. A.K.M. Rafiquz-zaman, Director General, NIPORT

Mr. Badal Rahman, Film Director, A D F I L M

Mr. M. Azizur Rahman, Joint Secretary (Hospital & Public Health) and Chairperson, IEC Technical Committee, Ministry of Health and Family Welfare, Bangladesh Secretariat, Dhaka

Mr. Mizanur Rahman, AVCom Productions

Mr. Waliur Rahman, Managing Director, Social Marketing Company

Khandokar Mizanur Rahman, Project Director, Bangladesh Integrated Nutrition Project (BINP)

Mr. Masum Reza, Creative Director, Stride Plus

Mr. Abdur Rouf, Executive, PSTC

Mr. Anis Salem, Chief, PCIS, UNICEF

India

Mr. S. M. Afsar, Deputy General Manager, IEC, SIFPSA.

Dr. Prem Agarwal, Hon. Gen. Secretary, Indian Medical Association

Ms. Vasudha Ambiye, Head of Dept., ASTHA, Xavier Institute of
Communications/St. Xavier's College

Dr. Dharam Anand, Director, Scientific Illustration and Education Technology

Ms. Feruzi Anjirbag, Head of Dept. AXIS, Xavier Institute of
Communications/St. Xavier's College

Dr. Akshay Bharadwaj, Jain Satellite Television Studios

Mr. Shivaji Bhattacharya, Vice-President and Manager, Thompson Social

Dr. Bimal Buch, Consultant

Mr. Ashoke Chatterjee, former Director, National Institute of Design, Consultant

Mr. Gerson daCunha, Consultant

Mr. Desmond D'Monte, Director, Xavier Institute of Communications/St.
Xavier's College

Dr. J. C. Doshi, Consultant

Dr. H. Helen, Director, National Institute for Health and Family Welfare

Dr. Ragini Jain, Managing Director, Jain Satellite Television Studios

Mr. Deepak Kapoor, Partner, Price Waterhouse (India)

Ms. Indu Kapoor, CHETNA, Ahmedabad

Mr. Kiran Karnik, CEO, Discovery Channel (India), Consultant

Mr. Ajai Lal, Director, Audio Visual Consultants

Prof. Rishikesh Maru, Director, Indian Institute of Health Management Research

Mrs. Adarsh Mishra, Joint Secretary, IEC, Ministry of Health

Mr. Alok Mukhopadhyaya, Executive Director, Voluntary Health Association of
India

Ms. Vinita Nanda, Project Smita Society

Dr. P. D. Nayer, Consultant

Mr. Vali Nijhawan, Partner, Price Waterhouse (India)

Dr. Ashish Panigrahi, Associate Vice President, Operations Research Group

Dr. B. R. Patil, Consultant

Mrs. Uma Pillai, former Executive Director, Society for Innovations in Family
Planning Services (SIFPSA)

Dr. N. Bhaskara Rao, Chairman, Center for Media Studies

Ms. Meera Shekar, Consultant

Ms. Meera Shiva, Head, Public Policy Division, Voluntary Health Association
of India

Mr. Dinesh Singh, Additional Executive Director, SIFPSA

Mr. Madan Singh, Director, Literacy House

Dr. J. C. Sobti, Indian Medical Association

Dr. Hemlorter Swaroop, AIWD/SO

Ms. Sudha Tewari, Director, Parivar Seva Sanstha

Mr. R. S. Tolia, Director, Uttar Pradesh Academy of Administration

Ms. Hema Vishwanathan, Senior Vice-President and General Manager, Social
and Rural Research Institute

Mr. Luv Verma, Secretary, Family Welfare, MOHFW, Government Of Uttar
Pradesh

Dr. J. S. Yadava, Director, Indian Institute of Mass Communications

Indonesia

Dr. Loet Afandi, Vice Chairman, State Ministry for Population/National Family
   Planning, Coordinating Board (BKKBN)
Dr. Andarus, Chief, International Training Center for Population/Family
   Planning
Dr. Azrul Azwar, Chairman, Indonesia Doctors Association (IDI)
Dr. Kartono Mohammad, Chairman, PKBI
Dr. Sunandar Ngaliun, Deputy for Family Planning, BKKBN
Dr. Sardin Pabbadja, Deputy for Program Analysis, BKKBN
Dr. Pudjo Raharjo, Deputy for Training and Program Development, BKKBN
Ishadi SK, Director, Televisi Republik Indonesia (TVRI)
Dr. Sudarmadi, Deputy for Management, BKKBN
Dr. Haryono Suyono, State Minister of Population/Chairman of BKKBN

Nepal

Mr. Khagendra N. Adhikari, Director, Nepal Contraceptive Retail Services
Mr. S. K. Alok, Country Director, UNFPA
Mr. L. R. Ban, Under Secretary, National Health Education Information
   Communication Center (NHEICC)
Mr. Hari Bandi, Section Officer, NHEICC
Dr. Indira Basnet, Maternal Health Service Officer, National Health Training
   Center (NHTC)
Mr. Chuda Mani Bhandari, Public Health Officer, Family Health Division
   (FHD)
Dr. Shyam P. Bhattarai, Director, NHEICC
Mr. Kuber Gartaula, CEO and Independent Scriptwriter/Producer, Educational
   AV
Mr. Sunil Gartaula, Producer, Educational AV
Mr. Binod Giri, Assistant Director/Producer, Educational AV
Dr. Shiva Shanker Jha., Regional Medical Director, Ministry of Health—Central
   Region
Mme. Vijaya K.C., Special Secretary, Ministry of Health
Mr. D. B. Lama, Assistant Resident Rapresentative, UNFPA
Dr. Marta Levitt, FP/MCH Advisor and Project Director for Redd Barna, NHTC
Mr. Radha Krishna Mainali, Minister of Health, Ministry of Health
Mr. Ashesh Malla, Director, Sarbanam Inc.
Mr. Shanta Lal Mulmi, Director, Resource Center for Primary Health Care
   (RECPHEC)
Mr. Arjun Narasingha, K.C., Former Minister of Health, Ministry of Health
Mr. Shailes Neupane, Director, Valley Research Group (VaRG)
Mr. Ghana Nath Ojha, Secretary of Health, Ministry of Health
Mr. Ananta Raj Pandey, Joint Secretary, Population Division, Ministry of
   Population and Environment (MOPE)

Mr. Charu Pandel, Assistant Resident Representative, UNFPA

Dr. Kalyan Raj Pandey, Director General, Department of Health Services, Ministry of Health

Dr. L. R. Pathak, Director, Family Health Division (FHD)

Mr. Prabhat S.J.B. Rana, Chief, Communication Division, Family Planning Association of Nepal (FPAN)

Dr. Peden Pradhan, PHECT

Mr. Shailendra Raj Sharma, Executive Director, Radio Nepal

Ms. Hasina Gyanu Shrestha, Consultant, UNFPA, NHEICC

Mr. Rameshwar Shrestha, Independent Scriptwriter

Mr. Krishna Raj Siri, Senior Health Education Officer (NHEICC)

Mr. Nanda Man Sthapit, Under Secretary, NHTC

Dhruba Thapa, Associate Director and Editor-in-Charge, Radio Nepal

The Philippines

Ms. Mercy Abad, President, Trends

Dr. Angelita Ago, Executive Vice-President and Dean, Ago Medical and Educational Center (AMEC)

Ms. Rowena O. Alvarez, Executive Director, Institute for Social Studies and Action (ISSA)

Ms. Teresita Marie P. Bagasao, Executive Director, Kabalikat

Ms. Sony Chin, Administrator, Davao Medical School Foundation Institute of Primary Health Care, Mindanao Training and Resource Center

Mr. J. Prospero E. de Vera, Jr., Former Executive Director, Philippine Legislators' Committee on Population and Development Foundation Inc. (PLCPD)

Undersecretary Benjamin Dideleon, Office of the President

Ms. Esperanza Dowling, Executive Director, Philippine Federation of Natural Family Planning (PFNFP)

Dr. Jovencia Dumindjin-Quintong, Director, Family Planning Services, Department of Health

Ms. Florina Dumlao, Former Director, Philippine NGO Council

Senator Juan M. Flavier

Mr. Romeo H. Gecolea, Director, Development Training & Communication Planning/UNDP (DTCP/UNDP)

Dr. Rebecca Infantado, Acting Assistant Secretary for Special Concerns, Department of Health

Cecile Joaquin-Yasay, Executive Director, Commission on Population, POPCOM

Mr. Billy Lacaba, President and General Manager, Raya Media Services, Inc.

Dr. Antonio Lopez, Undersecretary for Public Health Services, Department of Health

Mr. Romulo S. Maranan, President, Federation of Jeepney Operators and Drivers Association in the Philippines

Dr. Ceasar M. Mercado, Planner /Programmer, and Monitoring Evaluation
 Specialist, DCTP/UNDP
Senator Orlando Mercado
Bishop Javier Gil C. Montemayor, Former Executive Director, Family Planning
 Organization of the Philippines (FPOP)
Mr. Horacio R. Morales, Jr., President, Philippine Rural Reconstruction
 Movement
Mr. Jose Obordo, Former Executive Director, Integrated Maternal and Child
 Health (IMCH)
Ms. Yoly Ong, President, Campaigns, Inc.
Ms. Teresita Oreta, Co-Chairperson, PLCPD
Dr. Rebecca Ramos, Officer-in-Charge, Jose Fabella Memorial Hospital
Dr. Carmencita N. Reodica, Secretary of Health, Department of Health
Ms. Ana Lea Sarabia, Women's Media Circle
Senator Leticia Shahani
Ms. Aurora Silayan-Go, President, Foundation for Adolescent Development
Atty. Ramon Tagle, Jr., formerly with FPOP

LATIN AMERICA

Bolivia

Ms. Virginia Camacho, Reproductive Health Coordinator
Ms. Lupe Mendizabal, Director of SEAMOS
Mr. Oscar Sandoval Moron, National Secretary of Public Health
Ms. Carmen Beatriz Ruiz, National Director of Communication, Secretariat of
 Gender Affairs
Ms. Sietske Steneker, UNFPA Representative
Mr. Freddy Teodovich, Minister of Human Development
Mr. Javier Torrez Goitia, National Sub-Secretary of Public Health
Mr. Oscar Zuleta, National Director, Health & Nutrition for Mother and Child

Brazil

Mr. Flaminio Araripe, Local Newspaper Correspondent
Ms. Maria Auxiliadora Garcia da Costa, President, Ceara Council for Women
 Rights
Mr. Aureliano Biancareli, Editor, Cotidiano do Jornal Folha de Sao Paulo
Dra. Silvia Bomfim Hyppolito, Family Planning Coordinator, Ceara Federal
 University
Maria do Carmo Moreira, Trainer, Caera School of Public Health
Dra. Anamaria Cavalcante e Silva, Ex-Secretary, Ceara State Health Secretariat;
 currently Director of Children's Hospital Alberto Sabin
Mr. Claudio Csillag, Newspaper Editor in Sao Paulo

Dr. Marcos Paulo P. de Castro, Director, PRO-PATER
Bernadete de Castro, Project Manager, PRO-PATER
Mr. Jose M. De Magalhaes Neto, Health Secretary, Bahia State Health
  Secretariat
Neylar Lins, Superintendent, Foundation Emilio Odebrecht
Dra. Dirlene Mafalda da Silveira, Coordinator, Viva Mulher Program, Ceara
  State Health Secretariat
Dra. Silvia Mamede Studart Soares, Superintendent, Ceara School of Public
  Health
Mr. Jose Ferreira Nobre-Formiga, Chief Women's Health Assistance, Ministry
of Health
Ms. Balbina Pessoa Lemos, Project Coordinator for Reproductive Health, Bahia
  State Health Secretariat
Mr. Joe Pimentel, Video Maker, Ceara Federal University
Mr. Marcelo Pontes, Director, Sucursal do Jornal do Brasil
Dr. Anastacio Queiroz de Souza, Secretary of State, Health Secretariat
Dra. Jocileide Sales Campos, Health Director, Ceara State Health Secretariat
Mr. Ricardo Soares Gontijo, General Director, Foundation Roquete Pinto
Ms. Mari Travassos, Coordinator, Bahia Liceu de Artes e Oficios

Carribean

Brenda J. Grey, Jamaica Family Planning Association—JFPA
Elaine Perkins, Director, Concept Advertising Ltd.
Hetty Sarjeant, Executive Director, The Family Planning Association of Trinidad
  and Tobago—FPATT

Dominican Republic

Lic. Magaly Caram, Executive Director, Association for Dominican Family
  Welfare (Asociación Dominicana Pro Bienestar de la Familia—
  PROFAMILIA)
Paul Schendel, USAID

Ecuador

Dr. Juan Esteban Aguirre, UNFPA Director
Dr. Alejandro Alfonso, UNESCO Regional of State, Health Secretariat
Mr. Xavier Alvarado, ECUAVISA President
Mr. Hernan Cuellar, ASOCINE President
Dr. Asdrubal de la Torre, CIESPAL Director
Ms. Daniela del Castillo, ARCANDINA Director
Ms. Carmen de Vargas, Radio Director
Lic. Teresa de Vargas, APROFE Director
Dr. Francisco Huerta, Ex-Minister of Health

Dr. Jose Laso, Director, Andean University of Communication
Dr. Pablo Marangoni, APROFE Director
Dr. Nelson Oviedo, CEPAR Director
Ms. Yolanda Torres, TV Director
Dra. Magdalena Vanoni, Women's Network
Dra. Nila Velazquez, Editor/Ex-Vice Rector, Catholic University

El Salvador

Lic. Leonidas Aparicio, Local Coordinator, CENCAP
Ing. Antonio Cabrales, Minister, Ministry of Agriculture and Livestock—MAG
Brenda Doe, Deputy Director of Health Population and Nutrition, USAID
Dr. Delmy de Hernandez, Chief, Health Education Unit, Ministry of Public
    Health and Social Assistance
Jorge Hernández Isuzi, Executive Director, Salvadorean Demographic
    Association—ADS
Elba Velaseo, Executive Director, PROSAMI

Guatemala

Lic. Sandra Aguilar, Chief, Training Division, Guatemalan Association for
    Sexual Education (Asociación Guatemalteca de Educación Sexual—AGES)
Lic. Lucrecia Alegria, Population Official, UNFPA
Wende Skidmore Du Flon, Regional Advisor for Social Marketing,
    Interamerican Development Advisory Serivces, Ltd.—IDEAS
Magda Fischer, M.P. H., External Relations, INCAP
Dr. Roberto Santiso Gálvez, Executive Director, Guatemalan Family Welfare
    Association (APROFAM)
Mary McInerny, USAID
Dr. Paul Humberto Rosenberg Monzon, Chief, Family Planning Unit, The
    Populaiton Council (INOPAL Project)
Mary McInerny, USAID
Patricia O'Connor, USAID
Jorge Mario Ortega, Gerente General, Importer of Pharmaceutical Products
    (Importadora de Productos Farmacéuticos—IPROFASA)
Maria Cristina Rosales, Director, Regional Video Production Center in
    Guatemala (Centro Regional de Audiovisuales—CREA)
Lic. Eduardo Sacayón, Director, Guatemalan Association for Sexual Education
    (Asociación Guatemalteca de Educación Sexual—AGES)

Haiti

Dr. Jean André, Private Sector Assistance Organization (Association des
    Oeuvres Privées de Santé—AOPS)
Dr. Réginald Boulos, former Director, Centers for Development and Health

Dr. Jean Robert Brutus, Executive Director, Haitian Institute of Community Health

Dr. Clerisme Calixte, Researcher, Professional Management Services

Dr. Michel Cayemittes, Executive Director, Child Health Institute

Dr. Pierre P. Despagne, Executive Director, Centers for Development and Health (Centres pour le Développement et la Santé—CDS)

Fritz Moïse, Executive Director, Reproductive Health and Family Education Foundation (Fondation de Santé Reproductive and d'Education Familiale —FOSREF)

Dr. Serge Pintro, Executive Director, Association for the Promotion of the Family

Frantz Siméon, Director, Professional Management Services

Honduras

Dr. Wilfredo Alvarado, Minister of Health, Ministry of Health

Alejandro Flores Aguilar, Executive Director, ASHONPLAFA

Dra. Maria del Carmen Miranda, Population Advisor, USAID

Richard Monteth, HRD/HPN Officer, USAID

Dra. Olga Margarita Salgado, Clinic Director, IHSS

Mexico

Lucille Atkin, Program Officer, Ford Foundation

Lic. Luz Maria Chapela, Director of Population Education, National Population Council (CONAPO)

Art Danart, AID Country Representative Secretary, USAID

Esperanza Delgado, Mexico Representative, Pathfinder International

Luis de Llano, Producer and Director, TELEVISA, S.A. de C.V.

Dr. Javier Dominguez del Olmo, Head of Family Planning Services and Health Programs, ISSSTE

Lic. Gabriela Durazo, Executive Director, Mexican Federation of Private Family Planning Associations (FEMAP)

Dra. Celia Escandón, Medical Coordinator, IMSS/SOLIDARIDAD

Psic. Luz Amalia Esquivel, Head of Coordination and Technical Assistance

Dr. RodolfoTuirán Gutiérrez, Director General of Population Programs, National Populaiton Council (CONAPO)

Dr. Jesus Vasquez Hernandez, MEXFAM/Chiapas

Dr. Jose Ruben Jara, President, DELPHI and IBOPE, GAMMA

Emilio Ascarraga Jean, TELEVISA, S.A. de C.V.

Lic. Alfonso Lopez Juarez, Director, MEXFAM

Heriberto Lopez, TELEVISA

Heriberto López, Director General, GAMMA

Dra. Anameli Monroy López, Director/President, Council for Adolescents (CORA)

Dra. Ana Maria Goitia Marquez, Director of Public Works in Reproductive
  Health
Antonieta Martin, Local Coordinator, JHU/PCS Local Office
Dr. Jorge Martinez-Manautou, Director, Mexican Academy for the Study of
  Medical Demography (AMIDEM)
Marie McLeod, Population Advisor, USAID
Lic. Luis M. Moyano, Director, EMI Capitol de Mexico, S.A. de C.V.
Dr. Jorge Arturo Cardona Pérez, Chief, Family Planning and Rural Health
  Services
Dr. Gregorio Pérez Palacios, Director General of Reproductive Health
Rainer Rosenbaum, Director, United Nations Population Foundation of Mexico,
  Cuba, and the Dominican Republic (UNFPA)
Miguel Sabido, Secretary, TELEVISA
Maria Luisa Sánchez, GIRE
Raquel Schlosser, Director, Center for the Investigation and Study of Sexuality
Remy Basten Van der Meer, General Manager, NESA
Richard C. Vernon, Ph.D., Researcher, The Population Council—INOPAL

Nicaragua

Lic. Jorge Porto Carrero, Hilo Productions and Publications
Jairo Palacio Garcia, UNFPA Representative
Martha Fabiola Gomez, Social Communications Assistant, PROFAMILIA
Dra. Indiana Herrera, Director General, Information Systems, Ministry of Health
Ma. Auxiliadora Lacayo, Executive Director, PROFAMILIA
Marlene Landero, Director of Social Communication, PROFAMILIA
Francisco Mejia, Executive Director, Mejia Godoy Foundation
Dra. Azucena Maria Sabalos R., Director General, Ministry of Health
Veronica del Socorro Matus, IEC Director, PROFAMILIA
Adela Tapia, Director, Hilo Productions and Publications
Carolina Zuniga, Evaluation, PROFAMILIA

Peru

Ms. Michelle Alexander, Producer, IGUANA Productions
Mr. Jaime Althaus, Director, *Expreso* (newspaper)
Mr. Carlos Eduardo Aramburu, President, National Population Council
Dr. Daniel Aspilcueta, Director, INPPARES
Dr. Bruno Benavides, Project Peru 2000 Technical Assistance Deputy Director
Ms. Carola de Luque, APROPO General Manager
Ms. Susana Galdos, Head, Manuela Ramos Movementd
Mr. Alberto Isola, Theater Play Director
Mr. Rafael Leon, Advertising Creative, Humorist, Scriptwriter
Mr. Luis Llosa, Film Director and Director, IGUANA Productions
Ms. Margarita Morales, Manager, IGUANA Productions

Mr. John Nagahata, MINSA Reproductive Health and FP Director
Dr. Hugo Oblitas, Director, Project Peru 2000
Ms. Giovanna Peñaflor, IMASEN Manager and Public Opinion Analyst
Mr. Rafael Roncagliolo, Communication Researcher
Dr. Eduardo Salazar, Head PROCLAME, Cayetano Heredia University
Dr. Jorge Sanchez, Head PROCETS, Ministry of Health
Ms. Guisella Valcarcel, TV Host
Dr. Carlos Vidal, Dean, Cayetano Heredia University
Mr. Pedro Pablo Villanueva, UNFPA Representative
Ms. Marilu Wiegold, Publicist and Project Manager, APROPO

NEAR EAST

Near East Regional

Catherine Briggs, Population Initiatives for Peace
Hamouda Hanafi, Population Initiatives for Peace
Sitoo Mukerjee, Former Director of Research Utilization Programs, IDRC

Egypt

Dr. Samir Al Alfy, Consultant, State Information Service/Information Education
    and Communication Center
Mickey Aramati, Technical Assistance Manager, Pathfinder International
Ms. Sawsan El Bakly, former Director, State Information Service/Information
    Education and Communication Center
Dr. Safaa' El Baz, Director, Ain Shams University Regional Center for Training
    in Family Planning Faculty of Medicine
Dr. Hassan El Gebaly, Director, Systems Development Project II, Ministry of
    Health and Population
Dr. Mosheira El Shaffie, Undersecretary of Health, Ministry of Health
Mr. Waleed El-Khatib, Chief of Party, Pathfinder International
Mr. Farag Elkamel, Center for Development Communication
Dr. Badrawy M. Fahmy, Executive Director, Egyptian Family Planning
    Association
Nagwa Farag, Communication Officer, UNICEF
Dr. Soleiman Farah, Center for Development Services
Mr. Roger Hardister, Center for Development Services
Dr. Barbara Ibrahim, Senior Representative, the Population Council
Dr. Samir Khamis, UNFPA
Nabiha Loutfy, filmmaker
Dr. Sara Loza, President, Social Planning, Analysis & Administration
    Consultants

Prof. Dr. Maher Mahran, Director, National Population Council
Mr. Gamal Nahas, National Population Council
Tarek Noor, President, Americana Advertising Agency
Mr. Fathi Osman, Director, State Information Service/Information Education and
    Communication Center
Mr. Nabil Osman, Executive Director, State Information Service
Mr. Jestyn Portugill, Porter/Novelli Incorporated
Dr. Mostafa Sadek, Director, Health Insurance Organization
Dr. Ismail Sallam, Minister of Health
Dr. Amr Taha, Central Manager, Egyptian Junior Medical Doctors' Association
Dr. Mohamed Wafai, late Director, Wafai and Associates
Dr. Huda Zurayk, the Population Council

Jordan

Dr. Walid Abubaker, Resident Advisor, Quality Assurance Project, University
    Research Corporation
Rafik Al-Khateeb, Ministry of Islamic Affairs
Dr. Mo'tassem Awamleh, Director of Planning and Programs, Ministry of Health
Mr. Ahmad Batayneh, International Center for Studies and Research
Dr. Arif Batayneh, Minister of Health, Ministry of Health
Zahia Enab, Director of Programs, Jordan TV
Mr. Michel Farsoun, the Market Research Organization
Dr. Mona Hamza, Head of Department of Health Education, Ministry of Health
Dr. Fouad Hassan, Jordanian Association for Family Planning & Protection
Nina Jada', Noor Al Hussein Foundation
Dr. Hashem Jaddou', Secretary General, Ministry of Health
Mr. Mohammed Kamel, County Support Team Member, UNFPA
Abdel Halim Kharabshet, Department of Statistics
Ms. Nadine Khoury, the Market Research Organization
Dr. Issa Masarweh, University of Jordan
Ms. Lina Obeidat, Country Office Representative, UNFPA
Ms. Lina Qardan, Communication and Information Manager, National
    Population Commission
Mr. Nabih Salameh, General Secretariat, National Population Commission
Jordan H.R.H. Princess Basma Bint Talal, Queen Alia Fund for Social Work

Lebanon

Najwa Ksaifi, researcher, director, filmmaker, writer
Janane Mallat, director, filmmaker
Paul Mattar, director, writer, actor, producer
George Theodori, Chairman, Management, Planning and Research Consultants

Morocco

Dr. Khalid Alioua, ALCO Alternative Consultants
Prof. Khalil Amrani, Sociologist
Prof. Mohammed El Aouad, Sociologist
Dr. Amina Balafrej, Director, IEC Division, Ministry of Health
Ms. Farida Belyazid, scriptwriter
Dr. Jane Bertrand, Tulane University Evaluation Project
Dr. Najia Hajji, Director, Family Planning Division, Ministry of Health
Dr. Abderrahman Harouchi, former Minister, Ministry of Health
Ms. Nancy Harris, John Snow Inc.
H.R.H. Princess Lalla Meriem
Mr. Dick Moore, John Snow Inc.
Dr. Mostafa Tyane, Director of Population, Ministry of Health
Dr. A.W. Zerrari, Director, Maternal Child Health Division, Ministry of Health

Oman

Ms. Sabah Al-Bahlani, Director, Department of Health Education, Ministry of
   Health
Mr. Ibrahim Al Bashir, Advisor to the Minister, Ministry of Health
Mr. Saleh Al-Fahdi, Coordinator, Al-Seeb Sports Club
Dr. Ahmad Al-Ghassani, Undersecretary for Health Affairs, Ministry of Health
Dr. Souad Al-Lamki, MCH Coordinator for Muscat, Ministry of Health
Ms. Sawsan Al Rawass, Project Officer, UNICEF
Dr. Asya Al-Riyami, Director of Studies and Research Department, Ministry of
   Health
Dr. Msellem Saif El-Bually, Senior Pediatrician, National Women Child Care
   Commission
Ms. Fatima El-Ghazali, Director of International Relations, Ministry of Health
Dr. Yasmin Ja'afar, Director, Department of Family and Community Health
Dr. Ali Jaffer, Director General for Health Affairs, Directorate General of Health
   Affairs
Ms. Shahnaz Kianian, Country Representative, UNICEF
Dr. Ali Mousa, Minister of Health, Ministry of Health

Palestine

Azza El-Hassan, filmmaker

Tunisia

Fatma Skandrani, filmmaker

Turkey

Ugur Aytack, Deputy Director General, Ministry of Health
Feyyaz Berker, Chairman of Executive Board, Turkish Family and Health
    Planning Foundation
Turgut Denizel, former National Program Coordinator. UNFPA
Dr. Ayşe Akin Dervişoğlu, former Director General, Ministry of
    Health/Family Planning—MCH/FP
Nuray Fincancioğlu, former Executive Director, Human Resources Development
    Foundation
Vehbi Koç, former President, Turkish Family and Health Planning Foundation
Semral Koral, Executive Director, Family Planning Association of Turkey
Dr. Güntac Ozler, President, ZET Nielsen Turkey
Turkan Senkol, President, Turkish Midwife Association
Dr. Tandogan Tokgoz, former Ministry of Health Undersecretary
Dr. Ergül Tunçbilek, former Director of Hacettepe University/Haceteppe
    Institute for Population Studies
Dr. Sunday Üner, Hacettepe University/Hacceteppe Institute for Population
    Studies
Mr. Yasar Yaser, Executive Director, Turkish Family Health and Planning
    Foundation

NEW INDEPENDENT STATES

Kazakhstan

Dr. Tamara Djusubalieva, Director, Human Reproductive Center of Almaty
Dr. Aman Duisekeev, Deputy Minister for MCH, Ministry of Health (MOH)
Dr. Nina Kaiupova, Chief Ob/Gyn, MOH
Ms. Roslana Ramazanovna Taukina, Director, Totem Television-Radio
    Broadcasting
Mr. Alexander Ruzanov, President, BRIF: Social Marketing Research Agency

Kyrgyzstan

Mr. Adylbek T. Biynazarov, President, Pyramid Television-Radio Company
Dr. Bulashev, Chief Pediatrician, Ministry of Health (MOH)
Dr. Kalieva, Deputy Minister of Health, MOH
Mr. Vladislav Pototsky, Deputy Director, Republic Center for Public Opinion
    (RCPO)
Dr. Bektursun Tokubaev, Chief, Republic Health Center (RHC)

Russia

Dr. Inga Grebesheva, Director, Russian Family Planning Association
Dr. Lioudmila Kamisouk, Deputy Director, Russian Family Planning
    Association
Mr. Sergei Khovenko, Pygmalion
Vyacheslav Nedoshivin, Alter Ego
Dr. Elena Verobtsova, Moscow Youth Center

Turkmenistan

Dr. Khangel'di Mamedovich Mamedov, Deputy Minister, Ministry of Health

Ukraine

Dr. Elina Chaikovska, Family Planning Center at the Lviv Perinatal Institute
Dr. Svetlana Lashina, Odessa Women's Consultation Center No. 14, National
    Family Planning Center, Kiev Research Institute of Pediatrics and Ob/Gyn
Dr. Natalia Pryadko, Donetsk Regional Center for Maternal and Child Health
Ukrainian Social Surveys and Market Research
Dr. Irina Vouk, National Family Planning Center, Kiev Research Institute of
    Pediatrics & Obstetrics/Gynecology

Uzbekistan

Alisher Ilkhamov, Head of Center, Expert Sociological Research Center
Dr. Goulnara Jouldasheva, Chairman, Fund for a Healthy Generation
Mr. Rashid Malikov, Director, Flamingo Video (FLM)
Dr. Ahror Yarkulov, Deputy, Ministry of Health

JHU/PCS COLLABORATING CELEBRITIES, 1982–1996

AFRICA

Cameroon

Roger Milla, soccer player

Côte d'Ivoire

Cheikh Smith, singer and composer

Mali

Payi Camara, singer

Gimba, comedian
Djeneba Seck, singer

Nigeria

King Sunny Adé, singer
Onyeka Onwenu, singer and songwriter
Moses Adejumo, Baba Sala, comedian
Chief Zebudaya Chika Opalla, comedian
Femi Jarret, actor

Uganda

House Lane B, singing group, *Ray of Hope*
Philly Latoya, composer, *It's Not Easy*
Barry Nsibimana ("DJ Barry"), radio variety show host

Zimbabwe

Prudence Katomeni, actress, *More Time*
Thomas Mapfumo, singer
Oliver Mutukudzi, singer
Peter Ndlovu, singer

ASIA

Bangladesh

Mr. Humayan Ahmed, scriptwriter
Prof. Selim Al-Din, actor
Ms. Runa Laila, musician
Ms. Ferdousi Majumdar, actor
Mr. Asaduzzaman Noor, actor
Mr. Badal Rahman, film director
Mr. Khan Ataur Rahman, film director
Mr. Mamunur Rashid, actor
Ms. Sabina Yasmin, musician
Mr. Nasiruddin Yousuf, actor
Mr. Aly Zaker, actor

Indonesia

Teguh Karya, film director
Alex Komang, actor

Garin Nugroho, film director
Slamet Raharjo Djarot, film director
Ayu Ashari, actress
Maudy, actress
Titi D.J., actress

The Philippines

Joseph Estrada, Vice President, actor
Senator Juan M. Flavier, former Health Secretary
Senator Leticia Ramos-Shahani, Co-Chairperson, PLCPD
Lea Salonga, spokesperson, singer, actress, artist

LATIN AMERICA

Bolivia

Maria Elena Alcoreza, actress
Victor Hugo Cardenas, Vice President of Bolivia
Lidia Catari de Cardenas, Second Lady of Bolivia
Gonzalo Sanchez De Lozada, President of Bolivia
Ximena Sanchez De Lozada, First Lady of Bolivia
Javier Torrez Goitia (father), Senator
Jorge Ruiz, film director
Zulma Yugar, singer

Ecuador

Carmen de Vargas, radio director
Mercedes Erazo, TV and radio director
Yolanda Torres, TV director

Mexico

Tatiana Palacios, singer

Peru

Jaime Althaus, director, *Expreso* (newspaper)
Alberto Isola, theater play director
Rafael Leon, advertising creative, humorist, scriptwriter
Jean Franco Obrero, actor
Miguel Rubio, scriptwriter
Guisella Valcarcel, TV host

Actors

Milena Alba
Carlos Alcantara
Ivonne Barriga
Gianfranco Brero
Monchi Brugue
Katia Condos
Maria Pia Copello
Ana Correa
Adriana Davila
Javier Delgiudice
Fernando de Soria
Javier Echeverria
Ivonne Frayssinet
Jaime Lertora
Jose Enrique Mavila (Theater Director)
Marcelo Rivera
Hernan Romero
Monica Sanchez
Liliana Trujillo
Javier Valdes
Marco Zunnino

Graphic Artists

Juan Luis Gargurevich
Gredna Landolt
Francisco Sanchez
Walter Ventocilla

Puerto Rico

Edgardo Diaz, producer
Johny Lozada, singer
Charlie Masso, singer

NEAR EAST

Egypt

Fardous Abdul Hamid, actress
Mustapha Hussein, cartoonist

Ahmad Maher, actor
Karima Moukhtar, actress
Osama Anwar Okash, scriptwriter
Hesham Salim, actor
Sana' Younis, actress

Oman

Ibrahim Al Zadjali, actor

Turkey

Mr. Tarik Akan, actor
Mr. Bülent Bilgiç, actor
Prof. Dr. Tansu Ciller, Former Prime Minister of Turkey
Ms. Fusun Demirel, actress
Mr. Syleyman Demirel, Former President of Turkey
Mr. Kadir İnanir, actor
H.R.H. Princess Lalla Meriem
Bilge Olgac, director
Ms. Özlem Savaş, actor
Ms. Turkan Soray, actress
Ms. Gülseven G. Yaşer, President, Ultima TV Production Center and Producer
Atif Yilmaz, director
Uğur Yücel, actor

USAID MISSION COLLABORATORS

Benedicta Ababro
Carmela Abate
Lawrence Adnonum
Munira Al Batrani
Mohamed Ali Hassairi
Vathani
  Amirtanayagam
Jay Anderson
Maria Angelica
  Borneck
Felix Awantang
Dennis Baker
P. E. Balakrishnan
Victor Barbiero
Chris Barrett
Souleyman Barry
Wuleta Betamariam
Salwa Bitar

Dan Blumhagen
Lois Bradshaw
Susana Brems
Betsy Brown
John Burdick
Mona Byrkit
Perle Cambary
Deborah Caro
Carol Carpenter-
  Yaman
Lisa Carty
Jatinder Cheema
Eugene Chiavaroli
Sarah Clark
Sarah Clarke
Rebecca Cohn
Gary Cook
Thomas Cornell

Robert Cunnane
Leslie Curtin
Rabiha Dabbas
Lana Dakan
Art Dannart
Mercia Davids
Benoit de Marcken
Maria del Carmen
  Miranda
David Denman
Ephraim
  Despabiladeras
Brenda Doe
John Dumm
Paul Ehmer
Sameh El-Saharty
Sharon Epstein
Irina Eramova

Ilka Esquivel
Amina Essolbi
Michael Farbman
Kenneth Farr
Barbara Feringa
Maria Filomena Klin
Alan Foose
Matthew Friedman
Molly Gingerich
Joseph Goodwin
Michael Gould
James Graham
Richard Greene
Monty Harper
Paul Hartenberger
Karen Hilliard
Joyce Holfield
Millie Howard
James Hradsky
Ming Hung
John Paul James
William Jansen
Connie Johnson
William Johnson
Jerusha Karuthiru
Zareen Khair
Tawhida Khalil
Ray Kirkland
Peter Kolar
Hafid Lakhdar
Linda Lankanau
Joan LaRosa
Joanna Laryea
Earle Lawrence
Gary Leinen
Charles Lerman

Charles Lewellyn
Zohra Lhaloui
Malu Lins
Charles Llewellyn
Angela Franklin Lord
David Losk
Pancha Kumari-
     Manandhar
Cora Mandoto
Sara Pacqué Margolis
Richard Martin
Mark Matthews
Francis Mburu
Nancy McKay
Marie McLeod
Keys McManus
Elba Mercado
Gary Merrit
Carol Miller
Claude Milogo
Tom Morris
Michael Mushi
Nellie Mwanzia
Ursula Narodny
Margaret Neuse
Gary Newton
Gloria Nichtawitz
Nancy Nolan
Turhan Noury
Eilene Oldwine
David Oot
Shelagh O'Rourke
Doug Palmer
Carol Payne
Bill Pearson
Mark Pickett

David L. Piet
Shirlie Pinkham
Bonnie Pounds
David Puckett
Margarita Quevedo
Ken Randolph
Eugene (Gene) Rauch
Joy Riggs-Perla
Ricardo Roberto
Roxana Rogers
John Rogosch
Susan Ross
Bambang Samekto
Marilynn Schmidt
Amani Selim
Mary-Pat Selvaggio
Samaresh Sengupta
Pinar Senlet
Jinny Sewell
Liese Sherwood-Fabre
Shelley Snyder
Barbara Spaid
Steve Spielman
Carina Stover
Sherry Suggs
Siana Tackett
John Thomas
Rudy Thomas
Terry Tiffany
Raul Guillermo Toledo
Dana Vogel
Emmanuel
     Voulgaropoulos
Barbara Winkler
Holly Wise
Pamela Wolf

Bibliography

Ahmed, S. 1996. Contraceptive Use and Maternal-Child Health Care Utilization: A Search for Path of Joint Determination. Doctoral dissertation, Johns Hopkins School of Public Health, Department of Population Dynamics, Baltimore.

Ajiboye, J.K.T., I. George, S. Krenn, M. Soyoola, D. Phido, K. Kiragu, and S. Chapman. 1995. The Impact of Provider Training in Antenatal and Postnatal Clinics: Bauchi State, Nigeria. Paper prepared for the Nigeria Family Health Services Project, Lagos, Nigeria, and the Johns Hopkins Center for Communication Programs, Baltimore.

Ajzen, I. 1989. Attitude, Structure, and Behavior. In A. R. Pratkanis, S. J. Breckler, and A. G. Greenwald (eds.), *Attitude, Structure, and Function*. Hillsdale, NJ: Lawrence Erlbaum.

Alcalá, M. E. 1995. *Commitments to Sexual and Reproductive Health and Rights for All: Framework for Action*. New York: Family Care International.

Alcalay, R. 1980. The Impact of Mass Communication Campaigns in the Health Field. *Social Science and Medicine* 17 (2): 87–94.

Aldhous, P. 1995. A Local Dish. *New Scientist* 48 (1998): 36–37.

Altman, L., and P. T. Piotrow. 1980. Social Marketing: Does It Work? *Population Reports,* J (21). Baltimore: Johns Hopkins University, Population Information Program.

Amin, M. K. 1993. Indian Medical Association (IMA) Logo Promotes Doctors Providing Counseling Services. *USAID Weekly Highlights*, June 16. Baltimore: Johns Hopkins University, Population Communication Services.

Andreason, A. R. 1995. *Marketing for Social Change: Changing Behavior to Promote Health, Social Development, and the Environment*. San Francisco: Jossey-Bass.

Aristotle. *Poetics.* 1987. Translated by Stephen Halliwell. Chapel Hill: University of North Carolina Press.

Asch, S. E. 1955. Opinions and Social Pressure. *Scientific American* 193: 31–35.

Atkin, C. K. 1979. Research Evidence on Mass Mediated Health Communication Campaigns. In D. Nimmo (ed.), *Communication Yearbook 3*. New Brunswick, NJ: Transaction Books.

Atkin, C. K., and E. B. Arkin. 1990. Issues and Initiatives in Communicating Health Information. In C. Atkin and L. Wallack (eds.), *Mass Communication and Public Health*. Newbury Park, CA: Sage.

Babalola, S., and M. N. Jato. 1993. Burkina Faso Family Planning Expansion Project: 1992 Baseline Community Study. A final evaluation report for the Ministry of Health and Social Action/Directorate of Family Health, Burkina Faso, and the Johns Hopkins University, Population Communication Services, Baltimore.

Babalola, S., A. S. Lawal, I. V. Mako, J. G. Rimon, C. Corso, K. Kiragu, and C. Church. 1993. The Impact of a Mobile Drama on Family Planning Behavior in Ogun State, Nigeria. *Hygiene, Population and Education,* September: 42–45.

Backer, T. E., and E. M. Rogers (eds.). 1993. *Organizational Aspects of Health Communication Campaigns: What Works?* Newbury Park, CA: Sage.

Ball-Rokeach, S. J., and M. L. Defleur. 1976. A Dependency Model of Mass-Media Effects. *Communication Research* 3: 3–21.

Bandura, A. 1977. *Social Learning Theory*. Englewood Cliffs, NJ: Prentice-Hall.
———. 1986. *Social Foundations of Thought and Action*. Englewood Cliffs, NJ: Prentice-Hall.

Bandura, A. (ed.). 1995 *Self-Efficiacy in Changing Societies*. Cambridge, MA: Cambridge University Press.

Bangladesh Ministry of Health and Family Welfare. 1992. Family Planning in Bangladesh: An Emerging Success Story. Dhaka: Bangladesh Ministry of Health and Family Welfare.

Bankole, A., G. Rodríguez, and C. F. Westoff. 1993. The Mass Media and Reproductive Behavior in Nigeria. Paper presented at the annual meeting of the Population Association of America, Cincinnati, April 1–3.

Baron, D., O. M. Kumah, C. L. Lettenmaier, S. C. Krenn, M. E. Bashin, M. N. Jato, C. A. Church, Y. M. Kim, and P. F. Langlois. 1993. Qualitative Research for Family Planning Programs in Africa. *Occasional Paper Series No. 2.* Baltimore: Johns Hopkins Center for Communication Programs.

Bashin, M. E., and H. A. Allen, Jr. 1989. Family Planning Comes of Age in Niger: A Post-Project Survey of Family Planning Knowledge, Attitudes, and Practice in Niamey, Maradi, and Zinder. Report prepared for the Johns Hopkins University, Population Communication Services, Baltimore.

Becker, G. 1976. *Economic Approach to Human Behavior*. Chicago: University of Chicago Press.

Becker, G., and H. Lewis. 1973. Interaction Between Quantity and Quality of Children. *Journal of Political Economy* 81 (2): 141.

Bentler, P. M. 1995. *EQS Structural Equations Program Manual*. Encino, CA: Multivariate Software, Inc.

Berlo, D. K. 1960. *The Process of Communication: An Introduction to Theory and Practice.* New York: Holt, Rinehart and Winston.

Berry, G. 1991. The Story of Me and the Helaki: Street Theater in the Sale-Rabat Area [Morocco]. Manuscript. Boston: John Snow, Inc. (JSI).

Bertrand, J. T. 1988. Continuation and Expansion of Family Planning Operations Research in Zaire: 48 Months Progress Report and Workplan for Year V, October 1988 to September 1989. New Orleans: Tulane University, School of Public Health and Tropical Medicine.

Bertrand, J. T., and D. L. Kincaid. 1996. Evaluating Information, Education, and Communication (IEC) Programs for Family Planning and Reproductive Health. Final report of the IEC Working Group, the EVALUATION Project, Carolina Population Center, University of North Carolina at Chapel Hill.

Bertrand, J. T., P. Russell-Brown, and E. G. Landry. 1985. Evaluation of the Caribbean Contraceptive Social Marketing Project in Three Countries. Evaluation conducted for USAID under DPE 0632-C-00-2007-00 by Tulane University, New Orleans.

Blumler, J., and E. Katz. 1974. *The Uses of Mass Communication.* Beverly Hills, CA: Sage.

Bogue, D. J., and W. B. Johnson. 1969. Toward a Master Plan for Family Planning Communication. Paper presented at a Roundtable on Communication and Development at the Eleventh World Conference of the Society for International Development, New Delhi, November 15.

Bongaarts, J. 1992. Do Reproductive Intentions Matter? *International Family Planning Perspectives* 18 (3): 102–108.

———. 1995. The Role of Family Planning in Contemporary Fertility Transitions. *Research Division Working Paper* 71. New York: Population Council.

Bradac, J. J. (ed.). 1989. *Message Effects in Communication Science.* Newbury Park, CA: Sage.

Bradshaw, L. E., and C. P. Green. 1977. A Guide to Sources of Family Planning Program Assistance. *Population Reports,* J (15). Washington, DC: Population Information Program.

Brockerhoff, M. 1995. Fertility and Family Planning in African Cities: The Impact of Female Migration. *Journal of Biosocial Science* 27: 347–358.

———. 1996. Migration and the Fertility Transition in African Cities. Paper presented at the UNFPA Symposium on Internal Migration and Urbanization in Developing Countries: Implications for Habitat II, New York, January 24–26.

Bromham, D. R., A. Davey, L. Gaffikin, and C. A. Ajello. 1995. Materials, Methods and Results of the Norplant Training Program. *Advances in Contraception* 11 (3): 255–262.

Brown, L., H. Kane, and E. Ayres. 1993. *Vital Signs 1993: The Trends that Are Shaping Our Future.* New York: W. W. Norton.

Brown, L., J. Rice, M. Tyane, and J. Bertrand. 1995. Measuring the Effect of Quality of Services on Contraceptive Use in Morocco. Paper presented at the annual meeting of the Population Association of America, San Francisco, April 6–8.

Brown, W. J. 1994. Lessons Learned About the Entertainment-Education Strategy at Home and Abroad. Paper presented at the meeting of the Southern States Communication Association, Norfolk, VA, April 6–9.

Bruner, J. 1990. *Acts of Meaning*. Cambridge, MA: Harvard University Press.

Bryant, J. 1989. Message Features and Entertainment Effects. In J. Bradac (ed.), *Message Effects in Communication Science*. Newbury Park, CA: Sage, pp. 231–262.

Buana, Y. K., A. Sasongko, P. Richardson, and J. Eichner. 1990. Improving the Utilization and Self-Sufficiency of Private Urban Family Planning Clinics in Indonesia. Final report of the University Research Corporation, Family Planning Operations Research, Asia Project, Bethesda, MD.

Buchanan, D. R., S. Reddy, and Z. Hossain. 1994. Social Marketing: A Critical Appraisal. *Health Promotion International* 9 (1): 49–57.

Bulatao, R. A., A. Levin, E. R. Bos, and C. Green. 1993. *Effective Family Planning Programs*. Washington, DC: World Bank.

Bumin, C., and D. Boztok. 1995. Turkey Reproductive Health Services Situation Analysis Study 1994. Presentation of the Gazi University Department of Health and the Association for Voluntary Surgical Contraception study findings at the National Women Health and Family Planning Training-Communication Strategy Conference, Istanbul, March 16–18.

Burke, K. 1945. *A Grammar of Motives*. Englewood Cliffs, NJ: Prentice-Hall.

Cahill, L., B. Prins, M. Weber, and J. L. McGaugh. 1994. β-Adrenergic Activation and Memory for Emotional Events. *Nature* 371 (20): 702–704.

Caldwell, J. C. 1987. *Theory of Fertility Decline*. New York: Academic Press.

Campbell, D. T., and J. C. Stanley. 1963. *Experimental and Quasi-Experimental Designs for Research*. Boston: Houghton Mifflin.

Carr, D., and A. Way. 1994. *Women's Lives and Experiences*. Calverton, MD: Demographic and Health Surveys.

Casterline, J. B., A. E. Perez, and A. E. Biddlecom. 1996. Factors Underlying Unmet Need for Family Planning in the Philippines. *Research Division Working Paper* 84. New York: Population Council.

Center for International Research, Bureau of the Census. 1994. *Population of Developing Countries in 1994 by Age and Sex* [electronic data tape, 10/14/94]. Washington, DC: Bureau of the Census [producer and distributor].

Chaffee, S. H. 1982. Mass Media and Interpersonal Channels: Competitive, Convergent, or Complementary. In G. Gumpert and R. Cathcart (eds.), *Inter/Media: Interpersonal Communication in a Media World*. New York: Oxford University Press.

Chaudhuri, S. K. 1983. *Practice of Fertility Control: A Comprehensive Textbook*. Calcutta: Current Book Publishers.

Chen, H. 1990. *Theory-Driven Evaluations*. Newbury Park, CA: Sage.

Chen, H., and P. H. Rossi. 1983. Evaluating with Sense: The Theory-Driven Approach. *Evaluation Review* 7: 283–302.

———. 1987. The Theory-Driven Approach to Validity. *Evaluation and Program Planning* 10: 95–103.

Church, C. A., and M. E. Bashin. 1991. No Detail Is Minor: Steps to Assure Comprehension and Appropriateness in Family Planning Materials. Poster on the development of the Africa Norplant Flipchart shown at the American Public Health Association Annual Conference, Washington, DC, November 10–14.

Church, C. A., and J. S. Geller. 1989. Lights, Camera, Action! Promoting Family Planning with TV, Video, and Film. *Population Reports*, J (38). Baltimore: Johns Hopkins University, Population Information Program.

Ciszewski, R., and P. D. Harvey. 1991. The Effect of Price Increases on Contraceptive Sales in Bangladesh. *Journal of Biosocial Science* 26: 25–35.

Clark, M. S. (ed). 1992. Emotion and Social Behavior. *Review of Personality and Social Psychology 14.* Newbury Park, CA: Sage.

Cleland, J. 1985. Marital Fertility Decline in Developing Countries: Theories and the Evidence. In J. Cleland, J. Hobcraft, and B. Dinesen (eds.), *Reproductive Change in Developing Countries: Insights from the World Fertility Survey.* New York: Oxford University Press.

———. 1986. Fertility and Family Planning Surveys: Future Priorities in the Light of Past Experience. *International Family Planning Perspectives* 12 (1): 2–7.

Cleland, J. 1994. Different Pathways to Demographic Transition. In: F. Graham-Smith (ed.), *Population—The Complex Reality: A Report of the Population Summit of the World's Scientific Academies.* London: Royal Society, pp. 229–247.

Cleland, J., J. Hobcraft, and B. Dinesen (eds.). 1985. *Reproductive Change in Developing Countries: Insights from the World Fertility Survey.* New York: Oxford University Press.

Cleland, J., and C. Wilson. 1987. Demand Theories of Fertility Transition: An Iconoclastic View. *Population Studies* 41: 5–30.

Coale, A. J., and S. Watkins. 1986. *The Decline of European Fertility.* Princeton, NJ: Princeton University Press.

Cohen, J. E. 1995. *How Many People Can the Earth Support?* New York: W. W. Norton.

Cohen, S. I. 1993. Developing an Information, Education and Communication (IEC) Strategy for Population Programs. *United Nations Population Fund (UNFPA) Technical Paper No. 1.* New York: UNFPA.

Coleman, J. S., E. Katz, and H. Menzel. 1966. *Medical Innovation: A Diffusion Study.* New York: Bobbs Merrill.

Coleman, P. L. 1986a. Combining Mass Media and Interpersonal Communication. *Sex Education Coalition News*, June.

———. 1986b. Music Carries a Message to Youths. *Development Communication Report*, 53: 1–3.

———. 1996. (Johns Hopkins Center for Communication Programs) [Continuing corporate sponsorship of the Philippine Dial-A-Friend Project]. Personal communication to authors, November 5.

Coleman, P. L., and R. C. Meyer. 1990. *Entertainment for Social Change.* Proceedings of the Enter-Educate Conference. Baltimore: Johns Hopkins University, Center for Communication Programs

Conly, S. R. 1996. *Taking the Lead: The United Nations and Population Assistance.* Washington, DC: Population Action International (PAI).

Conly, S. R., and J. E. Rosen. 1996. International Population Assistance Update: Recent Trends in Donor Contributions. *PAI Occasional Paper No. 2.* Washington, DC: Population Action International.

Consumer Pulse Research Group. 1991. Project Star Final Report: Values and Lifestyles Study of Filipinos in the Lower Socioeconomic Sector. Prepared for the Johns Hopkins University, Center for Communication Programs, Baltimore.

Cook, T. D., and D. T. Campbell. 1979. *Quasi-Experimentation: Design and Analysis Issues for Field Studies.* Chicago: Rand McNally.

Cotten, N., J. Stanback, H. Maidouka, J. Taylor-Thomas, and T. Turk. 1992. Early Discontinuation of Contraceptive Use in Niger and the Gambia. *International Family Planning Perspectives* 18 (4): 1415–1419.

Critchlow, D. T. 1995. Birth Control, Population Control, and Family Planning: An Overview. *Journal of Policy History* 7 (1): 1–21.

Cronbach, L. J. 1982. *Designing Evaluations of Educational and Social Programs.* San Francisco: Jossey-Bass.

de Fossard, E. 1997. *How to Write a Radio Serial Drama for Social Development: A Script Writer's Manual.* Baltimore: Johns Hopkins University, Population Communication Services, Center for Communication Programs.

Debus, M. 1990. *Methodological Review: A Handbook for Excellence in Focus Group Research.* Washington, DC: Academy for Educational Development (AED/HEALTHCOM).

DeClerque, J. L., and A. O. Tsui. 1984. Contraceptive Discontinuation in Egypt: Differentials and Determinants of Length of Use. Research Report of the 1981–82 Egypt Follow-Up Survey on Family Life and Family Planning No. 4. Chapel Hill, NC: Carolina Population Center, University of North Carolina at Chapel Hill.

DeFleur, M. L. 1970. *Theories of Mass Communication.* 2nd ed. New York: David McKay.

DeFleur, M. L., and S. Ball-Rokeach. 1982. *Theories of Mass Communication.* 4th ed. New York: Longman.

Descouens, M., and R. Dow. 1986. Summary of the Study of Distribution of Contraceptive Products in Tunisia. Unpublished paper prepared for the Tunisian National Family Planning Organization, Tunis.

Destler, H., D. Liberi, J. Smith, and J. Stover. 1990. *Preparing for the 21st Century: Principles for Family Planning Service Delivery in the Nineties.* Report prepared for the U.S. Agency for International Development (USAID), Washington, DC.

Diggle, P. J., K. Y. Liang, and S. L. Zeger. 1994. *Analysis of Longitudinal Data.* New York: Oxford University Press.

Domestic Research Bureau (DRB) of Lever Brothers Pakistan, Limited. 1990. A Qualitative Study on Message Development for Population Communication Services. Study conducted by DRB for the Johns Hopkins University/ Population Communication Services, Pakistan.

Donaldson, P. J., and A. O. Tsui. 1990. The International Family Planning Movement. *Population Bulletin* 45 (3): 1–46.

Dwyer, J., J. Haws, G. Wambwa, M. Babawale, F. Way, and P. Lynam. 1991. COPE: A Self-Assessment Technique for Improving Family Planning Services. *Working Paper No. 1*. New York: Association for Voluntary Surgical Contraception (AVSC).

Easterlin, R. 1975. An Economic Framework for Fertility Analysis. *Studies in Family Planning* 6 (3): 54–63.

Eerola, M. 1994. *Probabilistic Causality in Longitudinal Studies*. New York: Springer-Verlag.

E-Land.com. [Internet statistics as of November 27, 1996. Number of net users and future projections] (http://www.e-land.com).

El-Bakly, S., and R. W. Hess. 1994. Mass Media Makes a Difference. *Integration* 41: 13–15.

El-Zanaty, F., E. M. Hussein, G. A. Shawky, A. A. Way, and S. Kishor. 1996. Egypt Demographic and Health Survey 1995. Calverton, MD: National Population Council [Egypt] and Macro International Inc.

Ezeh, A. C. 1993. The Influence of Spouses Over Each Other's Contraceptive Attitudes in Ghana. *Studies in Family Planning* 24: 163-174.

Family Planning Association of Kenya (FPAK). 1991. The Kenya Provider and Client IEC Project. Report prepared for the Johns Hopkins University, Population Communication Services, Baltimore.

Family Planning Association of Kenya (FPAK), the National Council for Population and Development (NCPD), and the Johns Hopkins Population Communication Services (JHU/PCS). 1995. Haki Yako: Developing the New with Lessons from the Past. The Kenya Provider and Client IEC Project, 1991–1994. Baltimore: Johns Hopkins University, Population Communication Services.

Family Planning Association of Uganda (FPAU). 1992. Family Planning: We Cannot Use What We Do Not Understand! Paper prepared for the Johns Hopkins University/Population Communication Services, Baltimore.

Farsoun, M., N. Khoury, and C. Underwood. 1996. In Their Own Words: A Qualitative Study of Family Planning in Jordan. *Information, Education, Communication (IEC) Field Report No. 6*. Baltimore: Johns Hopkins University, Center for Communication Programs.

Fayorsey, C. 1989. Family Planning in Africa: The Relevance of Gender Issues. In *Developments in Family Planning Policies and Programs in Africa*. Legon: University of Ghana, Regional Institute for Population Studies, pp. 194–229.

Fee, E. 1987. *Disease and Discovery: A History of the Johns Hopkins School of Hygiene and Public Health, 1916–1939*. Baltimore: Johns Hopkins University Press.

Ferguson, A., J. Gitonga, and D. Kabira. 1988. Family Planning Needs in Colleges of Education. Report of a study of 20 colleges in Kenya, prepared for the Ministry of Health, Division of Family Health-GTZ Support Unit, and the Family Planning Association of Kenya, Nairobi, Kenya.

Festinger, L. 1954. A Theory of Social Comparison Processes. *Human Relations* 7: 117–140.

Finkel, S. E. 1995. *Causal Analysis with Panel Data.* Thousand Oaks, CA: Sage.

Fishbein, M., and I. Ajzen. 1975. *Belief, Attitude, Intention and Behavior: An Introduction to Theory and Research.* Reading, MA: Addison-Wesley.

Fisher, A., B. Mensch, R. Miller, I. Askew, A. Jain, C. Ndeti, L. Ndhlovu, and P. Tapsoba. 1996. *Guidelines and Instruments for a Family Planning Situation Analysis Study.* Rev. ed. New York: Population Council.

Fisher, B. A. 1978. *Perspectives on Human Communication.* New York: Macmillan.

Fisher, R. A. 1956. *Statistical Methods and Scientific Inference.* Edinburgh: Oliver and Boyd.

Fisher, W. R. 1987. *Human Communication as Narration: Toward a Philosophy of Reason, Value, and Action.* Columbia: University of South Carolina Press.

Flay, B. R., and D. Burton. 1990. Effective Communication Strategies for Health Campaigns. In C. Atkin and L. Wallack (eds.), *Mass Communication and Public Health.* Newbury Park, CA: Sage.

Flay, B. R., D. Di Tecco, and R. P. Schlegel. 1980. Mass Media in Health Promotion: Analysis Using an Extended Information-Processing Model. *Health Education Quarterly* 7 (2): 127–147.

Foreit, K. G., M.P.P. de Castro, and E.T.D. Franco. 1989. The Impact of Mass Media Advertising on a Voluntary Sterilization Program in Brazil. *Studies in Family Planning* 20 (2): 107–116.

Foreit, K. G., and R. E. Levine. 1993. Cost Recovery and User Fees in Family Planning. *Options for Population Policy Paper Series No. 5.* Washington, DC: Options for Population Policy.

Fraser, C. 1987. *Education Through Entertainment: The British Radio Drama Series, "The Archers"—An Everyday Story of Country Folk.* Rome: Food and Agriculture Organization of the United Nations.

Freedman, R. 1984. The KAP-Gap: An Important Problem for Science and Social Policy. Manuscript prepared for Demographic and Health Surveys, Institute for Resource Development, Macro Systems, Inc., Columbia, MD.

———. 1987a. The Contribution of Social Science Research to Population Policy and Family Planning Program Effectiveness. *Studies in Family Planning* 18 (2): 57–82.

———. 1987b. The Social and Political Environment, Fertility, and Family Planning Program Effectiveness. In R. J. Lapham and G. B. Simmons (eds.), *Organizing Effective Family Planning Programs.* Washington, DC: National Academy Press, pp. 35–57.

———. 1990. Family Planning Programs in the Third World. *Annals of the American Academy of Political and Social Science* 510: 33–43.

Freedman, R., and B. Berelson. 1976. The Record of Family Planning Programs. *Studies in Family Planning* 7 (1): 1–40.

Freedman, R., and A. K. Blanc. 1992. Fertility Transition: An Update. *International Family Planning Perspectives* 18 (2): 44–50.

Freeman, L. C. 1979. Centrality in Networks: Conceptual Clarification. *Social Networks* 1: 215–239.

Gallen, M. E., C. L. Lettenmaier, and C. P. Green. 1987. Counseling Makes a Difference. *Population Reports*, J (35). Baltimore: Johns Hopkins University, Population Information Program.

Gallen, M. E., and W. Rinehart. 1987. Operations Research: Lessons for Policy and Programs. *Population Reports*, J (31). Baltimore: Johns Hopkins University, Population Information Program.

Gao, M. 1995. A Traveling Opera Troupe. *China Population Today* 12: 19.

Gardner, R., and R. Blackburn. 1996. Reproductive Health Care for Migrants. *Population Reports*, J (45). Baltimore: Johns Hopkins University, Population Information Program.

Gass, P. M., and R. Barber-Madden. 1990. Women's Health Services Utilization: Illustrative Examples of Under-utilization from Latin America and the Caribbean. Paper presented at the 118th Annual Meeting of the American Public Health Association, New York.

Gerbner, G. 1973. Cultural Indicators—The Third Voice. In G. Gerbner, L. Gross, and W. Melody (eds.), *Communications Technology and Social Policy*. New York: Wiley.

———. 1977. *Mass Media Policies in Changing Cultures*. New York: Wiley.

Gerbner, G., L. Gross, M. Morgan, and N. Signorelli. 1980. The Mainstreaming of America: Violence Profile No. 11, *Journal of Communication* 30: 10–27.

Ghana Ministry of Health/Health Education Unit (MOH/HEU) and the Johns Hopkins University/Population Communication Services (JHU/PCS). 1992. Partners in Family Health Communication. Summary report of the Johns Hopkins Center for Communication Programs, Baltimore.

———. 1993a. Family Planning Campaign Brief, 1993. Summary report of the Johns Hopkins Center for Communication Programs, Baltimore.

———. 1993b. The Launching of a Family Health Communication Strategy for Ghana, 1993–1994. Summary report of the Johns Hopkins Center for Communication Programs, Baltimore.

Ghana Statistical Service and Macro International, Inc. 1994. *Ghana Demographic and Health Survey 1993*. Calverton, MD: Macro International, Inc.

Gigerenzer, G., Z. Swijtink, T. Porter, L. Daston, J. Beatty, and L. Kruger. 1989. *The Empire of Chance*. New York: Cambridge University Press.

Gillespie, D. G. 1993. Family Planning Programs: The Challenge of Rising Expectations. In P. Senanayake and R. L. Kleinman (eds.). Proceedings of the IPPF Family Planning Congress, New Delhi, October 1992. *Family Planning: Meeting Challenges, Promoting Choices*. Carnforth, England.

Glanz, K., F. M. Lewis, and B. K. Rimer (eds.). 1990. *Health Behavior and Health Education*. San Francisco: Jossey-Bass.

Glass, W. 1992. Partners in Family Health Communication: Lessons Learned from the Ghana Health and Family Planning Information Program. Report prepared for the Johns Hopkins University/Population Communication Services, Baltimore.

———. 1993. The Launching of a Family Health Communication Strategy for Ghana for 1993–94: May 10–May 21, 1993. Workshop report prepared for the Ghana Health Education Unit/Ministry of Health, Accra, and the Johns Hopkins University/Population Communication Services, Baltimore.

Glass, W., and H. D. Smith. 1993. Family Planning Association of Uganda: The Radio Scriptwriters' Workshop in Kampala, Uganda, July 27–August 17, 1993. Trip report for the Johns Hopkins University/Population Communication Services, Baltimore.

Glymour, C., R. Scheines, P. Spirtes, and K. Kelly. 1987. *Discovering Causal Structure*. Orlando, FL: Academic Press.

Goffman, E. 1974. *Frame Analysis: An Essay on the Organization of Experience*. Cambridge, MA: Harvard University Press.

Government of Turkey and UNICEF. 1991. *The Situation Analysis of Mothers and Children in Turkey*. Country Program, 1991–1995, Series 2 Report. Government of Turkey and UNICEF Program of Cooperation. Ankara: UNICEF.

Govindasany, P., M. K. Stewart, S. O. Rutstein, J. T. Boerma, and A. E. Sommerfelt. 1993. High-Risk Births and Maternity Care. *Demographic and Health Surveys Comparative Studies No. 8*. Columbia, MD: Macro International.

Graeff, J. A., J. P. Elder, and E. M. Booth. 1993. *Communication for Health and Behavior Change: A Developing Country Perspective*. Publication of the HEALTHCOM Project, Academy for Educational Development (AED), funded by the U.S. Agency for International Development (USAID). San Francisco: Jossey-Bass.

Green, C. P. 1992. Strategic Management of Family Planning Programs. *World Bank Working Paper No. 976*. Washington, DC: World Bank.

Green, L. W., and M. W. Kreuter. 1991. *Health Promotion Planning: An Educational and Environmental Approach*. 2nd ed. Mountain View, CA: Mayfield Publishing.

Green, M. 1993. The Evolution of U.S. International Population Policy, 1965–92: A Chronological Account. *Population and Development Review* 19 (2): 303–321.

Greenberg, R. H., R. J. Williams, J. A. Yonkler, G. Saffitz, and J. G. Rimon. 1996. *How to Select and Work with an Advertising Agency*. Baltimore: Johns Hopkins Center for Communication Programs.

Greenhalgh, S. 1992. Negotiating Birth Control in Village China. *Working Paper No. 38*. New York: Population Council.

Gueye, M., T. Kane, M. Jato, S. Pacque-Margolis, I. Speizer, E. Sampara, and D. Baron. 1992. Modern and Traditional Media Project: Baseline IEC Survey on Family Planning in Bamako. Evaluation report for the Association for the

Promotion and Protection of the Family, the Center for Applied Research on Population and Development, and the Johns Hopkins Population Communication Services, Baltimore.

Gunby, P. 1995. International Electronic Link Solves Medical Puzzle. Medical News and Perspectives. *Journal of the American Medical Association* 247 (22): 1750.

Gushin, I., M. C. Hooper, and G. Saffitz. 1994. Technical Assistance to the Central Asian Republics: Almaty, Kazakhstan and Bishkek, Kyrgyzstan. Trip report, April 14–May 5, 1994. Johns Hopkins Population Communication Services, Baltimore.

Hagenaars, J. A. 1990. *Categorical Longitudinal Data: Log Linear Panel, Trend, and Cohort Analysis.* Newbury Park, CA: Sage.

Harper, P. B. 1991. Guidelines for Producing Training Films and Videos. *Development Communication Report* 73: 14–15.

Harper, P. B., S. Schneider, and K. Mworia. 1990. Producing Family Planning Training Films in Africa: Involving the Audience from A to Z. Paper presented at the 118th Annual Meeting of the American Public Health Association (APHA), New York, September 30–October 4.

Harvey, P. D. 1993. To Maximize Contraceptive Prevalence, Keep Prices Low. *DKT International Reports/Findings* 3 (August). Washington, DC: DKT International.

———. 1994. The Impact of Condom Prices on Sales in Social Marketing Programs. *Studies in Family Planning* 25 (1): 52–58.

———. 1996. Contraceptive Social Marketing Statistics. Washington, DC: DKT International.

Haryono, S. 1989. Give the People What They Want and Spread Their Satisfaction for Others to Follow: The Indonesia Family Planning Experience. Speech delivered at the 1989 Hugh Moore Award, Washington, DC, July 19.

Haryono, S., G. Saffitz, and J. G. Rimon II. 1990. Indonesia: The Blue Circle Campaign. Paper presented at the American Public Health Association (APHA) Conference, Chicago.

Hastings, G., and A. Haywood. 1991. Social Marketing and Communication in Health Promotion. *Health Promotion International* 6 (2): 135–145.

Hayduk, L. A. 1987. *Structural Equation Modeling with LISREL: Essentials and Advances.* Baltimore: Johns Hopkins University Press.

Health Education Division/Tanzania Ministry of Health and the Johns Hopkins University, Population Communication Services (JHU/PCS). 1991. Attitudes and Beliefs Regarding Child-Spacing: Focus Group Discussions with Men and Women from Six Regions of Tanzania. Study report of the Johns Hopkins Center for Communication Programs, Baltimore.

Heckert, K. A., Y. Karki, K. Onta, J. D. Storey, and A. Bhatt. 1996. Interpersonal Communication: The Unifying Factor in the Nepal Redline Strategy for Addressing the Unmet Need. Paper presented at the American Public Health Association Annual Conference, New York, November 17–21.

Henderson, N. R. 1994a. Summary Notes on 7 In-Depth Interviews and Two Mini-Groups in Denver, Colorado. Qualitative Market Research by Riva Market Research, Inc., for Johns Hopkins University, Baltimore, February 9.

———. 1994b. Topline Report on Three Focus Groups to Review Final Designs for the Immunize on Time . . . Your Baby's Counting on You Campaign. Qualitative Market Research by Riva Market Research, Inc., for Harvard University, Center for Health Communications, Boston, April 4.

Henshaw, S. K. 1990. Induced Abortion: A World Review—1990. *International Family Planning Perspectives* 22 (2): 76–81.

Hill, A. B. 1971. Statistical Evidence and Inference. In A. B. Hill (ed.), *Principles of Medical Statistics*. New York: Oxford University Press.

Hindin, M. J., D. L. Kincaid, O. M. Kumah, W. Morgan, Y. M. Kim, and J. K. Ofori. 1994. Gender Differences in Media Exposure and Action During a Family Planning Campaign in Ghana. *Health Communication* 6 (2): 117–135.

Hornik, R. C. 1988. *Development Communication*. New York: Longman.

———. 1989. Channel Effectiveness in Development Communication Programs. In R. E. Rice and C. K. Atkin (eds.), *Public Communication Campaigns*. 2nd ed. Newbury Park, CA: Sage, pp. 309–330.

Hovland, C. I. 1973. *Communication and Persuasion: Psychological Studies of Opinion Change*. New Haven, CT: Yale University Press.

Hovland, C. I., and I. L. Janis. 1959. *Personality and Persuasibility*. New Haven, CT: Yale University Press.

Hovland, C. I., A. A. Lumsdain, and F. D. Sheffield. 1949. *Experiments on Mass Communication*. New York: John Wiley and Sons.

Huntington, D., C. L. Lettenmaier, and I. Obeng-Quaidoo. 1990. User's Perspective of Counseling Training in Ghana: The "Mystery Client" Trial. *Studies in Family Planning* 21 (3): 171–177.

Huntington, D., and S. R. Schuler. 1993. The Simulated Client Method: Evaluating Client-Provider Interactions in Family Planning Clinics. *Studies in Family Planning* 24 (3): 187–193.

Huston, P. 1979. *Third World Women Speak Out: Interviews in Six Countries on Change, Development, and Basic Needs*. New York: Praeger.

Indian Medical Association (IMA). 1992. Strategic Debriefing Document: India. Project summary of the IMA and the Johns Hopkins University/Population Communication Services, Baltimore.

Indonesia Central Bureau of Statistics (CBS), National Family Planning Coordinating Board (NFPCB), and Institute for Resource Development/Westinghouse (IRD/W). 1989. *National Indonesia Contraceptive Prevalence Survey 1987*. Columbia, MD: IRD/Demographic and Health Surveys.

Indonesia Central Bureau of Statistics (CBS), State Ministry of Population/National Family Planning Coordinating Board (NFPCB), Ministry of Health, and Macro International, Inc. (MI). 1995. *Indonesia Demographic and Health Survey 1994*. Calverton, MD: CBS and MI.

Inkeles, A., and D. H. Smith. 1974. *Becoming Modern*. Cambridge, MA: Harvard University Press.

Institute for Adult Education, University of Ghana, and the Johns Hopkins Center for Communication Programs. 1995. Mass Media Support for Adult Population Education: A Community-Based Approach to Population Communication Activities. Project status report prepared for the United Nations Population Fund (UNFPA), New York.

International Bank for Reconstruction and Development/The World Bank. 1993. *Effective Family Planning Programs*. Washington, DC: The World Bank.

International Broadcasting Audience Research Library/British Broadcasting Company (IBAR/BBC). 1996. *World Radio and Television Receivers, 1996.* London: IBAR/BBC World Service.

International Science and Technology Institute (ISTI). 1988. Contraceptive Social Marketing Assessment, 1 & 2. Arlington, VA: ISTI. Mimeographed.

Jabre, B., L. Jaroudi, S. Khamis, and W. Rinehart. 1993. The Minya Initiative: A Step-by-Step Guide for Planning and Implementing Social Mobilization for Family Planning at the Local Level. Training manual prepared in collaboration with the National Population Council, State Information Service, Directorate of Health, with funding from the U.S. Agency for International Development (USAID). Baltimore: Johns Hopkins Center for Communication Programs.

Japan's ODA Growth Slows to a Record Low. 1996. *JOICFP News* 267. Tokyo: Japanese Organization for International Cooperation in Family Planning, Inc., September.

Jara, R. 1990. Evaluation of the Karina and Charlie Campaign for Young People. Evaluation report by the Institute for Communication Research, Mexico City, for the Johns Hopkins University/Population Communication Services, Baltimore, April.

Jato, M. N. 1996. (Johns Hopkins Center for Communication Programs) [Tanzania 1993 JHU/PCS materials evaluation]. Personal communication to authors, November 11.

Jato, M. N., O. M. Kumah, and D. Awasum. 1991. Cameroon Childspacing Promotion Project: Baseline Audience Survey Report. Final evaluation prepared for the Ministry of Public Health/Directorate Family and Mental Health, Cameroon, and the Johns Hopkins University/Population Communication Services, Baltimore.

Jato, M. N., and J. Moyo. 1994. Communication Strategies to Overcome Medical Barriers. Paper presented at the East and South Africa Regional Workshop, Improving Quality of Care and Access to Contraception: Reducing Medical Barriers, Harare, Zimbabwe, January 30–February 4.

Jato, M. N., C. Simbakalia, J. M. Tarasevich, and D. N. Awasum. 1996. The Impact of the Multimedia Family Planning Promotion on the Contraceptive Behavior of Women in Tanzania. Paper presented at the 124th Annual Meeting of the American Public Health Association, New York, November 17–21.

Jato, M. N., A. van der Straten, O. M. Kumah, C. Vondrasek, L. Tsitsol, and R. Seukap. 1993. Women Take Leadership in Health Development Communication in Cameroon: Results of Focus Group Discussion Research. Evaluation report prepared for the Ministry of Public Health and Ministry of

Women's Affairs, Cameroon, and the Johns Hopkins University/Population
Communication Services, Baltimore.

John Snow, Inc. (JSI). 1996. Overview of USAID Population Assistance: FY 1995.
Report by the Family Planning Logistics Management Project. Washington,
DC: JSI.

Johns Hopkins University/Center for Communication Programs (JHU/CCP). 1995.
Reaching Young People Worldwide: Lessons Learned from Communication
Projects, 1986–1995. *CCP Working Paper No. 2,* Baltimore: JHU/CCP.

Johns Hopkins University/Center for Communication Programs/Population
Communication Services/Population Information Program (JHU/CCP/
PCS/PIP). 1984. Basic Processes and Principles for Population/Family
Planning Communication (P Process booklet). Baltimore: JHU/CCP.

Johns Hopkins University/Population Communication Services (JHU/PCS). 1986a.
Final Report: Generic Condom Promotion in Colombia (LA-COL-01).
Baltimore: Johns Hopkins Center for Communication Programs.

————. 1986b. Review of the Information, Education, Communication (IEC)
Component of the Indonesia Population Program. Recommendations for IEC
Planning, 1987–1991. Baltimore: Johns Hopkins Center for Communication
Programs.

————. 1988. Final Report: The Brazilian Association of Family Planning
Agencies (ABEPF), Family Planning Activities (LA-BRA-01). Baltimore:
Johns Hopkins Center for Communication Programs.

————. 1989a. *Johns Hopkins University, Population Communication Services
1989 Annual Report.* Baltimore: Johns Hopkins Center for Communication
Programs.

————. 1989b. Final Report: Community Based Training Materials (AF-KEN-04).
Baltimore: Johns Hopkins Center for Communication Programs.

————. 1990a. Final Report: Bolivia Family Health Information, Education,
Communication Project (LA-BOL-01). Baltimore: Johns Hopkins Center for
Communication Programs.

————. 1990b. Final Report: Freedom Sells Condoms in Colombia (LA-COL-02
& 03). Baltimore: Johns Hopkins Center for Communication Programs.

————. 1990c. Final Report: Pakistan Focus Group Research for Message
Development (AS-PAK-01), August 15–October 31, 1990. Baltimore: Johns
Hopkins Center for Communication Programs.

————. 1990d. Final Report: Using Television to Influence Family Planning
Behavior: The Experience in Urban Nigeria with "In a Lighter Mood" (AF-
NGA-07 & 08). Baltimore: Johns Hopkins Center for Communication
Programs.

————. 1990e. Final Report: Using Male Motivators to Generate Demand for
Family Planning in a Male Farmer Organization (AS-PH1-01). Baltimore:
Johns Hopkins Center for Communication Programs.

————. 1990f. *Johns Hopkins University, Population Communications Services
1990 Annual Report.* Baltimore: Johns Hopkins Center for Communication
Programs.

————. 1991a. Final Report: Service Provider and Client Survey (AS-PAK-05), August 15, 1991–January 30, 1992. A project conducted by AFTAB Associates for the Johns Hopkins University/Population Communication Services, Center for Communication Programs, Baltimore.

————. 1991b. *Johns Hopkins University, Population Communications Services 1991 Annual Report.* Baltimore: Johns Hopkins Center for Communication Programs.

————. 1992a. *Center for Communication Programs Newsletter,* 1 (5). Dhaka: Johns Hopkins Center for Communication Programs/Population Communication Services.

————. 1992b. Family Planning Campaign "Breaks the Bank" in Ghana. *USAID Weekly Report,* September 2. Baltimore: Johns Hopkins Center for Communication Programs.

————. 1992c. Final Report: Building Support for Population Policy (LA-BOL-03). Baltimore: Johns Hopkins Center for Communication Programs.

————. 1992d. Final Report: Clinic Promotion for Indigenous People (LA-BOL-02). Baltimore: Johns Hopkins Center for Communication Programs.

————. 1992e. Final Report: El Salvador Motivators' Training Project (LA-ELS-02). Baltimore: Johns Hopkins Center for Communication Programs.

————. 1992f. Final Report: Family Planning IEC and Training Materials Project (AF-GAM-01). Baltimore: Johns Hopkins Center for Communication Programs.

————. 1992g. Final Report: Production of the Social Drama *Aahat* (AS-PAK-03), June 1, 1991–September 30, 1992. A project conducted by Pakistan Television Corporation for the Johns Hopkins University/Population Communication Services, Center for Communication Programs, Baltimore.

————. 1992h. Ghana Conference Highlights Dramatic Rise in Contraceptive Use, Radio Award. *USAID Weekly Report,* April 22. Baltimore: Johns Hopkins Center for Communication Programs.

————. 1992i. JHU/PCS Quarterly Reports on Activities in Pakistan. Tenth and Twelfth Quarters: October 1, 1992–June 30, 1993. Baltimore: Johns Hopkins Center for Communication Programs.

————. 1992j. *Johns Hopkins University, Population Communication Services 1992 Annual Report.* Baltimore: Johns Hopkins Center for Communication Programs.

————. 1993a. Bangladesh *Jiggasha* (Community Network) Approach Makes FP a Community Norm. *USAID Weekly Report,* March 3. Baltimore: Johns Hopkins Center for Communication Programs.

————. 1993b. Bauchi State MotherCare (Nigeria) IEC Project Overview. Baltimore: Johns Hopkins Center for Communication Programs.

————. 1993c. Haiti: Health/IEC Overview and Strategic Options Design. Baltimore: Johns Hopkins Center for Communication Programs.

————. 1993d. Mali Sings and Dances in Celebration of National Family Planning Logo. *USAID Weekly Report,* May 12. Baltimore: Johns Hopkins Center for Communication Programs.

————. 1993e. The Minya Initiative: Fruits of Collaboration. End-of-Project Seminar, December 22. A collaboration between the Minya Directorate of Health, Minya National Population Council, Minya State Information Service, and the Johns Hopkins Center for Communication Programs, Baltimore.

————. 1993f. Nigeria Family Health Services/Information, Education, Communication (FHS/IEC) Division Project at a Glance. Baltimore: Johns Hopkins Center for Communication Programs.

————. 1993g. *Johns Hopkins University, Population Communication Services 1993 Annual Report.* Baltimore: Johns Hopkins Center for Communication Programs.

————. 1993h. Philippine PLCPD Advocacy Project: Summary, Scope of Work and Conditions, February 1, 1993–January 31, 1994. Baltimore: Johns Hopkins University, Population Communication Services.

————. 1994a. Final Report: Communication for Young People II (LA-MEX-09) and Evaluation of Communication for Young People II (LA-MEX-10) [The Karina and Charlie projects in Mexico and Peru]. Baltimore: Johns Hopkins Center for Communication Programs.

————. 1994b. The Minya Initiative. *Integration* 41: 20–23.

————. 1994c. Monitoring Summary: The Public Service Announcement (PSA)/Logo Campaign, Nigeria FHS/IEC Project. Baltimore: Johns Hopkins Center for Communication Programs.

————. 1994d. Monitoring Summary: The Uganda Family Planning Promotion Program. Case study presented at the Advances in Family Health Communication Workshops, Program Monitoring session, Baltimore. Johns Hopkins Center for Communication Programs.

————. 1994e. *Johns Hopkins University, Center for Communication Programs 1994 Annual Report.* Baltimore: Johns Hopkins Center for Communication Programs.

————. 1994f. Project Proposal for the Population and Environment Education Project under the Indonesian Ministry of Population/BKKBN, April 1994–June 1995. Baltimore: Johns Hopkins University/Population Communication Services.

————. 1994g. Project Proposal: The Third Phase—Childspacing in Cameroon (AF-CAM-03), January 1994–June 1995. Baltimore: Johns Hopkins University, Population Communication Services.

————. 1994h. Technical Assistance and Media Support for Family Planning in India. Technical report for the Johns Hopkins Center for Communication Programs, Baltimore.

————. 1995a. Communication Design and Evaluation System (CODES). Evaluation framework developed by the JHU/PCS, Research and Evaluation Division, Baltimore.

————. 1995b. *Johns Hopkins University, Population Communication Services 1995 Annual Report.* Baltimore: Johns Hopkins Center for Communication Programs.

———. 1995c. Nepal Interpersonal Counseling Communication Guidebook. An interpersonal counseling training manual produced by the Johns Hopkins Center for Communication Programs, Baltimore.

———. 1996a. *Gold Star Opening in Luxor, Egypt: Elizabeth Maguire Visit* [Video]. Available through the Johns Hopkins Center for Communication Programs, Media/Materials Clearinghouse, Baltimore.

———. 1996b. *Johns Hopkins University, Population Communication Services 1996 Annual Report.* Baltimore: Johns Hopkins Center for Communication Programs.

Joreskog, K. G., and D. Sorbom. 1979. Advances in Factor Analysis and Structural Equation Models. Cambridge, MA: ABT.

Kaiser Family Foundation. 1996. The Uses of Mainstream Media to Encourage Social Responsibility: The International Experience. Report prepared by Advocates for Youth for the Henry J. Kaiser Family Foundation, Menlo Park, CA.

Kane, T., M. Gueye, D. Baron, I. Speizer, S. Pacque-Margolis, and E. Simpara. 1994. Use of Modern and Traditional Media IEC Interventions to Improve Contraceptive Knowledge, Attitudes, and Practice in Bamako, Mali. Paper presented at the annual meeting of the Population Association of America, Miami, May 5–7.

Katz, E., J. Blumler, and M. Gurevitch. 1974. Uses of Mass Communication by the Individual. In W. P. Davidson and F. Yu (eds.), *Mass Communication Research: Major Issues and Future Directions.* New York: Praeger.

Katz, K., K. Hardee, and M. T. Villinski. 1993. *Quality of Care in Family Planning: A Catalog of Assessment and Improvement Tools. A Manual of Assessment Indicators.* Durham, NC: Family Health International.

Katz, E., and P. F. Lazarsfeld. 1955. *Personal Influence.* Glencoe, IL: Free Press.

Kazungu, T. 1993. Tanzania Radio Soap Opera Treatment Design Mini-Workshop, March 15–19, 1993. Trip report, March 14–27, 1993, for the Johns Hopkins University, Population Communication Services, Baltimore.

Keeny, S. M. 1965. Korea and Taiwan: Two National Programs. *Studies in Family Planning* 1 (6): 1–6.

Kekevole, J., K. Kiragu, L. Muruli, and P. Josiah. 1996. The 1996 Kenya National Information, Education, and Communication (IEC) Situation Survey. Evaluation report prepared for the National Council for Population and Development, Central Bureau of Statistics, and the Johns Hopkins Center for Communication Programs, Baltimore. Forthcoming JHU/CCP IEC Field Report.

Keller, A., P. Severyns, A. Khan, and N. Dodd. 1989. Toward Family Planning in the 1990s: A Review and Assessment. *International Family Planning Perspectives* 15 (4): 127–135.

Kemprecos, L. F. 1994. Oman: Research Technical Assistance Visit for the Oman KAP Survey. Trip report, March 17–April 6, 1994, for the Johns Hopkins University/ Population Communication Services, Baltimore.

Kemprecos, L. F., J. D. Storey, B. Jabre, J. G. Rimon II, S. Khamis, and M. Wafai. 1994. Research Report: The Impact of the Minya IEC Initiative. Baltimore: Johns Hopkins University/Population Communication Services.

Khuda, B. E., A. Barkat, B. Robey, M. A. Mannan, J. Helali, A. Sultana, and S. A. Salam. 1994. Bangladesh Journalists Reporting on Population and Family Planning: Study Results. Johns Hopkins Center for Communication Programs and University Research Corporation, Bangladesh, *CCP Working Paper No. 1*. Baltimore: Johns Hopkins Center for Communication Programs.

Kihinga, C.N.B. 1993. Tanzania Family Planning Communication Project: The 1992 Baseline Clinic Study. Evaluation report for the Tanzania Ministry of Health, Health Education Division, and the Johns Hopkins University/ Population Communication Services, Baltimore.

Kim, C. H., and S. J. Lee. 1973. The Role of Husbands in Family Planning Behavior. *Psychological Studies in Population/Family Planning* 1 (5): 1–23.

Kim, Y. M. 1997. Indonesia Trip Report: December 17, 1996–January 14, 1997. Client-Provider Interaction Study. Baltimore: Johns Hopkins University, Population Communication Services.

Kim, Y. M., M. Amissah, J. K. Ofori, and K. White. 1994. Measuring the Quality of Family Planning Counseling: Integrating Observation, Interviews, and Transcript Analysis in Ghana. Evaluation report for the Ministry of Health/Health Education Unit, Accra, and the Johns Hopkins Center for Communication Programs, Baltimore.

Kim, Y. M., and D. Awasum. 1996. What Are the Particular Aspects of Counseling Male Family Planning Clients? A Case from Kenya. Paper presented at the 124th Annual Conference of the American Public Health Association, Men and Reproductive Health Task Force Workshop, New York.

Kim, Y. M. and A. Kols. 1996. Informed Choice and Decision Making: Family Planning Counseling in Kenya. Manuscript, Johns Hopkins Center for Communication Programs, Baltimore.

Kim, Y. M., O. M. Kumah, P. T. Piotrow, and W. B. Morgan. 1992. The Family Planning IEC Project in Ghana: Impact on Ghanaian Males. Paper presented at the 120th Annual Meeting of the American Public Health Association, Washington, DC.

Kim, Y. M., and C. L. Lettenmaier. 1995. Tools to Assess Family Planning Counseling: Observation and Interview. *IEC Research Tool*. Baltimore: Johns Hopkins Center for Communication Programs.

Kim, Y. M., C. L. Lettenmaier, D. Odallo, W. Sadomba, P. Chibatamoto, and R. Madzima. 1996. Haki Yako: A Client-Provider Information, Education, and Communication Project in Kenya. *IEC Field Report No. 8*. Baltimore: Johns Hopkins Center for Communication Programs.

Kim, Y. M., C. L. Lettenmaier, P. T. Piotrow, T. W. Valente, K. P. Böse, S. Yoon, O. Mugenda, A. Mugenda, and J. Mukolwe. 1992. Quality of Family Planning Counseling for Community Based Distribution Agents and Clinic Providers in Kenya. Paper presented at the 120th Annual Meeting of the American Public Health Association, New York, November 11.

Kim, Y. M., and C. Marangwanda. 1996. Attending Young Clients: Quality of Counseling in Zimbabwe. Baltimore: Johns Hopkins Center for Communication Programs, forthcoming.

Kim, Y. M., C. Marangwanda, and A. Kols. 1996. Involving Men in Family Planning: The Zimbabwe Male Motivation and Family Planning Method Expansion Project, 1993–1994. *IEC Field Report No. 3.* Baltimore: Johns Hopkins Center for Communication Programs.

Kim, Y. M., D. Odallo, M. Thuo, and A. Kols. 1997. Client Communication and the Quality of Family Planning Counseling: Interaction Analysis in Kenya. Forthcoming in *Health Communication.*

Kim, Y. M., and C. Olsen. 1992. Ghana Field Study and Trip Report: Monitoring and Evaluation of the Ghana Health and Family Planning Information Project. Analysis of Declining Issuance of Oral Contraceptives. Baltimore: Johns Hopkins University/Population Communication Services.

Kim, Y. M., J. G. Rimon II, K. Winnard, C. Corso, I. V. Mako, L. Sebioniga, S. Babalola, and D. Huntington. 1992. Improving the Quality of Service Delivery in Nigeria. *Studies in Family Planning* 23 (2): 117–126.

Kincaid, D. L. 1979. *The Convergence Model of Communication.* Paper 18. Honolulu: East-West Communication Institute, East-West Center.

———— (ed). 1987. *Communication Theory: Eastern and Western Perspectives.* New York: Academic Press.

————. 1988. The Convergence Theory of Communication: Its Implications for Intercultural Communication. In Y. Y. Kim (ed.), *Theoretical Perspectives on International Communication.* International and Intercultural Annual 8. Beverly Hills, CA: Sage.

————. 1992. Reaching Rural Women Through Their Own Community Information Centers: The *Jiggashas* of Trishal, Bangladesh. Paper presented at the National Council for International Health Conference, Arlington, VA, June 14–17.

————. 1993a. Changing High-Risk Behaviors: Family Planning—What Have We Learned? Paper presented to the National Academy of Sciences Committee on Population's Expert Meeting on Behavioral and Social Factors in Disease Prevention, Washington, DC, June 14.

————. 1993b. Computer Simulation of the Impact of Social Influence on Contraceptive Adoption in the Communication Network of a Bangladesh Village. Paper presented at the annual meeting of the Population Association of America, Miami, May 5–7.

————. 1993c. Using Television Dramas to Accelerate Social Change: The Enter-Educate Approach to Family Planning Promotion in Turkey, Pakistan, and Egypt. Paper presented at the annual meeting of the International Communication Association, Washington, DC, May 28.

————. 1995a. The Cumulative Impact of Family Planning in the Kenya National Family Planning Program. Evaluation report. Baltimore: Johns Hopkins Center for Communication Programs.

————. 1995b. The Impact of Social Influence on Contraceptive Adoption in the Communication Network of a Bangladesh Village. Paper presented at the annual meeting of the Population Association of America, Miami, May 5–7.

————. 1996. Evaluation of the *Jiggasha* Replication in Three Thanas of Bangladesh: Key Findings. Evaluation report. Baltimore: Johns Hopkins Center for Communication Programs.

Kincaid, D. L., P. L. Coleman, and J. G. Rimon II. 1995. Image and Adoption of Contraceptive Behavior: Impact of the Philippine National Communication Campaign in 1993. Paper presented at the annual meeting of the International Communication Association, Albuquerque, May 25–29.

Kincaid, D. L., A. Das Gupta, S. N. Mitra, E. Whitney, M. Senior, S. H. Yun, and E. Massiah. 1993. Community Networks and Family Planning Promotion: Impact of the *Jiggasha* Approach in Trishal, Bangladesh. Paper presented at the annual meeting of the American Public Health Association, San Francisco, October 27.

Kincaid, D. L., M. J. Hindin, and R. K. Foreman. 1993. Selected Figures and Tables from the Evaluation of the Family Planning Communication Project in Ghana, December 1989 to November 1991. Baltimore: Johns Hopkins Center for Communication Programs.

Kincaid, D. L., J. R. Jara, P. L. Coleman, and F. Segura. 1988. Getting the Message: The Communication for Young People Project. *Special Study No. 56.* Washington, DC: U.S. Agency for International Development.

Kincaid, D. L., N. Kapadia-Kundu, A. Das Gupta, and E. Whitney. 1994. The Influence of Social Networks on Health Behavior: The Case of Shahidpur Village, Bangladesh. Paper presented at the annual meeting of the American Public Health Association, Washington, DC, November 2.

Kincaid, D. L., Y. M. Kim, J. G. Rimon II, S. Babalola, K. Winnard, S. Krenn, and J. Daves. 1991. Using Popular Music to Promote Family Planning in Nigeria: Evaluation of the Initial Phase. Paper presented at the 119th Annual Meeting of the American Public Health Association, Atlanta, November 10–14.

Kincaid, D. L., E. Massiah, A. Das Gupta, and N. S. Mitra. 1993. Communication Networks, Ideation, and Family Planning in Trishal, Bangladesh. Paper presented at the annual meeting of the Population Association of America, Cincinnati, April 1–3.

Kincaid, D. L., A. Payne Merritt, and N. Castellon. 1988. The Bolivian National Family Planning Communication Campaign: Results of the Final Evaluation. Paper presented at the 116th Annual Meeting of the American Public Health Association, Boston, November 13–17.

Kincaid, D. L., A. Payne Merritt, L. Nickerson, S. de Castro Buffington, M.P.P. de Castro, and B. M. de Castro. 1996. Impact of a Mass Media Vasectomy Promotion Campaign in Brazil. *International Family Planning Perspectives* 2 (4): 169–175.

Kincaid, D. L., P. T. Piotrow, P. L. Coleman, and J. G. Rimon II. 1986. Evaluating Family Planning Print Materials Cross-Nationally: The Mexico-Nigeria

Experience. Paper presented at the 114th Annual Meeting of the American Public Health Association, Las Vegas, October 1.

Kincaid, D. L., J. G. Rimon II, P. T. Piotrow, and P. L. Coleman. 1992. The Enter-Educate Approach: Using Entertainment to Change Health Behavior. Paper presented at the annual meeting of the Population Association of America, Denver, April 24.

Kincaid, D. L., and W. Schramm. 1975. *Fundamental Human Communication: A Professional Development Module.* Honolulu: East-West Communication Institute, East-West Center.

Kincaid, D. L., T. W. Valente, A. Payne Merritt, H. Zhang, R. Jara, and H. Lopez. 1992. Sex and Contraceptive Use Among Adolescents in Lima and Mexico City. Paper presented at the 120th Annual Meeting of the American Public Health Association, Washington, DC, November 8–12.

Kincaid, D. L., S. H. Yun, P. T. Piotrow, and Y. Yaser. 1992. The Power of Mass Media Rediscovered: The Family Planning Communication Campaign of Turkey. Paper presented at the 42nd Annual Conference of the International Communication Association, Miami, May 21–25.

————. 1993. Turkey's Mass Media Family Planning Campaign. In T. E. Backer and E. M. Rogers (eds.), *Organizational Aspects of Health Communication Campaigns: What Works?* Newbury Park, CA: Sage.

Kincaid, D.L., S. H. Yun, P. T. Piotrow, Y. Yaser, and G. Ozler. 1990. The National Family Planning IEC Campaign of Turkey. Case study presented at Impact of Organizations on Mass Media Health Behavior Campaigns Workshop, Bethesda, MD, April 10.

Kincaid, D. L., H. Zhang, M. Senior, S. H. Yun, E. Whitney, A. Das Gupta, A. Barua, and N. Kapadia-Kundu. 1991. Family Planning and the Empowerment of Women in Bangladesh. Paper presented at the 119th Annual Meeting of the American Public Health Association, Atlanta, November 10–14.

Kiragu, K. 1991. *The Correlates of Sexual and Contraceptive Behavior Among In-School Adolescents in Kenya.* Ann Arbor, MI: University Microfilms International.

————. 1993a. Family Planning Needs in Uganda: Key Findings from a Baseline Survey of Selected Urban and Peri-urban Areas. Prepared by the Johns Hopkins University/Population Communication Services, Baltimore, in collaboration with the Family Planning Association of Uganda, Kampala.

————. 1993b. Key Findings: The Nigeria PSA/Logo Campaign. Results of the Evaluation. Prepared by the Johns Hopkins University, Population Communication Services, Baltimore, in collaboration with the IEC Division of the Nigeria Family Health Services Project, Lagos.

————. 1997. The Kenya Youth Variety Show. Paper presented at the CEDPA Symposium, Washington, DC, April 26.

Kiragu, K., S. Chapman, and G. L. Lewis. 1995. The Nigeria Family Planning Facility Census. *IEC Field Report No. 1.* Baltimore: Johns Hopkins Center for Communication Programs.

Kiragu, K., M. K. Galiwango, H. M. Mulira, and E. Sekatawa. 1996. Promoting Reproductive Health in Uganda: Evaluation of a National IEC Program. The Uganda Family Planning Promotion and Delivery of Improved Health Services Projects. *IEC Field Report No. 7*. Baltimore: Johns Hopkins Center for Communication Programs.

Kiragu, K., D. L. Kincaid, C. Church, J. G. Rimon II, H. Zhang, S. C. Krenn, J.K.T. Ajiboye, I. George, B. Kusimeju, O. Kalu, A. Adewuyi, A. K. Omideye, and M. O. Raimi. 1993. Impact of Complementary Multi-Media Campaigns on Family Planning Behavior in Nigeria. Paper presented at the 121st Annual Meeting of the American Public Health Association, San Francisco, October 24–28.

Kiragu, K., S. C. Krenn, B. Kusemiju, J.K.T. Ajiboye, I. Chidi, and O. Kalu. 1996. Promoting Family Planning Through the Mass Media in Nigeria: Campaigns Using Public Service Announcements and a National Logo. *IEC Field Report No. 5*. Baltimore: Johns Hopkins Center for Communication Programs.

Kiragu, K., R. Nyonyintono, J. Sengendo, M. Galiwango, D. Baron, and C. L. Lettenmaier. 1994. Family Planning Use in the Context of the AIDS Epidemic in Uganda. Paper presented at the 122nd Annual Meeting of the American Public Health Association. Washington, DC, October 31–November 3.

Kiragu, K., and B. A. Omotara. 1992. Key Findings: The Impact of a Mass Media Campaign on Family Planning Use in Borno State, Nigeria. Prepared by the Johns Hopkins University/Population Communication Services, Baltimore, in collaboration with the IEC Division of the Nigeria Family Health Services Project, Lagos.

Kiragu, K., and L. Zabin. 1993a. The Correlates of Premarital Sexual Activity Among School-Age Adolescents in Kenya. *International Family Planning Perspectives* 19: 92–97, 109.

———. 1993b. The Social Context of Contraceptive Use Among High School Adolescents in Kenya. Paper presented at the 121st Annual Meeting of the American Public Health Association, San Francisco, October 24–28.

Kiragu, K. H. Zhang, S. C. Krenn, J.K.T. Ajiboye, and G. Ibiba. 1994. The Impact of a Family Planning Mobile Drama in Benue State, Nigeria. Unpublished report for the Information, Education, and Communication Division of the Nigeria Family Health Services Project and Johns Hopkins Population Communication Services.

Klapper, J. 1960. *The Effects of Mass Communication*. New York: Free Press.

Knowles, J. 1991. *75 Years of Family Planning in America: A Chronology of Major Events*. New York: Planned Parenthood Federation of America.

Kone, H., and R. K. Yao. 1989. Panafrican Project on Printed Aids in Family Planning. *Center for Teaching and Research in Communication (CERCOM) Study No. 1*. Abidjan: Ivory Coast National University.

Kotler, P. 1982. *Marketing for Non-Profit Organizations*. Englewood Cliffs, NJ: Prentice-Hall.

Kotler, P., and E. Roberto. 1989. *Social Marketing: Strategies for Changing Public Behavior*. New York: Free Press.

Kotler, P. and G. Zaltman. 1971. Social Marketing: An Approach to Planned Social Change. *Journal of Marketing* 33: 10–15.

Krenn, S. C., and B. Kusemiju. 1992. Project Summary: The Nigerian National Family Planning Logo Project. Baltimore: Johns Hopkins Center for Communication Programs.

Kumah, O. M. 1986. Family Planning Communication in Ghana: Retrospect and Prospect. Paper presented at the Ghana Population Conference, Accra, April 7–10.

Kumah, O. M., D. L. Kincaid, I. A. Tweedie, W. B. Morgan, W. Glass, Y. M. Kim, and G. L. Lewis. 1993. Family Planning Audience Segmentation Plan: Ghana Family Planning and Health Project. Project design document of the Johns Hopkins University/Population Communication Services, Center for Communication Programs, Baltimore.

Kumah, O. M., D. Odallo, C. Shefner, N. Muturi, J. Karueru, F. Gachanja, and N. Nwanzia. 1992. Kenya Youth Needs Assessment. Baltimore: Johns Hopkins University/Population Communication Services, Center for Communication Programs.

Kuseka, I., and T. Silberman. 1990. The Zimbabwe Male Motivation Impact Evaluation Survey. Evaluation report by the Zimbabwe National Family Planning Council Evaluation and Research Unit, Harare, Zimbabwe.

Lacey, L., and N. Rutenberg. 1993. Nigeria FOS Quarterly Survey Results and Technical Assistance Needs. Preliminary findings report for the EVALUATION Project, Chapel Hill, NC.

Lande, R. E. 1993. Controlling Sexually Transmitted Diseases. *Population Reports*, L (9). Baltimore: Johns Hopkins University, Population Information Program.

Lande, R. E., and J. S. Geller. 1991. Paying for Family Planning. *Population Reports*, J (39). Baltimore: Johns Hopkins University, Population Information Program.

Lapham, R. J., and W. P. Mauldin. 1972. National Family Planning Programs: Review and Evaluation. *Studies in Family Planning* 3 (3): 29–52.

———. 1984. The KAP-Gap: An Important Problem for Science and Social Policy. Manuscript prepared for Demographic and Health Surveys, Arlington, VA.

———. 1985. Contraceptive Prevalence: The Influence of Organized Family Planning Programs. *Studies in Family Planning* 16 (3): 117–137.

Laswell, H. D. 1948. The Structure and Function of Communication in Society. In L. Bryson (ed.), *The Communication of Ideas*. New York: Harper.

Latane, B. 1981. The Psychology of Social Impact. *American Psychology* 36: 343–365.

Latzko, W. J., and D. M. Saunders. 1995. Four Days with Dr. Deming: *A Strategy for Modern Methods of Management*. Reading, MA: Addison-Wesley.

Lazarsfeld, P. F., B. Berelson, and H. Gaudet. 1948. *The People's Choice*. 2nd ed. New York: Columbia University Press.

Lefebre, R. C., and J. A. Flora. 1988. Social Marketing and Public Health Interventions. *Health Education Quarterly* 15: 299–315.

Lerner, D. 1963. Toward a Communication Theory of Modernization. In L. W. Pye (ed.), *Communication and Political Development*. Princeton, NJ: Princeton University Press.

Lettenmaier, C. L. 1995. (The Johns Hopkins Center for Communication Programs) [Uganda launch logistics]. Personal communication to authors, June.

Lettenmaier, C. L., and M. Gallen. 1987. Counseling Guide. *Population Reports*, J (36). Baltimore: Johns Hopkins University, Population Information Program.

Lettenmaier, C. L., R. Lovich, Y. M. Kim, and L. Botsh. 1993. Coached Client Evaluation of Family Planning Counseling Training in Zimbabwe. Paper presented at the annual meeting of the American Public Health Association, San Francisco, October 27.

Liskin, L. S. 1990. Using Mass Media for Aids Prevention. *AIDS Care* 2: 419–420.

Liskin, L. S., C. A. Church, P. T. Piotrow, and J. A. Harris. 1989. AIDS Education—A Beginning. *Population Reports*, L (8). Baltimore: Johns Hopkins University, Population Information Program.

Liskin, L. S., C. Wharton, R. Blackburn, and P. Kestelman. 1990. Condoms—Now More than Ever. *Population Reports*, H (8). Baltimore: Johns Hopkins University, Population Information Program.

Lissance, D. M., and W. P. Schellstede. 1993. Evaluating the Effectiveness of a Family Planning IEC Program in Bangladesh. *PSI Special Reports No. 2*. Washington, DC: Population Services International (PSI).

Lozare, B. V. 1988. Development Communication: Can Broadcasting Make a Difference? *Media Asia* 2: 2.

Lozare, B. V., R. Hess, S. H. Yun, A. Gill-Bailey, C. Valmadrid, A. Livesay, S. R. Khan, and N. Siddiqui. 1993. Husband-Wife Communication and Family Planning: Impact of a National Television Drama. Paper presented at the annual meeting of the American Public Health Association, San Francisco, October 25.

Lozare, B. V., S. Loza, M. Farag, M. Hashem, J. G. Rimon II, K. Treiman, and D. L. Kincaid. 1991. An Evaluation of Clinic Promotion Activities in Egypt: The CSI Experience. Paper presented at the 119th Annual Meeting of the American Public Health Association, Atlanta, November 13.

Lynam, P. F., J. C. Dwyer, and J. Bradley. 1994. Inreach: Reaching Potential Family Planning Clients Within Health Institutions. *AVSC Working Paper No. 5*. New York: Association for Voluntary Surgical Contraception (AVSC).

MacFarquhar, N. 1996. With Iran Population Boom, Vasectomy Receives Blessing. *New York Times*, September 8, p. A1.

Mager, R. F. 1984. *Preparing Instructional Objectives*. Rev. 2nd ed. Belmont, CA: Lake Publishing.

Maguire, E. 1996. (U.S. Agency for International Development) [Egypt Gold Star launch and "Doctora Kareema"]. Personal communication to Phyllis T. Piotrow.

Manoff, R. K. 1985. *Social Marketing, New Imperative for Public Health*. New York: Praeger.

Marketing and Social Research Institute (MSRI), Ltd. 1993. *Ghana Family Planning and Health Project: Consumer Baseline Study. A Nationwide KAP Survey on Contraceptives, AIDS, Malaria, and Childhood Diarrheal Disease.* Accra, Ghana: MSRI.

Massiah, E. 1993. *Multi-level Analysis of Contraceptive Use in Trishal, Bangladesh: The Role of Communication Networks.* Ann Arbor, MI: University Microfilms International.

Massiah, E., D. L. Kincaid, S. H. Yun, M. Senior, E. Whitney, A. Barua, and A. Das Gupta. 1992. The Role of Social Networks in Developing Community-Based Interventions in Bangladesh. Paper presented at the 120th Annual Meeting of the American Public Health Association, Washington, DC, November 8–12.

Mauldin, W. P., and J. A. Ross. 1991. Family Planning Programs: Efforts and Results, 1982–89. *Studies in Family Planning* 22 (6): 350–367.

————. 1994. Prospects and Programs for Fertility Reduction, 1990–2015. *Studies in Family Planning* 25 (2): 77–95.

Mauldin, W. P., and S. W. Sinding. 1993. Review of Existing Family Planning Policies and Programs: Lessons Learned. *Research Division Working Paper No. 50.* New York: Population Council.

Mbunda, W., M. N. Jato, Y. M. Kim, T. W. Valente, and C. L. Lettenmaier. 1991. Tanzania Family Planning Communication Project Baseline Audience Survey Report. A collaborative study with the Tanzania Family Planning Association, Dar es Salaam, Tanzania, and Johns Hopkins University, Population Communication Services, Baltimore.

McCauley, A., N. Kapadia-Kundu, and L. G. Clemmons. 1992. Using Women's Groups to Promote Healthy Communities. Paper presented at the 120th Annual Meeting of the American Public Health Association, Washington, DC, November 8–12.

McCauley, A., B. Robey, A. K. Blanc, and J. S. Geller. 1994. Opportunities for Women Through Reproductive Choice. *Population Reports*, M (12). Baltimore: Johns Hopkins University, Population Information Program.

McCauley, A., and C. Salter. 1995. Meeting the Needs of Young Adults. [Population Reports], J (41). Baltimore: Johns Hopkins University, Population Information Program.

McCombie, S., and R. Hornik. 1992. Evaluation of a Workplace-Based Peer Education Program Designed to Prevent AIDS in Uganda. *Working Paper 1011.* University Park: University of Pennsylvania, Annenberg School of Communication.

McDevitt, T. M. 1996. *World Population Profile: 1996.* U.S. Bureau of the Census, Report WP/96. Washington, DC: U.S. Government Printing Office.

McGuire, W. J. 1969. Theory-Oriented Research in Natural Settings: The Best of Both Worlds of Social Psychology. In M. Sherif and C. W. Sherif (eds.), *Interdisciplinary Relationships in the Social Sciences.* Chicago: Aldine.

————. 1986. The Myth of Massive Media Impact: Savagings and Salvagings. In G. Comstock (ed.), *Public Communication and Behavior* 1. Orlando, FL: Academic Press.

————. 1989. Theoretical Foundations of Campaigns. In R. R. Rice and C. K. Atkin (eds.), *Public Communication Campaigns*. 2nd ed. Newbury Park, CA: Sage.

McQuail, D. 1987. *Mass Communication Theory*. London: Sage.

————. 1994. *Mass Communication Theory: An Introduction*. 3rd ed. Thousand Oaks, CA: Sage.

McWilliam, J., and E. M. Rogers. 1989. Evaluation of the Population Communication Services Project, 1986–1989. Report No. 88-011-095. Prepared for the Office of Population, Bureau for Science and Technology, U.S. Agency for International Development by the Population Technical Assistance Project, Dual and Associates, Inc., and International Science and Technology Institute, Inc., Arlington, VA.

Media Dynamics, Inc. 1995. *TV Dimensions 1995*. New York: Media Dynamics.

Mitra, S. N., C. Lerman, and S. Islam. 1992. Bangladesh Contraceptive Prevalence Survey, 1991. Survey conducted and published by Mitra and Associates, Dhaka, Bangladesh.

Mitra, S. N., M. Nawab Ali, S. Islam, A. R. Cross, and T. Saha. 1994. *Bangladesh Demographic and Health Survey 1993–1994*. Calverton, MD: National Institute of Population Research and Training (NIPORT), Mitra and Associates, and Macro International, Inc.

Moffitt, R. 1991. Program Evaluation with No Experimental Data. *Evaluation Review* 15 (3): 291–314.

Mohr, L. B. 1992. *Impact Analysis for Program Evaluation*. Newbury Park, CA: Sage.

Morris, L. 1992. Sexual Behavior and Use of Contraception Among Young Adults: What Have We Learned from the Young Adult Reproductive Health Surveys in Latin America? Paper presented at the First Inter-African Conference on Adolescent Health, Nairobi.

Moscovici, S. 1976. *Social Influence and Social Change*. London: Academic Press.

Mosley, W. H. 1996. (Johns Hopkins School of Public Health, Population Dynamics) [Use of maternal child health and family planning services]. Personal communication to authors, July 11.

Mumford, S. D. 1983. The Vasectomy Decision-Making Process. *Studies in Family Planning* 14 (3): 83–88.

Mwarogo, P., Y. M. Kim, and A. Kols. 1996. Reaching Out to Men—The Forgotten 50 Percent: The Kenya Male Involvement Project Formative Research and Strategy. Paper presented at the Africa Regional Conference on Men's Participation in Family Planning and Reproductive Health, Harare, Zimbabwe, December 1–6.

National Institutes of Health (NIH). 1992. Making Health Communication Programs Work: A Planner's Guide. Bethesda, MD: U.S. Department of Health, Public Health Service, NIH, Office of Cancer Communications, National Cancer Institute.

Ndumbu, A. 1993. Vasectomy Ethnographic Study in Kenya. Report prepared for the Johns Hopkins University/Population Communication Services, Baltimore.

Nepal Ministry of Health/Family Health Division. 1995. *National Medical Standard for Reproductive Health: Contraceptive Services*. Vol. 1. Manual developed by the Nepal Ministry of Health/Family Health Division, the Nepal Fertility Care Center with assistance from the Johns Hopkins University/Population Communication Services and support from the Office of Population and Health/United States Agency for International Development and used at the Contraceptive Technology Update Workshop, January 15–21, Kathmandu, Nepal.

Nesselroad, J. R., and S. L. Hershberger. 1993. Intraindividual Variability: Methodological Issues for Population Health Research. In K. Dean (ed.), *Population Health Research: Linking Theory and Methods*. Thousand Oaks, CA: Sage.

Nickerson, L., A. Payne Merritt, P. Poppe, and N. Castellon. 1992. The Trickle Up Approach: Uniting for Reproductive Health in Bolivia. Paper presented at the 120th Annual Meeting of the American Public Health Association, Washington, DC, November 8–12.

Njau, W. 1994. Kenya Youth Initiative Project: A Review of Youth Reproductive Health with Special Attention to Legislative and Policy Environment for Adolescents in Kenya. Report presented to the Family Planning Association of Kenya (FPAK) on behalf of the collaborating youth-serving organizations under the auspices of the National Council for Population and Development. Compiled by the Center for the Study of Adolescence, Nairobi, Kenya.

———. 1995. The Kenya Youth Initiative Project: A Report on In-Depth Interviews with Policy-Makers and Leaders in Kenya. Prepared for the Johns Hopkins University/Population Communication Services by the Center for the Study of Adolescence, Nairobi, Kenya.

Noel-Nariman, H. 1993. *Soap Operas for Social Change: Toward a Methodology for Entertainment-Education Television*. Media and Society Series. Westport, CT: Praeger.

Noelle-Neumann, E. 1993. *The Spiral of Silence*. 2nd ed. Chicago: University of Chicago Press.

Nortman, D. L. 1972. *Population and Family Planning Programs: A Factbook*. 4th ed. Reports on Population/Family Planning No. 2. New York: Population Council.

Norton, M., and S. P. Benoliel. 1987. Guidelines for Data Collection, Monitoring, and Evaluation Plans for A.I.D.-Assisted Projects. *A.I.D. Program Design and Evaluation Methodology Report No. 9*. Washington, DC: U.S. Agency for International Development.

Notestein, F. W. 1946. Population—The Long View. In T. W. Schultz (ed.), *Food for the World*. Chicago: University of Chicago Press, pp. 36–57.

Novelli, W. 1988. Marketing Health and Social Issues: What Works? In R. Dunmire (ed.), *Social Marketing: Accepting the Challenge in Public Health*. Atlanta: Centers for Disease Control, Public Health Service, U.S. Department of Health and Human Services.

Ogilvy, D. 1963. *Confessions of an Advertising Man*. New York: Atheneum.

Olaleye, D. O., and A. Bankole. 1992a. The Impact of Mass Media Family Planning Promotion on Family Planning in a Sub-Saharan African Country. Paper presented at the annual meeting of the Population Association of America, Denver, April 30–May 2.

————. 1992b. The Impact of Mass Media Family Planning Promotion on Family Planning in Ghana. Paper presented at the annual meeting of the Population Association of America, Denver, April 30–May 2.

Oman Ministry of Health and Johns Hopkins University, Population Communication Services. 1995. Birth Spacing Knowledge, Attitudes, and Practices in the Sultanate of Oman. Draft report of the Johns Hopkins Center for Communication Programs, Baltimore.

Pakistan Ministry of Population Welfare, U.S. Agency for International Development (Pakistan), U.S. Agency for International Development (Washington, DC) and the Johns Hopkins University, Population Communication Services. 1993. Pakistan: Report on Technical Assistance to the Ministry of Population Welfare, Government of Pakistan. August, 1990–June 30, 1993. A joint technical assistance visit to Pakistan.

Palda, K. S. 1966. The Hypothesis of a Hierarchy of Effects: A Partial Evaluation. *Journal of Marketing Research* 3: 13–24.

Palmore, J. A. 1968. Awareness Sources and Stages in the Adoption of Specific Contraceptives. *Demography* 5 (2): 960–972.

Payne Merritt, A. 1992. Family Planning Goes Public. *Integration* June (32): 41–43.

————. 1993. Preliminary Needs Assessment and Trip Report: Brazil, January 19–30, 1993. Baltimore: Johns Hopkins University, Population Communication Services.

————. 1996. (The Johns Hopkins Center for Communication Programs) [Local monitoring of television broadcasts in Honduras]. Personal communication to authors, April 1.

Payne Merritt, A., P. L. Coleman, and L. D. Nickerson. 1990. Freedom Sells Condoms in Colombia. Paper presented at the 118th Annual Meeting of the American Public Health Association, New York, September 30–October 4.

Payne Merritt, A., D. L. Kincaid, and N. Castellon. 1989. Communication as a Process. Bolivia—Family Planning Goes Public. Paper presented at the 117th Annual Meeting of the American Public Health Association, Chicago, October 23–26.

Payne Merritt, A., and E. Lawrence. 1990. A Strategic Approach to Family Communication in Ecuador. Johns Hopkins University, Population Communication Services report for the U.S. Agency for International Development, Washington, DC.

Payne Merritt, A., and P. Poppe. 1991. Foundations Toward a National Communication Strategy: Four Institutional Communication Strategies. A Ten Year Communication Strategy for the USAID National Family Health Program in Guatemala. Prepared by the U.S. Agency for International Development in collaboration with the Johns Hopkins University, Population Communication Services, the Guatemalan Sexual Education Association, the Guatemalan Family Welfare Association, the Importer of Pharmaceutical Products, and the Family Planning Unit of the Guatemalan Ministry of Health.

Payne Merritt, A., and M. Raffaelli. 1993. Creating a Model HIV Prevention Program for Youth. *The Child, Youth, and Family Services Quarterly* (Division 37, American Psychological Association) 16 (2): 709.

Philippine Legislators' Committee on Population and Development (PLCPD). 1994. Project Summary, Scope of Work and Conditions, February 1, 1993–January 31, 1994. Manila: PLCPD Advocacy Project.

Phillips, J. F., and J. A. Ross (eds.). 1992. *Family Planning Programmes and Fertility*. Oxford: Clarendon Press.

Piotrow, P. T. 1992. Toward a Household Word and a Community Norm: Cost-Effective Communication Strategies in Four Countries. Paper presented at the International Workshop on Child Health Interventions, Baltimore, November 30–December 2.

————. 1994. Entertainment-Education: An Idea Whose Time Has Come. *Population Today: News, Numbers, and Analysis* 22 (3): 4–5.

Piotrow, P. T., and P. L. Coleman. 1992. The Enter-Educate Approach. *Integration* March (31): 4–6.

Piotrow, P. T., D. L. Kincaid, M. J. Hindin, C. L. Lettenmaier, I. Kuseka, T. Silberman, A. Zinanga, and Y. M. Kim. 1992. Changing Men's Attitudes and Behavior: The Zimbabwe Male Motivation Project. *Studies in Family Planning* 23 (6): 365–375.

Piotrow, P. T., J. G. Rimon II, and K. Kiragu. 1993. Nigeria's New Baby: The 1992 National Family Planning Logo Campaign. Paper presented at U.S. Agency for International Development, Washington, DC, April.

Piotrow, P. T., J. G. Rimon II, K. Winnard, D. L. Kincaid, D. Huntington, and J. Convisser. 1990. Mass Media Family Planning Promotion in Three Nigerian Cities. *Studies in Family Planning* 21 (5): 265–274.

Piotrow, P. T., K. A. Treiman, J. G. Rimon II, S. H. Yun, and B. V. Lozare. 1994. Strategies for Family Planning Promotion. *World Bank Technical Paper No. 223*. Washington, DC: World Bank.

Planned Parenthood Federation of Nigeria (PPFN). 1992. Report on Sexual Responsibility Music Public Service Announcements (PSA) Broadcast in Nigeria, June–November, 1992. A PPFN report for the Johns Hopkins University/Population Communication Services Nigeria PSA Project.

Poppe, P. R. 1995. (The Johns Hopkins Center for Communication Programs) [Peru, Villa el Salvador broadcasts]. Personal communication to authors, November 13.

―――. 1996a. (The Johns Hopkins Center for Communication Programs) [Working with advertising agencies in Peru]. Personal communication to authors, June 5.

―――. 1996b. (The Johns Hopkins Center for Communication Programs) [Peru, data collection]. Personal communication to authors, November 14.

Poppe, P. R., and R. Leon. 1993. Las Tromes: Dispelling Myths and Rumors of Modern Family Planning. A Peru Case Study. Baltimore: Johns Hopkins Center for Communication Programs.

Poppe, P. R., G. Rodriguez, and A. Payne Merritt. 1991. Attitudes and Perceptions of Family Planning Practices in Rural Mexico: Focus Group Results from Chiapas. Paper presented at the annual meeting of the American Public Health Association, Atlanta, November 13.

Population Action International (PAI). 1994. Financing the Future: Meeting the Demand for Family Planning [wall chart]. Washington, DC: PAI.

Population Council. 1994. Guidelines and Instruments for a Family Planning Situation Analysis Study. February draft. Population Council, New York.

Population Information Project—Ghana. 1987. *Population Growth and Socio-Economic Development in Ghana: A RAPID Analysis of Long-Term Growth.* RAPID 3 report of the Ghana Population Information Project. Washington, DC: Futures Group.

Population Reference Bureau (PRB). 1976. *World Population Growth and Response: 1965–75. A Decade of Global Action.* Washington, DC: PRB.

―――. 1993. 1993 World Population Data Sheet: Demographic Data and Estimates for the Countries and Regions of the World [wall chart], Washington, DC: PRB.

―――. 1996. 1996 World Population Data Sheet: Demographic Data and Estimates for the Countries and Regions of the World [wall chart]. Washington, DC: PRB.

―――. 1997. 1997 World Population Data Sheet: Demographic Data and Estimates for the Countries and Regions of the World [wall chart]. Washington, DC: PRB.

Population Services International (PSI). 1996. PSI Annual Report 1995–1996. Washington, DC: PSI.

Potter, S. H., and J. M. Potter. 1990. *China's Peasants: The Anthropology of a Revolution.* Cambridge: Cambridge University Press.

Prochaska, J. O., C. C. DiClemente, and J. C. Norcross. 1992. In Search of How People Change: Applications to Addictive Behaviors. *American Psychologist* 47 (9): 1102–1112.

Quest Research Services. 1987. Report on the Zimbabwe Audience Analysis for the Johns Hopkins University, Population Communication Services (JHU/PCS). Research study for JHU/PCS, Center for Communication Programs, Baltimore.

Ramlow, R. 1994. SOMARC Reaches Record Numbers: Theater Events in Uganda Promote "Protector" Condoms and "Pilplan" Oral Contraceptives. *SOMARC III Highlights*, September (12): 1–2.

Ranganath, H. K. 1980. *Using Folk Entertainers to Promote National Development*. New York: UNESCO.

Retherford, R. D. 1985. A Theory of Marital Fertility Transition. *Population Studies* 39 (2): 249–268.

Rimon, J. G. II. 1986. IEC Strategy for the Urban Family Planning Program in Indonesia. Baltimore: Johns Hopkins University, Center for Communication Programs.

————. 1989. Leveraging Messages and Corporations: The Philippine Experience. *Integration*, December (22): 37–44.

Rimon, J. G. II, D. L. Kincaid, A. Silayan-Go, K. Treiman, and R. Abejuela. 1991. Leveraging Messages and Corporations: Fertility Program in the Philippines. Paper presented at the 119th Annual Meeting of the American Public Health Association, Atlanta, November 13.

Rimon, J. G. II, and M. Lediard. 1993. Nepal IEC Needs Assessment: Findings and Recommendations. Report prepared by the Johns Hopkins University, Population Communication Services and the Academy for Educational Development for the U.S. Agency for International Development in Nepal.

Rimon, J. G. II, R. C. Meyer, D. L. Kincaid, and P. J. Allen. 1992. Emerging Issues in Public Health Education: Changing Behavior Through Mass Media. Paper presented at the 120th Annual Meeting of the American Public Health Association, Washington, DC, November 8–12.

Rimon, J. G. II, F. Reed, B. Deolalikar, R. Griffin, and R. Pereira. 1986. Review of the IEC Component of the Indonesian Population Program and Recommendations for IEC Planning: 1987–1991. Document commissioned by USAID and the Indonesian National Family Planning Coordinating Board (BKKBN), in preparation for the "privatization" campaign in Indonesia. Baltimore: Johns Hopkins University, Center for Communication Programs.

Rimon, J. G. II, K. A. Treiman, D. L. Kincaid, A. Silayan-Go, M. S. Camacho-Reyes, R. M. Abejuela, and P. L. Coleman. 1994. Promoting Sexual Responsibility in the Philippines Through Music: An Enter-Educate Approach. *Occasional Paper Series No. 3*. Baltimore: Johns Hopkins Center for Communication Programs.

Rimon, J. G. II, K. E. Winnard, and C. Kazi. 1986. Nigeria: A Case Study of Managing Communication Programs in a Multi-ethnic Society. Paper presented at the 114th Annual Meeting of the American Public Health Association, Las Vegas, September 28–October 2.

Rimon, J. G. II, and M. Zimmerman. 1987. Print Materials Review and IEC Needs Assessment of Four Egyptian Agencies. Trip report, October 4–2, 1987. Baltimore: Johns Hopkins Center for Communication Programs.

Robey, B., P. T. Piotrow, and C. Salter. 1994. Family Planning Lessons and Challenges: Making Programs Work. *Population Reports*, J (40). Baltimore: Johns Hopkins University, Population Information Program.

Robey, B., J. A. Ross, and I. Bhushan. 1996. Meeting Unmet Need: New Strategies. *Population Reports*, J (43). Baltimore: Johns Hopkins University, Population Information Program.

Robey, B., S. O. Rutstein, and L. Morris. 1993. The Fertility Decline in Developing Countries. *Scientific American* 269 (6): 60–67.

Robey, B., S. O. Rutstein, L. Morris, and R. Blackburn. 1992. The Reproductive Revolution: New Survey Findings. *Population Reports*, M (11). Baltimore: Johns Hopkins University, Population Information Program.

Robey, B., and P. Stauffer. 1995. Helping the News Media Cover Family Planning. *Population Reports*, J (42). Baltimore: Johns Hopkins University, Population Information Program.

Rogers, E. M. 1962. *Diffusion of Innovations*. New York: Free Press.

———. 1973. *Communication Strategies for Family Planning*. New York: Free Press.

———. 1983. *Diffusion of Innovations*. 3rd ed. New York: Free Press.

———. 1994. *A History of Communication Study: A Biographical Approach*. New York: Free Press.

———. 1995. *Diffusion of Innovations*. 4th ed. New York: Free Press.

———. 1996. The Field of Health Communication Today: An Up-to-Date Report. *Journal of Health Communication: International Perspectives* 1 (1): 15–23.

Rogers, E. M., S. Aikat, S. Chang, P. Poppe, and P. Sopory. 1989. Proceedings of the Conference on Entertainment-Education for Social Change. Los Angeles: Annenberg School of Communications, University of Southern California, March 29–April 1.

Rogers, E. M., and L. Antola. 1985. Telenovelas in Latin America: A Success Story. *Journal of Communication* 35: 24–35.

Rogers, E. M., and D. L. Kincaid. 1981. *Communication Networks: A Paradigm for New Research*. New York: Free Press.

Rogers, E. M., and F. F. Shoemaker. 1971. *Communication of Innovations: A Cross-Cultural Approach*. New York: Free Press.

Rosenkrantz, B. G. 1972. *Public Health and the State: Changing Views in Massachusetts*, 1842–1936. Cambridge, MA: Harvard University Press.

Ross, J. A., and E. Frankenberg. 1993. *Findings from Two Decades of Family Planning Research*. New York: Population Council.

Ross, J. A., and W. P. Mauldin. 1996. Family Planning Programs: Efforts and Results, 1972–94. *Studies in Family Planning* 27 (3): 137–147.

Rossi, P. H., and H. E. Freeman. 1989. *Evaluation: A Systematic Approach*. Newbury Park, CA: Sage.

Roter, D., and J. Hall. 1992. *Doctors Talking with Patients, Patients Talking with Doctors: Improving Communication in Medical Visits*. Westport, CT: Auburn House.

Rudy, S. 1996. (The Johns Hopkins Center for Communication Programs) [Use of IEC training materials in Kenya]. Personal communication to authors, June.

Ryan, B., and N. C. Gross. 1943. The Diffusion of Hybrid Seed Corn in Two Iowa Communities. *Rural Sociology* 8: 15–24.

————. 1950. Acceptance and Diffusion of Hybrid Corn Seed in Two Iowa Communities. *Rural Sociology* (Research Bulletin 372). Ames: Iowa Agricultural Experiment Station.

Ryerson, W. N. 1994. Population Communications International: Its Role in Family Planning Soap Operas. *Population and Environment* 15 (4): 255–264.

Saba, W. 1993. Final Report and Evaluation of the Mass Media Campaign: Peru AIDS Project. Baltimore: Johns Hopkins Center for Communication Programs.

————. 1996. (The Johns Hopkins Center for Communication Programs) [Peru commercial strategy]. Personal communication to authors, November 12.

Saba, W., T. W. Valente, A. Payne Merritt, D. L. Kincaid, M. Lujan, and J. Foreit. 1994. The Mass Media and Health Beliefs: Using Media Campaigns to Promote Preventive Behavior. Manuscript Johns Hopkins University, Center for Communication Programs, Baltimore, MD.

Sabido, M. 1981. Towards the Social Use of Soap Operas: Mexico's Experience with the Reinforcement of Social Values Through TV Soap Operas. Paper presented at the annual conference of the International Institute of Communications, Strasbourg.

Saffitz, G. 1992. IEC Technical Assistance to the Minya [Egypt] Project. Trip report, July 8–23, 1992. Prepared for the Johns Hopkins University, Population Communication Services, Center for Communication Programs, Baltimore.

Saffitz, G., and J. G. Rimon II. 1992. 80/20 Vision: The Indonesia Blue Circle Campaign. Project overview. Baltimore: Johns Hopkins University, Population Communication Services, Center for Communication Programs.

Salway, S. 1994. How Attitudes Toward Family Planning and Discussion Between Wives and Husbands Affect Contraceptive Use in Ghana. *International Family Planning Perspectives* 20 (2): 44–47.

Schlesselman, J. 1982. *Case-Control Studies: Design, Conduct, and Analysis.* New York: Oxford University Press.

Schramm, W. 1971. Communication in Family Planning. *Studies in Family Planning* 7: 1–43.

————. 1973. *Men, Messages, and Media: A Look at Human Communication.* New York: Harper and Row.

Schuler, S. R., E. N. McIntosh, M. C. Goldstein, and B. R. Pande. 1985. Barriers to Effective Family Planning in Nepal. *Studies in Family Planning* 15 (5): 260–270.

Schultz, D. E., D. Martin, and W. P. Brown. 1987. *Strategic Advertising Campaigns.* 2nd ed. Lincolnwood, IL: NTC Business Books.

Schultz, T. W. (ed.). 1974. *Economics of the Family.* Chicago: University of Chicago Press.

Seidel, R. E. (ed.). 1993. Notes from the Field in Communication for Child Survival. Washington, DC: Academy for Educational Development for the U.S. Agency for International Development, Bureau for Research and Development, Office of Health.

Senanayake, P. 1992. Positive Approaches to Education for Sexual Health with Examples from Asia and Africa. *Journal of Adolescent Health* 13 (5): 351–354.

Senanayake, P., and R. L. Kleinman (eds.). 1993. *Family Planning: Meeting Challenges, Promoting Choices.* Proceedings of the IPPF Family Planning Congress, New Delhi, October 1992. Carnforth, England: Parthenon.

Serlemitsos, E. 1994. Project Close-Out for the Cameroon Child-Spacing Promotion Project, Phase 3 (AF-CAM-03). Trip report, April 13–May 18, 1994. Baltimore: Johns Hopkins University, Population Communication Services, Center for Communication Programs.

Shadish, W. R. Jr., T. D. Cook, and L. C. Leviton. 1991. *Foundations of Program Evaluation: Theories of Practice.* Newbury Park, CA: Sage.

Shedlin, M.G., and P. E. Hollerbach. 1981. Modern and Traditional Fertility Regulation in a Mexican Community: The Process of Decision Making. *Studies in Family Planning* 12 (6–7): 278–296.

Shelton, J. D., M. A. Angle, and R. A. Jacobstein. 1992. Medical Barriers to Access to Family Planning. *Lancet* 340 (8831): 1334–1335.

Sherrard, C., and G. Heinz. 1976. *Social Influence and Social Change.* New York: Academic Press.

Sherris, D., B. B. Ravenhold, and R. Blackburn. 1985. Contraceptive Social Marketing: Lessons from Experience. *Population Reports*, J (30). Baltimore: Johns Hopkins University, Population Information Program.

Shrestha, A., J. Stoeckel, and J. M. Tuladhar. 1988. Factors Related to Non-use of Contraception Among Couples with an Unmet Need for Family Planning in Nepal. Final report of an in-depth study conducted by New Era, Kathmandu, Nepal, under a Population Council subcontract with Demographic and Health Surveys Project/IRD/Westinghouse, Arlington, VA.

Sinding, S. W. 1993. Getting to Replacement: Bridging the Gap Between Individual Rights and Demographic Goals. In P. Senanayake and R. Kleinman (eds.), *Family Planning: Meeting Challenges, Promoting Choices.* Proceedings of the IPPF Family Planning Congress, New Delhi, October 1992. Carnforth, England: Parthenon.

Sinding, S. W., J. A. Ross, and A. G. Rosenfeld. 1994. Seeking Common Ground: Unmet Need and Demographic Goals. *International Family Planning Perspectives* 20 (1): 23–27.

Singhal, A. and E. M. Rogers. 1989. Prosocial Television for Development in India. In R. E. Rice and C. K. Atkin (eds.), *Public Communication Campaigns.* 2nd ed. Newbury Park, CA: Sage.

Snyder, L. 1990. Channel Effectiveness over Time: Knowledge, Attitudes and Behavior Gaps. *Journalism Quarterly* 67 (4): 875–886.

Snyder, S. R. 1993. Oman Family Spacing Needs Assessment. Manuscript prepared for the Oman Ministry of Health and the Omani American Joint Commission under the auspices of the USAID Office of Population, Near East Bureau.

Social Planning, Analysis, and Administration Consultants (SPAAC). 1988. Final Evaluation Report: SIS/IEC Impact Evaluation Study, Cairo, Egypt. Report for the SIS/IEC project of the Johns Hopkins University/Population Communication Services, Center for Communication Programs, Baltimore.

Social Weather Stations, Inc. 1992. Social Attitudes of Filipinos Towards Family Planning Interest Groups. Report commissioned by the Philippine Legislators' Committee on Population and Development (PLCPD) with funding from the Population Crisis Committee, Manila.

Starr, P. 1982. *The Social Transformation of American Medicine*. New York: Basic Books.

Storey, J. D., S. Chhabra, and H. Viswanathan. 1995. Perceptual Mapping of Service Providers and Contraceptive Methods in Uttar Pradesh, India: Key Findings. Report prepared for the State Innovations in Family Planning Services Agency, Lucknow, India and the U.S. Agency for International Development, New Delhi, India by the Johns Hopkins University, Population Communication Services, Baltimore, MD.

Storey, J. D., A. Ilkhamov, I. Pogrebov, and B. Jabre. 1994. Clients' Perspectives on Contraceptive Technology and Practices in the Tashkent Region of Uzbekistan: A Report of Focus Group Research Findings. Report for the Johns Hopkins University, Population Communication Services, Center for Communication Programs, Baltimore.

Storey, J. D., A. Ilkhamov, and B. Saksvig. 1997. Perceptions of Family Planning and Reproductive Health Issues: Qualitative Studies in Kazakhstan, Turkmenistan, Kyrgyzstan, and Uzbekistan. *IEC Field Report Number 10*. Baltimore: Johns Hopkins Center for Communication Programs.

Storey, J. D., J. G. Rimon II, M. Amin, J. Williams, and J. Sobti. 1994. Promoting Private Sector Family Planning Services: Initial Impact of the Blue Triangle Campaign in India. Paper presented at the annual meeting of the American Public Health Association, Washington, DC, October 28–November 3.

Stycos, J. M. 1962. Experiments in Social Change: The Caribbean Fertility Studies. In C. V. Kiser (ed.), *Research in Family Planning*. Princeton, NJ: Princeton University Press.

———. 1973. *Clinics, Contraception, and Communications Evaluation Studies of Family Planning*. New York: Appleton-Century-Crofts.

Suls, J. M. 1977. Social Comparison Theory and Research. In J. M. Suls and R. L. Miller (eds.), *Social Comparison Processes*. New York: John Wiley.

Suyono, H., G. Saffitz, and J. G. Rimon II. 1990. Indonesia: The Blue Circle Campaign. Paper presented at the annual meeting of the American Public Health Association, Chicago, November 13.

Tanzania Ministry of Health, Health Education Division, and the Johns Hopkins University, Population Communication Services. 1991. Attitudes and Beliefs Regarding Child-Spacing: Focus Group Discussions with Men and Women from Six Regions of Tanzania. Baltimore: Johns Hopkins University, Population Communication Services.

Thaddeus, S. 1994. Oman: Technical Assistance Visit. Trip report, March 27–April 7, 1994. Baltimore: Johns Hopkins University, Population Communication Services.

Tobias, A. 1976. *Fire and Ice: The Story of Charles Revson, the Man Who Built the Revlon Empire.* New York: Morrow.

Traylor, W., B. Kearl, L. Leonard, and J. Wickstorm. 1992. Evaluation of the Population Information Program. Arlington, VA: Population Technical Assistance Project.

Trends–MBL, Inc. 1992. Final Report on Project Platypus. Evaluation study prepared for Johns Hopkins University, Population Communication Services, Baltimore, and the Department of Health, Manila.

Trout, J., and A. Ries. 1972a. The Positioning Era Cometh. *Advertising Age,* Features Section (Part 1 of 3), April 24.

———. 1972b. Positioning Cuts Through Chaos in Marketplace. *Advertising Age,* Features Section (Part 2 of 3), May 1.

———. 1972c. How to Position Your Product. *Advertising Age,* Features Section (Part 3 of 3), May 8.

Tsui, A. O. 1985. The Rise of Modern Contraception. In J. Cleland and J. Hobcraft (eds.), *Reproductive Change in Developing Countries: Insights from the World Fertility Survey.* Oxford: Oxford University Press.

Turkish Family Health and Planning Foundation (TFHPF) Annual Reports (1988; 1989–1990; 1991–1992; 1992–1993; and 1995–1996). Istanbul: TFHPF.

Turner, R. 1993. Operations Researchers Share Findings, Problems and Goals. *International Family Planning Perspectives* 19 (1): 29–30.

Turner, V. 1982. *From Ritual to Theater: The Human Seriousness of Play.* New York: Performing Arts Journal Publications.

Tweedie, I. A. 1995. Ghana Situation Analysis Preliminary Findings and Research Activities. Evaluation summary. Baltimore: Johns Hopkins Center for Communication Programs.

Tweedie, I. A., O. M. Kumah, D. L. Kincaid, W. Morgan, W. Glass, and Y. M. Kim. 1994. How Formative Research Can Improve Health Communication: An Innovative Strategy Used for Audience Segmentation in Ghana. Paper presented at the annual meeting of the American Public Health Association, Washington, DC, October 30–November 3.

Udry, J. R. 1974. *The Media and Family Planning.* Chapel Hill, NC: Carolina Population Center.

Underwood, C. 1994. (The Johns Hopkins Center for Communication Programs) [Knowledge, attitudes, and practices in Oman]. Personal communication to Lamia Jaroudi of JHU/CCP, June 28.

Underwood, C., L. F. Kemprecos, B. Jabre, and M. Wafai. 1994. And the Nile Flows On: The Impact of a Serial Drama in Egypt. Project report. Baltimore: Johns Hopkins Center for Communication Programs.

United Nations. 1973. *The Determinants and Consequences of Population Trends: New Summary Findings on the Interaction of Demographic, Economic, and*

Social Factors. Population Studies No. 50, Vol. 1. New York: Department of Economic and Social Affairs, United Nations.

————. 1977. *World Population Prospects as Assessed in 1973*. Population Studies No. 60. New York: Department of Economic and Social Affairs, United Nations.

————. 1989. *Levels and Trends of Contraceptive Use as Assessed in 1988*. Population Studies No. 110. New York: Department of International Economic and Social Affairs, United Nations.

————. 1992a. *Long Range World Population Projections: Two Centuries of Population Growth. 1950–2150*. New York: United Nations.

————. 1992b. *World Population Monitoring 1991: With Special Emphasis on Age Structure*. New York: United Nations.

————. 1992c. *World Population Prospects: The 1992 Revision. Annex Tables*. New York: United Nations.

————. 1994. *Report of the International Conference on Population and Development (ICPD), Cairo, September 5–13, 1994*. New York: United Nations Population Division, Department of Economic and Social Information and Policy Analysis.

————. 1995a. *Concise Report on the World Population Situation in 1995*. New York: Department for Economic and Social Information and Policy Analysis, Population Division, United Nations.

————. 1995b. Urban and Rural Areas 1994 [wall chart]. New York: Department for Economic and Social Information and Policy Analysis, Population Division, United Nations.

————. 1996. UN World Population Growth from Year 0 to Stabilization, data table, 1996. New York: Department for Economic and Social Information and Policy Analysis, Population Division, United Nations. Forthcoming.

United Nations Population Fund (UNFPA). 1995. *National Perspectives on Population and Development: Synthesis of 168 National Reports Prepared for the International Conference on Population and Development, 1994*. New York: United Nations.

United States Agency for International Development (USAID). 1993a. Philippine Population Assistance Strategy, 1993–1998. USAID program planning document, Washington, DC.

————. 1993b. The Substance Behind the Images: AID and Development Communication. USAID report, Washington, DC.

————. 1995. Synopsis: Population and Health Customer Appraisal, June 1995. Summary of Bangladesh study findings. Washington, DC: USAID.

United States Bureau of the Census. 1993. World Population Ages 10–24 as of July 1993 [data tables]. Washington, DC: United States Bureau of the Census.

"Usiniharakishe"—A Show of Rare Educational Value. 1986. *Daily Nation* [Kenya], News Analysis column, October 23.

Valente, T. W. 1995. *Network Models of the Diffusion of Innovations*. Cresskill, NJ: Hampton Press.

————. 1996. (The Johns Hopkins School of Public Health) [Peru wave data collection]. Personal communication to authors, November 21.

————. 1997. On Evaluating Mass Media Impact. *Studies in Family Planning Letters Section*, 28 (2), June.

Valente, T. W., Y. M. Kim, C. L. Lettenmaier, W. Glass, and Y. Dibba. 1994. Radio Promotion of Family Planning in the Gambia. *International Family Planning Perspectives* 20: 96–100.

Valente, T. W., L. D. Nickerson, M. Mérida, M. E. Coca, L. Solares, and R. Caballero. 1993. First Things First: The Bolivia National Reproductive Health Program Print Materials Evaluation. Evaluation report. Baltimore: Johns Hopkins Center for Communication Programs.

Valente, T. W., P. R. Poppe, M. E. Alva, R. V. de Briceño, and D. Cases. 1995. Street Theater as a Tool to Reduce Family Planning Misinformation. *International Quarterly of Community Health Education* 15 (3): 279–289.

Valente, T. W., P. R. Poppe, and A. Payne Merritt. 1996. Mass-Media-Generated Interpersonal Communication as Sources of Information About Family Planning. *Journal of Health Communication* 1: 247–265.

Valente, T. W., W. P. Saba, A. Payne Merritt, M. L. Fryer, T. Forbes, A. Pérez, and L. R. Beltrán. 1996. Reproductive Health Is in Your Hands: Impact of the Bolivia National Reproductive Health Program Campaign. *IEC Field Report No. 4* [Spanish-English edition]. Baltimore: Johns Hopkins Center for Communication Programs.

van de Walle, E., and J. Knodel. 1980. Europe's Fertility Transition: New Evidence and Lessons for Today's Developing World. *Population Bulletin* 34 (6): 3–44.

van den Borne, F., I. A. Tweedie, and W. B. Morgan. 1996. Family Planning and Reproductive Health in Zambia Today. *IEC Field Report No. 2*. Baltimore: Johns Hopkins Center for Communication Programs.

Van Hulzen, C. 1995. Technical Assistance to JHU/PCS/PIP Projects: Kenya Youth Initiatives Project (AFD-KEN-10), IPPF Male Involvement Project (FPAK/CCP-MOU-1), and Follow-Up on Kenya Office Issues. Trip report, July 10–August 4, 1995. Baltimore: Johns Hopkins Center for Communication Programs.

Vondrasek, C. 1994. (The Johns Hopkins Center for Communication Programs) [Pretesting the Cameroon Norplant flipchart]. Personal communication to authors, May.

Vriesendorp, S., L. K. Cobb, S. Helfenbein, J. A. Levine, and J. Wolff. 1989. A Framework for Management Development of Family Planning Program Managers. Paper presented at the 117th Annual Meeting of the American Public Health Association, Chicago, October 22–24.

Wafai, M. 1988. Zannana Campaign Evaluation: A Summary of Survey Results. Cairo: Wafai and Associates. Mimeographed.

————. 1992. Entertainment Educates: Using Music and Drama for Social Marketing. Paper presented at the Advista Arabia III Conference, Cairo, April 10–14.

———. 1994. Yielding Impressive Results: The Egyptian Experience in Family Planning Communication Campaign Has Been an Exemplary Model for Many Developing Countries. *Integration* 41: 8–11.

Wafai and Associates. 1993. The Private Practitioners' Family Planning Project: Media Campaign Evaluation [Egypt]. Prepared for the Johns Hopkins University, Population Communication Services, Center for Communication Programs, Baltimore.

Walton, M. 1986. *The Deming Management Method.* New York: Dodd, Mead and Co.

Warner and Associates. 1994. Report of Findings on Proposed Tag Lines for an Immunization Advertising Campaign. Report prepared for Burrell Advertising on behalf of the Centers for Disease Control and Prevention, Harvard University, the Ad Council, and the Johns Hopkins Center for Communication Programs.

Watson, W. B. (ed.). 1977. *Family Planning in the Developing World: A Review of Programs.* New York: Population Council.

Wawer, M. J., R. McNamara, T. McGinn, and D. Lauro, 1991. Family Planning Operations Research in Africa: Reviewing a Decade of Experience. *Studies in Family Planning* 22 (5): 289–293.

Weinstein, K. I., S. Ngallaba, A. R. Cross, and F. M. Mburu. 1994. The Tanzania Knowledge, Attitudes and Practices Survey, 1994. Bureau of Statistics Planning Commission, Dar es Salaam, Tanzania. Calverton, MD: Macro International, Inc.

Westoff, C. F. 1981. Unwanted Fertility in Six Developing Countries. *International Family Planning Perspectives* 7 (2): 43–52.

———. 1988. Is the KAP-Gap Real? *Population and Development Review* 14 (2): 225–232.

Westoff, C. F., and A. Bankole. 1995. Unmet Need: 1990–1994. *Demographic and Health Surveys Comparative Studies* 16. Calverton, MD: Macro International, Inc.

———. 1996. The Potential Demographic Significance of Unmet Need. *International Family Planning Perspectives* 22 (1): 16–20.

Westoff, C. F., L. Moreno, and N. Goldman. 1989. The Demographic Impact of Changes in Contraceptive Practice in Third World Populations. *Population and Development Review* 15 (1): 91–106.

Westoff, C. F., and L. H. Ochoa. 1991. The Demand for Family Planning: Highlights from a Comparative Analysis. In *Demographic Health Surveys 1991 World Conference Proceedings* 1. Calverton, MD: Macro International, Inc., pp. 575–598.

Westoff, C. F., and G. Rodriquez. 1995. The Mass Media and Family Planning in Kenya. *International Family Planning Perspectives* 21 (1): 26–31, 36.

Whitney, E. E., and T. N. Hamid. 1993. Jiggasha: A Community Network Approach to Family Planning. *South Asia Population Communication Conference Proceedings, February, 1993.* Dhaka, Bangladesh: Johns Hopkins University Center for Communication Programs.

Whitney, E. E., D. L. Kincaid, J. G. Rimon II, S. H. Yun, A. Silayan-Go, and E. Taguinin. 1989. Male Farmers as Family Planning Motivators: A New Strategy for the Philippines. Paper presented at the 117th Annual Meeting of the American Public Health Association, Chicago, October 22–24.

Williams, J. R. 1992. Increasingly Artful: Applying Commercial Marketing Techniques to Family Planning Communication. *Integration* 33 (August): 70–72.

Williams, L. B. 1990. *Development, Demography and Family Decision-Making: The Status of Women in Rural Java.* Brown University Studies in Population and Development. Boulder: Westview Press.

Winslow, C.E.A. 1923. *The Evolution and Significance of the Modern Public Health Campaign.* New Haven, CT: Yale University Press.

Woelfel, J., and E. Fink. 1980. *The Measurement of Communication Processes.* New York: Academic Press.

Wood, C., and B. Suitters. 1970. *The Fight for Acceptance: A History of Contraception.* Aylesbury, UK: Medical and Technical Publishing Co., Ltd.

World Health Organization (WHO). 1995. *National AIDS Program Management: A Training Course. 6. Condom Procurement and Distribution.* Rev. ed. Geneva: WHO, Global Program on AIDS.

Yassa, A. 1995. (Oman Ministry of Health) [Draft of quarterly report]. Personal communication to Lamia Jaroudi of JHU/CCP, January 11.

Yoder, P. S., R. Hornik, and B. C. Chirwa. 1996. Evaluating the Program Effects of Radio Drama About AIDS in Zambia. *Studies in Family Planning* 27 (4): 188–203.

Yun, S. H., and G. L. Lewis. 1994. Turkey: Moving Toward a National Strategy for Family Planning IEC: A Needs Assessment. Prepared by the Johns Hopkins Center for Communication Programs, Baltimore, with funding from USAID, for the U.S. Embassy, Ankara, in collaboration with the Ministry of Health, Maternal and Child Health/Family Planning Directorate.

Yun, S. H., P. T. Piotrow, D. L. Kincaid, Y. Yaser, and G. Olzer, 1989. Better Communication Makes a Difference in the Use of Family Planning—The Turkish Experience. Paper presented at the 117th Meeting of the American Public Health Association, Chicago, October 24.

Zabin, L. S., P. T. Piotrow, L. S. Liskin, E. Shadigian, and R. Seinick. 1990. Lessons from Family Planning and Their Application to AIDS Prevention. Prepared for the World Health Organization Global Program on AIDS by the Johns Hopkins University, Baltimore.

Zajonc, R. B. 1984. On the Primacy of Affect. *American Psychologist* 39 (2): 117–123.

Zajonc, R. B., S. T. Murphy, and M. Inglehart. 1989. Feeling and Facial Efference: Implications of the Vascular Theory of Emotion. *Psychological Review* 96 (3): 395–416.

Zander, A. 1971. *Motives and Goals in Groups.* New York: Academic Press.

ZET-Medya Research, Publishing and Consultancy Co. 1992. Audience Research for "Berdel." Rev. ed. Turkish audience research study report prepared for the Johns Hopkins University, Population Communication Services, Baltimore.

Zimmerman, M., and G. Perkins. 1982. Print Materials for Nonreaders: Experiences in Family Planning and Health. *Program for the Introduction and Adaptation of Contraceptive Technology (PIACT) Paper No. 9*. Seattle: PIACT.

Zimmerman, M., and L. Steckel. 1985. Formative Research: Pretesting, Revising, and More Pretesting. *Development Communication Report* No. 51: 9, 12.

Index

About the Authors

PHYLLIS TILSON PIOTROW is Director, Johns Hopkins Center for Communication Programs and Principal Investigator, Population Communications Services Project and Population Information Program. She is also Senior Associate, Department of Population Dynamics in the Johns Hopkins School of Public Health.

D. LAWRENCE KINCAID is Associate Director for Research, Johns Hopkins Center for Communication Programs and Associate Scientist, Department of Health Policy and Management in the Johns Hopkins School of Public Health.

JOSE G. RIMON II is Project Director, Population Communication Services; Deputy Director, Johns Hopkins Center for Communication Programs; and Associate, Department of Population Dynamics in the Johns Hopkins School of Public Health.

WARD RINEHART is Project Director, Population Information Program, a project of the Center for Communication Programs at the Johns Hopkins School of Public Health.

All have written extensively on reproductive health and family planning issues.

ISBN 0-275-95577-X

9 780275 955779

HARDCOVER BAR CODE